RELAPSE PREVENTION

RELAPSE PREVENTION

Maintenance Strategies in the
Treatment of Addictive Behaviors

Second Edition

Edited by

G. ALAN MARLATT
DENNIS M. DONOVAN

THE GUILFORD PRESS
New York London

© 2005 The Guilford Press
A Division of Guilford Publications, Inc.
72 Spring Street, New York, NY 10012
www.guilford.com

Printed in the United States of America

This book is printed on acid-free paper.

Last digit is print number: 9 8 7 6 5 4 3 2 1

Library of Congress Cataloging-in-Publication Data

Relapse prevention : maintenance strategies in the treatment of addictive
behaviors / edited by G. Alan Marlatt and Dennis M. Donovan.— 2nd ed.
        p. cm.
    Includes bibliographical references and index.
    ISBN 1-59385-176-6 (alk. paper)
 1. Substance abuse—Relapse—Prevention. 2. Substance abuse—Treatment. 3.
 Behavior therapy. I. Marlatt, G. Alan. II. Donovan, Dennis M. (Dennis
 Michael)
    RC564.R45 2005
    616.86′06—dc22

                                                             2005000834

About the Editors

G. Alan Marlatt, PhD, Director of the Addictive Behaviors Research Center and Professor of Psychology at the University of Washington, is renowned for his innovative theoretical and clinical work in the addictions field. Over the past two decades, he has made significant advances in developing programs for both relapse prevention and harm reduction for a range of addictive behaviors. In addition to coediting the first editions of *Relapse Prevention: Maintenance Strategies in the Treatment of Addictive Behaviors* (1985) and *Assessment of Addictive Behaviors* (1988), Dr. Marlatt is the editor of *Harm Reduction: Pragmatic Strategies for Managing High-Risk Behaviors* (1998), coeditor of *Changing Addictive Behavior: Bridging Clinical and Public Health Strategies* (1999), and coauthor of *Brief Alcohol Screening and Intervention for College Students (BASICS): A Harm Reduction Approach* (1999), all published by The Guilford Press. He is a Fellow of both the American Psychological Association and the American Psychological Society, and is a former president of the Association for Advancement of Behavior Therapy. He served as a member of the National Advisory Council on Drug Abuse at the National Institute on Drug Abuse from 1996 to 2002, and served on the National Advisory Council on Alcohol Abuse and Alcoholism Subcommittee on College Drinking from 1998 to 2001. Dr. Marlatt currently holds a Senior Research Scientist Award from the National Institute on Alcohol Abuse and Alcoholism, and received the Innovators Combating Substance Abuse Award from the Robert Wood Johnson Foundation in 2001. Previously, he was presented with the Jellinek Memorial Award for Alcohol Studies (1990), the Distinguished Scientist Award from the American Psychological Association's Society of Clinical Psychology (2000), the Visionary Award by the Network of Colleges and Universities Committed to the Elimination of Drug and Alcohol Abuse (2002), and the Distinguished Researcher Award from the Research Society on Alcoholism (2004).

Dennis M. Donovan, PhD, was affiliated with the Addictions Treatment Center at the Seattle Department of Veterans Affairs Medical Center for over 20 years, while engaging in clinical, administrative, training, and research activities. During that time he was also instrumental in the development of, and served as the Associate Director of, the first Center of Excellence in Substance Abuse Treatment and Education (CESATE) within the national Department of Veterans Affairs. He currently serves as the Director of the University of Washington's Alcohol and Drug Abuse Institute and holds the faculty ranks of Professor in the Department of Psychiatry and Behavioral Sciences, and Adjunct Professor in the Department of Psychology at the University of Washington in Seattle. He has written over 120 journal articles, 30 book chapters, and 3 books in the area of alcoholism and addictive behaviors, with emphases on social learning theory and biopsychosocial approaches to the etiology, maintenance, and treatment of addictions; the clinical assessment process and assessment measures; treatment of entrance and engagement; evaluation of treatment process and outcome; relapse prevention; and patient–treatment matching. Dr. Donovan's research has been funded by the National Institute on Alcohol Abuse and Alcoholism (NIAAA), the National Institute on Drug Abuse (NIDA), and the Center for Substance Abuse Treatment (CSAT). He has served as Associate Editor and as a member of the editorial boards for the *Journal of Studies on Alcohol*, *Psychology of Addictive Behaviors*, and *Addiction*. He has also been a member of the Clinical and Treatment Research Review Committee of NIAAA and the Behavioral AIDS Research Review Committee of NIDA. Dr. Donovan is a member of a number of national professional organizations and served as President of the Society of Psychologists in Addictive Behaviors. He has also been elected a Fellow of Division 50 (Division on Addictions) of the American Psychological Association.

Contributors

Arthur W. Blume, PhD, Department of Psychology, University of Texas at El Paso, El Paso, Texas

Kathleen M. Carroll, PhD, Department of Psychiatry, Division of Substance Abuse, Yale University School of Medicine, New Haven, Connecticut, and VA Connecticut Healthcare Center, West Haven, Connecticut

R. Lorraine Collins, PhD, Research Institute on Addictions, University at Buffalo, State University of New York, Buffalo, New York

Ned L. Cooney, PhD, Yale University School of Medicine, New Haven, Connecticut, and VA Connecticut Healthcare Center, West Haven, Connecticut

Jessica M. Cronce, BS, Department of Psychology, Yale University, New Haven, Connecticut

Berenice García de la Cruz, MA, Department of Special Education, University of Texas at Austin, Austin, Texas

Dennis M. Donovan, PhD, Department of Psychiatry and Behavioral Sciences and the Alcohol and Drug Abuse Institute, University of Washington School of Medicine, Seattle, Washington

William H. George, PhD, Department of Psychology, University of Washington, Seattle, Washington

Valerie A. Gruber, PhD, MPH, Department of Psychiatry, University of California, San Francisco, San Francisco, California

Chad Gwaltney, PhD, Center for Alcohol and Addiction Studies, Brown University, Providence, Rhode Island

Nancy A. Haug, PhD, Department of Psychiatry, University of California, San Francisco, San Francisco, California

Ronald M. Kadden, PhD, Department of Psychiatry, University of Connecticut School of Medicine, Farmington, Connecticut

Jon Kassel, PhD, Department of Psychology, University of Illinois at Chicago, Chicago, Illinois

Jason R. Kilmer, PhD, Addictive Behaviors Specialist, Evergreen State College, Olympia, Washington, and Saint Martin's College, Lacey, Washington

Debi A. LaPlante, PhD, Division on Addictions, Harvard Medical School, Boston, Massachusetts

G. Alan Marlatt, PhD, Department of Psychology and Addictive Behaviors Research Center, University of Washington, Seattle, Washington

Dennis McChargue, PhD, Department of Psychology, University of Illinois at Chicago, Chicago, Illinois

Rebekka S. Palmer, PhD, Department of Psychiatry, Division of Substance Abuse, Yale University School of Medicine, New Haven, Connecticut

Richard A. Rawson, PhD, UCLA Integrated Substance Abuse Programs, Department of Psychiatry and Biobehavioral Sciences, David Geffen School of Medicine, Los Angeles, California

Roger A. Roffman, DSW, School of Social Work, University of Washington, Seattle, Washington

Howard J. Shaffer, PhD, CAS, Division on Addictions, Harvard Medical School, Boston, Massachusetts

Saul Shiffman, PhD, Smoking Research Group, University of Pittsburgh, Pittsburgh, Pennsylvania

Yong S. Song, PhD, Department of Psychiatry, University of California, San Francisco, at San Francisco Veterans Affairs Medical Center, San Francisco, California

James L. Sorensen, PhD, Department of Psychiatry, University of California, San Francisco, San Francisco, California

Robert S. Stephens, PhD, Department of Psychology, Virginia Polytechnic Institute and State University, Blacksburg, Virginia

Susan A. Stoner, PhD, Department of Psychology and the Alcohol and Drug Abuse Institute, University of Washington, Seattle, Washington

Jennifer G. Wheeler, PhD, Sex Offender Treatment Program, Department of Corrections, Office of Correctional Operations, Monroe, Washington

Katie Witkiewitz, PhD, Department of Psychology and Addictive Behaviors Research Center, University of Washington, Seattle, Washington

Tina M. Zawacki, PhD, Department of Psychology, University of Texas at San Antonio, San Antonio, Texas

Preface

In the two decades since the first edition of this book was published in 1985, much has happened in the relapse prevention field. Many of these new developments and areas of application are described in this new edition. In the opening paragraph of the first edition, we stated that "Relapse Prevention (RP) is a self-management program designed to enhance the maintenance stage of the habit-change process. The goal of RP is to teach individuals who are trying to change their behavior how to anticipate and cope with the problem of relapse. In a very general sense, relapse refers to a breakdown or setback in a person's attempt to change or modify any target behavior." This definition of RP still applies and is consistent with the book's subtitle, "Maintenance Strategies in the Treatment of Addictive Behaviors." As can be seen in the contents of this edition, the range of application has expanded beyond substance use problems to include disorders associated with eating, gambling, and high-risk sexual behavior. Broadly conceived, RP is a cognitive-behavioral treatment (CBT) with a focus on the maintenance stage of addictive behavior change that has two main goals: to prevent the occurrence of initial lapses after a commitment to change has been made, and to prevent any lapse that does occur from escalating into a full-blown relapse (relapse management).

This new edition differs from the original 1985 volume in several important ways. The first edition consisted of two main sections: Part I, which provided a general theoretical overview of the RP model (Chapters 1 to 5), including coverage of high-risk situations for relapse, cognitive and behavioral coping skills, and lifestyle modification; and Part II, which contained four chapters describing application of RP with specific target behaviors (alcoholism, problem drinking, smoking, and weight management). The current edition contains chapters that extend the coverage of this approach to other addictive behaviors. The first chapter is designed to provide a summary of the RP approach in the treatment of alcohol and other drug problems, to provide an overview of treatment outcome studies that have evaluated the effectiveness of RP, and to describe recent updates in the theoretical underpinnings of the model. The second chapter provides an important discussion of issues that need to be considered when using RP programs with diverse client populations. The remaining 10 chapters are devoted to applications of RP and related CBT interventions for a variety of high-risk behaviors. Six chapters are devoted to substance use problems associated with the use of alcohol, tobacco/nicotine, stimulants, opioids, cannabis, and other substances (club drugs, hallucinogens, inhalants, and steroids). The final four chapters cover non-substance use problem behaviors, including eating disorders/obesity, gambling disorders, sexual offending, and sexually risky behaviors.

The most important change for readers to note is that this new edition of the RP book is designed to be used in conjunction with the second edition of our companion volume, *Assessment of Addictive Behaviors* (Donovan & Marlatt, 2005). Originally published in 1988, the new edition of *Assessment* contains chapters that are matched with content areas covered in the RP book. For example, readers who are seeking information on both assessment and RP intervention methods for alcohol problems can consult parallel chapters in both books. The same authors were invited to provide both the assessment and RP chapters, so as to enhance congruence of coverage and cross-referenced materials.

There are additional changes and updates in the current RP book that are also noteworthy. As described in Chapter 1, the original cognitive-behavioral model of the relapse process has been updated with the recent development of a dynamic model that incorporates both distal and proximal risk factors for relapse. This first chapter also describes the recent addition of mindfulness meditation as a metacognitive coping strategy to enhance client awareness of relapse risk and to facilitate coping with urges and cravings. Another new topic that is discussed in many chapters is how to develop an integrated RP intervention program for the treatment of co-occurring disorders (e.g., working with clients who have problems with both depression and excessive alcohol use). Since relapse is a potential risk for clients with both mental health and substance use problems, therapists who can provide an integrated RP assessment and treatment approach will benefit from this material.

Many chapters also describe how RP methods can be integrated with other intervention programs to enhance treatment effectiveness. Since the advent and influence of the motivational "stages of change" model, many treatment experts have recommended matching treatment interventions to the client's current stage of change. Based on this perspective, clients who are unmotivated (precontemplation stage) or ambivalent about changing their problem behavior (contemplation stage) may benefit most from motivational enhancement therapy (e.g., motivational interviewing). For clients who have already made a commitment to a specific action plan for change (e.g., to quit smoking), RP would be an appropriate intervention during the maintenance stage of habit change. Similarly, treatment engagement and adherence may be enhanced by the implementation of contingency management (CM) programs that provide reinforcement for successful progress, particularly in the early stages of treatment. Other behavioral approaches, including cue exposure, marital and family therapy, and acupuncture, are also mentioned by several authors as important treatment adjuncts to RP. Finally, the combination of pharmacotherapy with RP and other CBT programs is also recommended in several chapters. Since pharmacotherapy often has a beneficial effect in the early stages of treatment, and RP appears to have maximum benefits later in the maintenance stage (gradual improvement in coping capacity over time), the combination of the two treatment methods may be a promising treatment combination.

Readers will also note that RP programs have been developed to help clients in their pursuit of treatment goals, including both abstinence and moderation. Although abstinence is often the preferred goal for many substance use problems (e.g., quitting smoking), moderation is required for eating behavior and may be an alternative goal for other problems (e.g., moderate drinking or gambling). In the current text, RP methods are described for client goals that include both abstinence and harm reduction. For clients who are pursuing abstinence, coping with lapses involves similar relapse management strategies that are used in harm reduction programs (working with active users to minimize the risk of harmful consequences or escalation of the relapse process). An important basic principle of RP is to follow and support clients' treatment outcome goals, including abstinence or harm reduction, to help keep them on track on the challenging journey of habit change.

We would like to conclude by extending our sincere thanks and gratitude to our many colleagues who have contributed in important ways to the material presented in this book. First and foremost, we would like to thank the authors who contributed their time and efforts in writing chapters for our two books. We are delighted that we were able to include writings from the leading contributors and experts in each of the topic areas. As such, we feel we have included authors who are all at the "cutting edge" of their respective fields of expertise. We would also like to extend our sincere thanks and gratitude to two of our graduate students here at the University of Washington: Katie Witkiewitz and Ursula Whiteside, who both provided extensive reviews and editorial suggestions for all chapters. Katie Witkiewitz also served as coauthor on Chapter 1 and has made important contributions to the development of our new dynamic model of the relapse process. We would also like to thank The Guilford Press for its continued support of our work, with special gratitude extended to our editor, Jim Nageotte, and to our production editor, Jeannie Tang. Finally, we extend our sincere thanks to Judith Gordon, coeditor of the first edition of the RP book, who helped develop and disseminate what many people refer to as the "Marlatt and Gordon" approach to RP.

REFERENCE

Donovan, D. M., & Marlatt, G. A. (Eds.). (2005). *Assessment of addictive behaviors* (2nd ed.). New York: Guilford Press.

Contents

CHAPTER 1

Relapse Prevention for Alcohol and Drug Problems

G. Alan Marlatt
Katie Witkiewitz

The major goal of relapse prevention (RP) is to address the problem of re-lapse and to generate techniques for preventing or managing its occur-rence. Based on a cognitive-behavioral framework, RP seeks to identify high-risk situations in which an individual is vulnerable to relapse and to use both cognitive and behavioral coping strategies to prevent future re-lapses in similar situations. RP can be described as a tertiary prevention strategy with two specific aims: (1) preventing an initial lapse and main-taining abstinence or harm reduction treatment goals, and (2) providing lapse management if a lapse occurs, to prevent further relapse. The ulti-mate goal is to provide the skills to prevent a complete relapse, regardless of the situation or impending risk factors. In this chapter we summarize the major tenets of RP and the cognitive-behavioral model of relapse, in-cluding hypothesized precipitants and determinants of relapse. These latter topics are covered in greater detail in the second edition of *Assessment of Addictive Behaviors* (Donovan & Marlatt, 2005). We also provide a brief discussion of meta-analyses and reviews of the treatment outcome litera-ture and controlled clinical trials incorporating RP techniques. Finally, we describe a re-conceptualization of the relapse process and propose future directions for clinical applications and research initiatives.

MODELS OF RELAPSE

In 1986, Brownell and colleagues (Brownell, Marlatt, Lichtenstein, & Wilson, 1986) published an extensive, seminal review on the problem of relapse in addictive behaviors. At that time, addictive behaviors researchers were moving away from the disease model of addiction, and toward more cognitive and behavioral definitions of addictive disorders. Relapse has been described as both an outcome—the dichotomous view that the person is either ill or well, and a process—encompassing any transgression in the process of behavior change (Brownell, Marlatt, Lichtenstein, & Wilson, 1986; Wilson, 1992). The origins of the term "relapse" derive from a medical model, indicating a return to a disease state after a period of remission, but this definition has been diluted and applied to a variety of behaviors, from alcohol abuse to schizophrenia. Essentially, when individuals attempt to change a problematic behavior, a lapse (or instance of a previously cessated behavior) is highly probable. One possible outcome, following the initial setback, is a return to the previous problematic behavior pattern (relapse). Another possible outcome is the individual getting "back on track" in the direction of positive change (prolapse). Regardless of how relapse is defined, a general reading of the psychotherapy outcome literature from a variety of the behavior disorders reveals that "relapse" may be the common denominator in the treatment of psychological problems. That is, most individuals who make an attempt to change their behavior in a certain direction (e.g., lose weight, reduce hypertension, stop smoking, etc.), will experience lapses that often lead to relapse (Polivy & Herman, 2002).

The Cognitive-Behavioral Model of Relapse

Twenty-seven years ago, Marlatt (1978) obtained detailed, qualitative information from 70 chronic male alcoholics regarding the primary situations that led them to initiate drinking alcohol during the first 90 days following their release from an abstinence-based inpatient treatment facility. Based on the information obtained from this clinical data, Marlatt (1978) subsequently developed a detailed taxonomy of high-risk situations based on eight subcategories of relapse determinants. Drawing from this taxonomy of high-risk situations, Marlatt proposed the first cognitive-behavioral model of the relapse process (Cummings, Gordon, & Marlatt, 1980; Marlatt, 1996b; Marlatt & George, 1984; Marlatt & Gordon, 1985). Shown in Figure 1.1, the cognitive-behavioral model centers on an individual's response in a high-risk situation. The components include the interaction between the person (affect, coping, self-efficacy, outcome expectancies) and environmental risk factors (social influences, access to substance, cue exposure). If the individual lacks an effective coping response and/or confidence to deal with the situation (low self-efficacy; Bandura, 1977), the tendency is to "give in to temptation." The "decision" to use or not use is then mediated by the individual's outcome expectancies for the initial effects of using the substance (Jones, Corbin, & Fromme, 2001).

Individuals who choose to indulge may be vulnerable to the "abstinence violation effect" (AVE), which is the self-blame, guilt, and loss of perceived control that individuals often experience after the violation of self-imposed rules (Curry, Marlatt, & Gordon, 1987). The AVE contains both an affective and a cognitive component. The affective component is related to feelings of guilt, shame, and hopelessness (Marlatt, 1985), often triggered by the discrepancy between one's prior identity as an abstainer and one's present lapse behavior. The cognitive component, based on attributional theory (Weiner, 1974), assumes that if the individual attributes a lapse to factors that are internal, global and uncontrollable, then relapse risk is heightened. If, however, the individual views the lapse as external, unstable, and controllable, then the likelihood of a relapse is decreased (Marlatt & Gordon, 1985). For example, if an individual views a lapse as an irreparable failure or due to chronic disease determinants, then the lapse is more likely to progress to a relapse (Miller, Westerberg, Harris, & Tonigan, 1996); however, if the same individual views the lapse as a transitional learning experience, then the progression to relapse is less probable (Laws, 1995; Marlatt & Gordon, 1985; Walton, Castro, & Barrington, 1994). The individual who views a lapse as a learning experience is more likely to experiment with alternative coping strategies in the future, which may lead to more effective responses in high-risk situations. Several studies have demonstrated the role of the AVE in predicting relapse in alcoholics (Collins & Lapp, 1991), smokers (Curry, Marlatt, & Gordon, 1987), dieters (Mooney, Burling, Hartman, & Brenner-Liss, 1992), and marijuana users (Stephens, Curtin, & Roffman, 1994).

RELAPSE PREVENTION

The phrase "relapse prevention" may usefully stimulate thought, break old molds, get the adrenalin flowing, give the title to a book, but at the end of the day it can be an invitation to artificial segmentation of the interaction, total and fluctuating process of change. (Edwards, 1987, p. 319)

In his criticism of the first edition of Relapse Prevention (Marlatt & Gordon, 1985), Edwards (1987) suggested that RP would not provide an adequate account of the idiosyncrasies of change, and in doing so he highlighted the importance of the relapse process as an interactive, fluctuating process that may never be interrupted in certain individuals. Yet, as we will show, RP has been an adjunct to the treatment of several behavior disorders and a useful tool for navigating the rough waters of maintaining behavior change.

The cognitive-behavioral model and the taxonomy of relapse precipitants were originally developed as the basis for an intervention designed to prevent and manage relapse in individuals who received treatment for alcohol use disorders (Chaney, O'Leary, & Marlatt, 1978). The RP model has since provided an important heuristic and treatment framework for clinicians working with several types of addictive behavior (Carroll, 1996). Treatment approaches based on the model rely on the initial assessment of potentially high-risk situations for relapse (e.g., environmental stressors, personality characteristics). Once situations are identified, the therapist works with the client to monitor the individual's coping skills, self-efficacy, and lifestyle factors (e.g., lifestyle imbalance), which may increase the probability of the individual being in a high-risk situation (Daley, Marlatt, & Spotts, 2003; Larimer, Palmer, & Marlatt, 1999).

RP combines behavioral skills training with cognitive interventions designed to prevent or limit the occurrence of relapse episodes. RP treatment begins with the assessment of the potential interpersonal, intrapersonal, environmental, and physiological risks for relapse and the factors or situations that may precipitate a relapse (Marlatt, 1996a). Specific assessment strategies based on a biopsychosocial model are discussed in the second edition of *Assessment of Addictive Behaviors* (Donovan & Marlatt, 2005). Once potential relapse triggers and high-risk situations are identified, cognitive and behavioral approaches are implemented that incorporate both specific interventions and global self-management strategies. Specific interventions include teaching effective coping strategies, enhancing self-efficacy, and encouraging mastery over successful outcomes.

As in most cognitive-behavioral treatments, RP incorporates a large educational component, including cognitive restructuring of misperceptions and maladaptive thoughts. Challenging myths related to positive outcome expectancies and discussing the psychological components of substance use (e.g., placebo effects) provide the client with opportunities to make more informed choices in high-risk situations. Likewise, discussing the AVE and preparing clients for lapses may also serve to prevent a major relapse episode. Lapse management is presented as an emergency procedure to be implemented in the event a lapse occurs. It is critical that clients are taught to restructure their negative thoughts about lapses, not to view them as a "failure" or an indication of a lack of willpower. Education about the relapse *process* and the likelihood of a lapse occurring may better equip clients to navigate the rough terrain and slippery slope of cessation attempts.

After providing education and intervention strategies specific to the immediate high-risk situation, RP focuses on the implementation of global lifestyle self-management strategies. Lifestyle balance is a critical factor in the maintenance of goals following treatment, and RP incorporates the assessment of lifestyle factors that may relate to an increased probability of relapse. Oftentimes clients are experiencing several daily stressors, and the therapist should work with a client to either reduce stressors or increase pleasurable activities, such that a balance between daily negatives and positives may be achieved. In addition, specific cognitive-behavioral approaches, such as relaxation training, stress management, or a time management exercise, can be implemented. Recently, mindfulness techniques and meditation exercises have been incorporated into the treatment of several behavior disorders (e.g., borderline personality disorder, depression, anxiety), and preliminary results demonstrate that mindfulness meditation may be a viable, effective adjunct to the treatment of alcohol and drug abuse (Marlatt, 1998; Marlatt & Kristeller, 1999; Witkiewitz, Marlatt, & Walker, in press).

Bringing it all together, the therapist and the client can work together in the development of "relapse road maps," analyses of possible outcomes that may be associated with different choices in high-risk situations. Mapping out possible scenarios can help prepare clients for navigating situations and utilizing the appropriate coping responses. The exercise of identifying and rehearsing possible high-risk situations and effective coping strategies is designed to enhance client self-efficacy and prevent the incidence of a lapse.

Effectiveness and Efficacy of Relapse Prevention

Chaney and colleagues (1978) provided the first randomized trial of RP techniques in an inpatient population of problem drinkers. Forty individuals receiving inpatient alcohol treatment at a Veterans Administration hospital were randomly assigned to either group-based skills training, an insight-oriented discussion group, or treatment as usual. The skills training RP-type intervention incorporated modeling, behavioral rehearsal, coaching, and identifying and coping with high-risk situations. The results demonstrated that the skills training group had significantly fewer days drunk, less alcohol consumption, and shorter drinking periods than the two comparison groups. The authors concluded "that problem drinkers' responses to situations that present a high risk of relapse can be improved through training" (Chaney et al., 1978, p. 1101).

Since 1978, several studies have evaluated the effectiveness and efficacy of RP approaches for substance use disorders (Carroll, 1996; Irvin, Bowers, Dunn, & Wang, 1999), and there is evidence supporting RP for depression (Katon et al., 2001), sexual offending (Laws, Hudson, & Ward, 2000), obesity (Brownell & Wadden, 1992; Perry et al., 2001), obsessive–compulsive disorder (Hiss, Foa, & Kozak, 1994), schizophrenia (Herz et al., 2000), bipolar disorder (Lam et al., 2003), and panic disorder (Bruce, Spiegel, & Hegel, 1999). Carroll (1996) conducted a narrative review of 24 randomized, controlled trials utilizing RP or coping skills training techniques directly invoking the procedures recommended by Marlatt and Gordon (1985). Incorporating studies of RP for smoking, alcohol, marijuana, and cocaine addiction, Carroll concluded that RP was more effective than no-treatment control groups and equally effective as other active treatments (e.g., supportive therapy, social support group, interpersonal psychotherapy) in improving substance use outcomes. Several of the reviewed studies demonstrated that RP techniques reduced the intensity of relapse episodes, when compared to no-treatment or active treatment (Davis & Glaros, 1986; O'Malley et al., 1996; Supnick & Colletti, 1984). In addition, several studies identified sustained main effects for RP, suggesting that RP may provide continued improvement over a longer period of time (indicating a "delayed emergence effect"), whereas other treatments may only be effective over a shorter duration (Carroll, Rounsaville, & Gawin, 1991; Carroll, Rounsaville, Nich, & Gordon, 1994; Goldstein, Niaura, Follick, & Abrahms, 1989; Hawkins, Catalano, Gillmore, & Wells, 1989; Rawson et al., 2002).These findings suggest a lapse/relapse learning curve, in which incremental changes in coping skills lead to a decreased probability of relapse. Anyone who has attempted to water ski, snowboard, or ride a bicycle understands that most people rarely can avoid falling on their first attempt; for most it takes repeated trials of falling, adjusting, and trying again before a person masters these activities.

Irvin and colleagues (1999) conducted a meta-analysis of RP techniques in the treatment of alcohol, tobacco, cocaine, and polysubstance use. Twenty-six studies representing a sample of 9,504 participants were included in the review. The results demonstrated that RP was a successful intervention for reducing substance use and improving psychosocial adjustment. In particular, RP was more effective in treating alcohol and polysubstance use than it was in the treatment of cocaine use and smoking, although these findings need to be interpreted with caution due to the small number of studies ($n = 3$) evaluating cocaine use. RP was equally effective across different treatment modalities, including individual, group, and marital treatment delivery, although all of these methods were most effective in treating alcohol use. Considering RP was originally developed as an adjunct to treatment for alcohol use, it is not surprising that this meta-analysis found it was most effective for individuals with alcohol problems. This finding suggests that certain characteristics of alcohol use are particularly amenable to the current RP model and that scientist–practitioners should continue to modify/enhance RP procedures to incorporate the idiosyncrasies of other substance use (e.g., cocaine, smoking, heroin) and nonsubstance (e.g., depression, anxiety) relapse. For example, Roffman has developed a marijuana-specific RP intervention, which has produced greater reductions in marijuana use than a comparison social support treatment (Roffman & Stephens, Chapter 7, this volume; Roffman, Stephens, Simpson, & Whitaker, 1990).

Relapse Replication and Extension Project

The National Institute on Alcohol Abuse and Alcoholism (NIAAA) provided funding for a group of researchers to conduct a modern replication of Marlatt's original taxonomy for classifying relapse episodes. The Relapse Replication and Extension Project (RREP), initiated by the Treatment Research Branch of the NIAAA, was specifically designed to investigate the cognitive-behavioral model of relapse developed by Marlatt and colleagues (Lowman, Allen, Stout, & the Relapse Research Group, 1996). Three research centers—Brown University, Research Institute on Addiction, and University of New Mexico—recruited 563 individuals who were seeking treatment for alcohol abuse and dependence. These participants were recruited from several treatment programs, including both inpatient and outpatient programs, which represented a variety of approaches to alcohol treatment (although all treatment programs required an abstinence goal). All three research sites utilized several measurement instruments and received similar training, from Marlatt and his colleagues, on the scoring instructions for the relapse taxonomy. In addition to the initial assessment of relapse episodes and participant experiences, each site conducted follow-up assessments in bimonthly intervals for 12 months. The results from the RREP and commentaries are provided in a special issue of *Addiction* (1996, Volume 91, issue 12s).

The RREP focused on the replication and extension of the high-risk situation in relation to relapse, and the reliability and validity of the taxonomic system for classifying relapse episodes. The results from the RREP, provided in the 1996 supplement to the journal *Addiction*, are summarized here. Information on drinking behavior during the 12-month period following treatment supported previous findings on relapse rates (Hunt, Barnett, & Branch, 1971) with 82% and 73% of participants, outpatients and inpatients, respectively, having at least one drink. As in Marlatt's original studies of relapse episodes in alcoholics, the RREP found that negative emotional states and exposure to social pressure to drink were most commonly identified as high-risk situations for relapse (Lowman et al., 1996).

In general, the data and research questions used in the RREP raised significant methodological issues concerning the predictive validity of Marlatt's relapse taxonomy and coding system. Based on the findings in this set of studies, a major reconceptualization of the relapse taxonomy was recommended (Donovan, 1996; Kadden, 1996). Longabaugh and colleagues (Longabaugh, Rubin, Stout, Zywiak, & Lowman, 1996) suggested a revision of the taxonomy categories (to include more distinction between the inter- and intrapersonal determinants, more emphasis on craving, and less focus on hierarchical classification). In suggesting a modification of the relapse precipitant theory, the authors recommend identifying other factors that may be used in the prediction of relapse, including more emphasis on the "relapse occasion" (p. 87), wherein some individuals are more likely to relapse regardless of the specific situational context. Donovan (1996) concluded that the RREP did not adequately test the assumptions of the broader cognitive-behavioral model of relapse, on which several RP intervention strategies are based. Many of the RREP findings, including the influence of negative affect, the AVE, and the importance of coping in predicting relapse are in fact quite supportive of the original RP model (Marlatt, 1996b). More generally, all of the researchers for the RREP relied solely on statistical analyses that are grounded in the general linear model. Yet the major theories of the relapse process, as well as clinical case studies, suggest that relapse is "random," "complex," and "dynamic" (Brownell et al., 1986; Donovan, 1996; Litman, 1984; Marlatt, 1996a; Shiffman, 1989).

Working from the criticisms provided by the researchers in the RREP (Donovan, 1996; Kadden, 1996; Longabaugh et al., 1996), as well as other critiques of RP and the cognitive-behavioral model of relapse (Allsop & Saunders, 1989; Heather & Stallard, 1989; Sutton, 1979), the remainder of this chapter is devoted to a review of relapse risk factors and a proposal for a reconceptualization of the relapse taxonomy and relapse process. Although no single model of relapse could ever encompass all individuals attempting all types of behavior change, a more thorough understanding of the critical determinants of relapse and the underlying processes may provide added insight into the treatment and prevention of relapsing disorders.

DETERMINANTS OF LAPSE AND RELAPSE

Intrapersonal Determinants

Self-Efficacy

Self-efficacy is defined as the degree to which an individual feels confident and capable of performing a certain behavior in a specific situational context (Bandura, 1977). As described in the cognitive-behavioral model of relapse (Marlatt, Baer, & Quigley, 1995), higher levels of self-efficacy are predictive of improved alcoholism treatment outcomes (Annis & Davis, 1988; Burling, Reilly, Moltzen, & Ziff, 1989; Connors, Maisto, & Zywiak, 1996; Greenfield et al., 2000; Project MATCH Research Group, 1997; Rychtarik, Prue, Rapp, & King, 1992; Solomon & Annis, 1990). Connors and colleagues (1996) studied self-efficacy and treatment outcomes one year after inpatient and outpatient treatment. The authors found that self-efficacy was positively related to the percentage of days abstinent, and negatively related to the number of drinks per drinking day. Greenfield and colleagues (2000) considered the relationship between self-efficacy and relapse survival in a group of male and female alcoholic patients receiving inpatient treatment. The results from this prospective study supported the finding that self-efficacy is predictive of survival functions of abstinence. This finding suggests that a person's self-efficacy score was predictive of both the amount of time to first drink and time to relapse within the first 12 months following treatment. Self-efficacy, as measured by the Alcohol Abstinence Self-Efficacy Scale (AASE; DiClemente, Carbonari, Montgomery, & Hughes, 1994), was also shown to predict 3-year alcohol treatment outcomes (Project MATCH Research Group, 1998).

The measurement of self-efficacy continues to be a challenge, especially considering the context-specific nature of the construct. Annis and colleagues have created two self-report questionnaires that aim to measure self-efficacy. The Inventory of Drinking Situations (IDS; Annis, 1982a) and the Situational Confidence Questionnaire (SCQ; Annis, 1982b) measure past and current self-efficacy, respectively, in 100 situations. As described earlier, DiClemente and colleagues (1994) developed the AASE to evaluate an individual's confidence in abstaining and perceived temptation to drink in 20 situations. For all of these self-report measures, when removed from the contexts provided by these questionnaires an individual may report being very confident (high self-efficacy) in abstaining, but the true assessment of self-efficacy occurs in the real-time environment during an actual high-risk situation. For example, Curry, Marlatt, and Gordon (1987) found that prospectively predicted attributions of smoking lapses in hypothetical situations were not significantly associated with the attributions for lapses during actual smoking episodes. Annis and Davis (1988) maintain that the purpose of self-report measures in the treatment of alcohol dependence is to identify high-risk situations and to increase awareness of *where* and *when* the strongest coping skills might be needed. In addition, further consideration should be given to the measurement of self-efficacy in real situations (Shiffman et al., Chapter 4, this volume), such as through self-monitoring techniques (e.g., the ecological momentary assessment [EMA] technique developed by Stone and Shiffman, 1994).

A study by Shiffman and colleagues (2000) using EMA demonstrated that baseline differences in self-efficacy were as predictive of the first lapse as were daily measurements of self-efficacy, demonstrating the stability of self-efficacy during abstinence. However, daily variation in self-efficacy was a significant predictor of smoking relapse progression following a first lapse, above and beyond baseline self-efficacy and pretreatment smoking behavior. Using the same methodology, Gwaltney and colleagues (2002) showed that both individuals who experience a smoking lapse and those who abstain from smoking following treatment are capable of discriminating nonrisk from high-risk situations, with situations that are rated as high risk (e.g., negative affect contexts) receiving the lowest self-efficacy ratings.

Outcome Expectancies

Alcohol outcome expectancies are the anticipated effects that an individual expects will occur as a result of alcohol or drug consumption (Jones et al., 2001; Leigh & Stacy, 1991; Stacy, Widaman, & Marlatt, 1990). An individual's expectancies may be related to the physical, psychological, or behavioral effects of alcohol; the expected drug effects do not necessarily correspond with the actual effects experienced after consumption. For example, an individual may *expect* to feel more relaxed (physical), happier (psychological), and outgoing (behavioral) after drinking alcohol, but the individual's *actual* experience may include increased tension (physical), sadness (psychological), and withdrawal (behavioral). Treatment outcome studies have demonstrated that positive outcome expectancies (e.g., "A cigarette would be relaxing") are associated with poorer treatment outcomes (Connors, Tarbox, & Faillace, 1993) and negative outcome expectancies (e.g., "I will have a hangover") are related to improved treatment outcomes (Jones & McMahon, 1996).

Expectancies are typically measured using self-report questionnaires that have an underlying factor structure representing different expectancy types (e.g., the Alcohol Expectancy Questionnaire by Brown, Goldman, & Christiansen, 1985). The major criticism of this approach has been the reliance on measures of "expectancies," which may actually be assessing general attitudes toward drinking or drugging (Leigh & Stacy, 1991; Stacy et al., 1990). In response to these criticisms, network models of expectancy have been developed that incorporate the importance of long-term memory and cognitive processes in the prediction of current and future consumption (Goldman, Brown, Christiansen, & Smith, 1991).

Based on a network model of expectancies, Jones and colleagues (2001) concluded that although expectancies are strongly related to outcomes of treatment and prevention programs, there is very little evidence that targeting expectancies in treatment leads to changes in posttreatment alcohol consumption. Reductions in positive outcome expectancies do not always lead to reductions in alcohol consumption (Connors et al., 1993), and the role of expectancies in predicting treatment outcome may depend on the targeted population and motivational frameworks. From a simplistic view, positive expectations may provide the individual with motivation to drink, while negative expectations may provide motivation to restrain from drinking (Cox & Klinger, 1988).

Based on operant conditioning, the motivation to use in a particular situation is based on the expected positive or negative reinforcement value of a specific outcome in that situation (Bolles, 1972). For example, if an individual is in a highly stressful situation and holds the positive outcome expectancy that smoking a cigarette will reduce his or her level of stress, then the incentive of smoking a single cigarette has high reinforcement value. Baker and colleagues (Baker, Piper, McCarthy, Majeskie, & Fiore, 2004) have demonstrated that perceived or expected reductions in negative affect and withdrawal severity (Piasecki et al., 2000) provide negative reinforcement, which may enhance positive outcome expectancies.

Recently, more complex accounts of expectancies, based on implicit cognitive and affective processing models, have been proposed (Baker et al., in press; Ostafin, Palfai, & Wechsler, 2003). Experimental investigations have demonstrated that responses to explicit measures of expectancies may vary greatly from implicit measures, which could indicate automatic responding to alcohol-related stimuli and consequences (Kelly & Witkiewitz, 2003; Palfai & Ostafin, 2003). Kelly & Witkiewitz (2003) studied reaction time to attitudes about alcohol-expectancy domains (e.g., tension reduction) in heavy- and light-drinking college students. The results demonstrated slower responding in the heavy drinkers, which was interpreted to mean that heavy drinkers have more complex associations with alcohol-expectancy information. Palfai and Ostafin (2003) demonstrated that implicit attitudes toward the anticipation of drinking (i.e., alcohol-approach tendencies) were significantly correlated with global positive expectancies and reliably predicted stronger urges and more heightened arousal in the anticipation of drinking. These findings highlight the automatic processes underlying alcohol expectancies (Stacy, Ames, & Leigh, 2004). From a behavioral economics perspective it is postulated that, for heavy drinkers, the explicit weighing of negative expectancies for substance use consequences in high-risk situations is highly unlikely; rather, the consideration of current versus delayed reinforcers may lead to automatic pilot reactions (Vuchinich & Tucker, 1996).

Motivation

Cox and Klinger (1988, p. 168) proposed that the "common, final pathway to alcohol use is motivational." This idea was inherently tied to the idea of positive expectations for the effects of alcohol, as described by expectancy theory, but it also stimulated the notion that motivation for drinking was a key component in predicting behavior change. Motivation may relate to the relapse process in two distinct ways, the motivation for positive behavior change and the motivation to engage in the problematic behavior. The *Oxford English Dictionary* (2002) defines motivation as "the conscious or unconscious stimulus for action towards a desired goal provided by psychological or social factors; that which gives purpose or direction to behavior." Using the example of alcohol use we could define the first type of motivation (*motivation to change*) as the stimulus for action toward abstinence or reduced use of alcohol, and the second type of motivation (*motivation to use*) as the stimulus for engaging in drinking behavior.

The ambivalence toward change is often highly related to both self-efficacy (e.g., "I really want to quit shooting up, but I do not think that I'll be able to say no") and outcome expectancies (e.g., "I would quit drinking, but then I would have a really hard time meeting people"). Prochaska and DiClemente (1984) have proposed a transtheoretical model of motivation, incorporating five stages of readiness to change: precontemplation, contemplation, preparation, action, and maintenance. Each stage characterizes a different level of motivational readiness, with precontemplation representing the lowest level of readiness (DiClemente & Hughes, 1990). During preparation there is very little motivation to change, but as the individual moves toward contemplation there is an increase in ambivalence and "change talk."

Interventions that focus on resolving ambivalence (e.g., evaluating the pros and cons of change vs. no change) may increase intrinsic motivation by allowing clients to explore their own values and how they may differ from actual behavioral choices (e.g., "I want to be an effective employee, but I often spend my daytime hours hung-over and my evening hours getting drunk."). Motivational interviewing (MI), developed by Miller and Rollnick (1991, 2002), is a client-centered interviewing style with the goal of resolving conflicts regarding the pros and cons of change, enhancing motivation and encouraging positive behavior change. Originally developed to work with patients presenting for alcohol disorders, MI has demonstrated efficacy for reducing alcohol consumption and frequency of drinking in this population (Bien, Miller, & Boroughs, 1993; Miller, Benefield, & Tonigan, 1993). A recent meta-analysis of 30 different clinical trials of MI demonstrated that it is more effective than no treatment or placebo controls, and as effective as other active treatments for alcohol and drug problems, diet, and exercise (Burke, Arkowitz, & Menchola, 2003). With regard to MI for alcohol problems, the review demonstrated that the pooled effect of MI across studies indicated a 56% reduction in drinking. MI has also been successfully adapted and applied to work with a variety of other health behaviors, including use of illicit substances (Budney, Higgins, Radonovich, & Novy, 2000; Stephens, Roffman, & Curtin, 2000), smoking (Butler et al., 1999), and HIV risk reduction (Carey et al., 2000).

Coping

Based on the cognitive-behavioral model of relapse, the most critical predictor of relapse is the individual's ability to utilize effective coping strategies in dealing with high-risk situations. Coping includes both cognitive and behavioral strategies designed to reduce danger or achieve gratification in a given situation (Lazarus, 1966). Litman, Stapleton, Oppenheim, Peleg, and Jackson (1983) first emphasized the importance of coping strategies in preventing alcohol relapse in dangerous situations. Litman proposed a model of relapse that incorporated an interaction between the situation, the availability and effectiveness of coping behaviors, and the individual's self-efficacy in dealing with the situation.

Several types of coping have been proposed, which differ by function and topography. Shiffman (1984) described the distinctions between *stress coping*, which functions to diminish the impact of stressors, and *temptation coping*, which is intended to resist the temptation to use drugs, independent from stress. The relationship between stress or temptation coping and the individual's response has been described as transactional, whereby individuals make a cognitive appraisal of their ability to cope with the stressor or temptation, and that appraisal determines the response (Lazarus & Folkman, 1984). Either stress or temptation coping can take the form of *cognitive coping*, using mental processes and "willpower" to control behavior, and *behavioral coping*, which involves some form of action. An example of cognitive temptation coping is thinking about the negative consequences of using, whereas behavioral temptation coping may be the active avoidance of drug cues to prevent use. Cognitive stress coping might include mindfulness meditation as a stress management technique, and behavioral stress coping might include going for a walk to get out of a stressful situation, such as a family quarrel.

Moos (1993) highlighted the distinction between approach and avoidance coping. Approach coping may involve attempts to accept, confront, or reframe as a means of coping, whereas avoidance coping may include distraction from cues or engaging in other activities. Chung and colleagues (Chung, Langenbucher, Labouvie, Pandina, & Moos, 2001) predicted 12-month treatment outcomes in alcoholic patients by focusing on the distinctions between the behavioral and cognitive components of approach and avoidance coping. Utilizing the Coping Responses Inventory (CRI; Moos, 1993), they defined cognitive approach coping as attempts to gain insight on a stressor or positively reframe the stressor, cognitive avoidance coping as avoiding thinking about the stressor or acceptance of the stressor; behavioral approach coping as support seeking and problem solving, and behavioral avoidance coping as incorporating emotional discharge and alternative pleasurable activities. Results suggested that avoidance coping, particularly cognitive avoidance coping, was predictive of fewer alcohol (including alcohol problem severity and alcohol-dependence symptoms), interpersonal, and psychological problems at the 12-month follow-up. Behavioral approach coping also predicted decreased alcohol problem severity at 12 months. In general, the alcohol patients reduced their use of avoidance coping and increased their use of approach coping.

Although these studies have demonstrated that coping is a critical factor in predicting and preventing relapse, issues of definition and measurement remain: What is coping? And, how do we measure it? Coping is commonly operationally defined as scores on a self-report questionnaire, such as the Coping Behavior Inventory (CBI; Litman, Stapleton, Oppenheim, & Peleg, 1983), or as responses to specific situations (Chaney et al., 1978; Monti et al., 1993). The Situational Competency Test, originially developed by Chaney and colleagues (1978), demonstrated that latency in responding to a high-risk situation was predictive of relapse. Monti and colleagues (1993) developed the Alcohol-Specific Role Play Test, which incorporates observer ratings of demonstrated coping skills in general and in alcohol-specific situations. While this procedure may provide more objective information than a self-report questionnaire, the generalizability of a role play to a real-world high-risk situation is questionable. More importantly, the use of coping skills while "in role" as part of a treatment program or research study may actually be a measure of either demand characteristics (e.g., wanting to please treatment staff or the experimenter), self-efficacy (e.g., the client is confident in his or her ability to abstain), or readiness to change (e.g., the client is highly motivated to practice and utilize coping strategies).

The role of coping skills, self-efficacy, and motivation in the prediction of alcohol treatment outcome was investigated by Litt and colleagues (2003). The results demonstrated that self-efficacy and coping independently predicted successful treatment outcomes. Motivation was related to treatment outcome via its relationship with coping skills, such that higher levels of readiness enhance the use of coping skills, resulting in more successful outcomes. Litt and colleagues (2003) examined the effectiveness of cognitive-behavioral therapy (CBT), which included coping skills training, versus a treatment based on interactional/interpersonal therapy (IPT) that did not include coping skills training. Both treatments yielded good outcomes, based on percentage of days abstinent and proportion of heavy drinking days, and improvements in coping skills. Availability of coping skills following treatment was a significant predictor of outcome, yet neither CBT nor IPT led to substantially greater increases in coping skills. These results are consistent with a recent review conducted by Morganstern and Longabaugh (2000), which found that improvements in coping skills was not a mediating mechanism of improved outcomes following cognitive-behavioral interventions. The finding that coping skills do not mediate the effectiveness of CBT has led these authors to conclude that research has not yet determined the active mechanisms of CBT.

One explanation for these findings is the dynamic interaction between coping, self-efficacy, and motivation (Litt et al., 2002; Shiffman et al., 2000). A second explanation is the operationalization of coping in previous studies: Are we accurately measuring how "coping" is experienced by the individual? The definitions of coping described earlier involve an *ac-*

tive, conscious response (Monti et al., 1993; Moos, 1993; Shiffman, 1984). Paradoxically, the act of engaging in substance use, in the presence of stress, negative affect, or substance cues, could be described as an ineffective and over-learned *active* coping strategy.

Coping may also be experienced as *inaction*. Inaction has typically been interpreted as the acceptance of substance cues (e.g., Litman, 1984; Marlatt, 2002), which can be described as "letting go" and not acting on an urge. This view of inactive coping is consistent with the Buddhist notion of skillful means (Marlatt, 2002)—the acceptance of the present moment and observation of logical, sensory, physical, and intuitive experiences, without analyzing, judging, or emotional responding. The focus is not about "doing what's right" or making good decisions, but rather the goal is to "just do." An example of a coping strategy that is consistent with skillful means is the use of "urge surfing" (Marlatt & Kristeller, 1999). Using a wave metaphor, urge surfing is an imagery technique to help clients gain control over impulses to use drugs or alcohol. In this technique, the client is first taught to label internal sensations and cognitive preoccupations as an urge, and to foster an attitude of detachment from that urge. The focus is on identifying and accepting the urge, not acting on the urge or attempting to fight it.

In a recent study on the effectiveness of a mindfulness meditation technique (of the Vipassana tradition) in reducing substance abuse in an incarcerated population, participants reported that "staying in the moment" and being mindful of urges were helpful coping strategies (Marlatt et al., 2004). Mindfulness meditation is also a major component of dialectical behavior therapy for the treatment of borderline personality disorder (Linehan, 1993) and mindfulness-based cognitive therapy for depression (Segal, Williams, & Teasdale, 2002). Borderline personality disorder (BPD), depression, and substance abuse are similar in that individuals with these disorders utilize ineffective and maladaptive learned coping strategies in stressful life situations. It has been proposed that meditation may provide an alternative coping strategy in response to stress, negative affect, and anxiety (Marlatt, Pagano, Rose, & Marques, 1984). In describing the use of meditation as a coping strategy for addictive behavior, Groves and Farmer (1994) state: "In the context of addictions mindfulness might mean becoming aware of triggers for craving . . . and choosing to do something else which might ameliorate or prevent craving, so weakening this habitual response" (p. 189). Focusing on the present moment and silently observing and accepting the distress associated with craving, stress, or negative affect, may provide addicts with an effective and adaptive coping strategy.

Emotional States

In the original qualitative investigation of relapse episodes (Marlatt & Gordon, 1980), negative emotional state was the strongest predictor of relapse in a sample of male alcoholics (37% of the sample reported that negative affect was the primary relapse trigger). Several other studies have reported a strong link between negative affect and relapse to substance use (e.g., Brandon, Tiffany, Obremski, & Baker, 1990; Cooney, Litt, Morse, Bauer, & Guapp, 1997; Hodgins, el Guebaly, & Armstrong, 1995; Litman, 1984; Litt, Cooney, Kadden, & Gaupp, 1990; McKay, Rutherford, Alterman, Cacciola, & Kaplan, 1995; Shiffman, Paty, Gnys, Kassel, & Hickcox, 1996). Baker and colleagues (2003) have recently identified negative affect as the primary motive for drug use. According to this affective model of drug motivation, excessive substance use is motivated by affective regulation, both positive and negative. Substance use is often reinforcing for clients, leading the individual to engage in future substance use. Oftentimes substance use provides negative reinforcement via the amelioration of an unpleasant affective state, such as physical withdrawal symptoms (Baker et al., 2004). For example, McKay and colleagues (1995) found that cocaine addicts experienced loneliness (62.1%), depression (55.8%), tension (55.8%), and anger (40%) on the day of a relapse; a smaller percentage of the sample experienced feeling extremely good (37.9%) and extremely excited (33.7%).

In response to the high comorbidity of substance use and mood disorders, it has been proposed that substance dependence may be a form of self-medication (Khantzian, 1974). According to this theory, individuals who are experiencing severe affective disturbance may be utilizing addictive drugs as a coping mechanism, albeit a strategy that is only effective in the short-term, but can oftentimes be maladaptive in the long run. In other words, individuals are using substances to relieve symptoms of preexisting mood disorders. Alternatively, it has been proposed that drug taking as self-medication is an attempt to relieve substance-induced affective disturbances (Raimo & Schuckit, 1998), which further substantiates the finding that lapses are often predicted by self-reported negative affect (Hodgins et al., 1995). A recent study using ecological momentary assessment (EMA) provided support for this model, with alcohol consumption being prospectively predicted from nervous mood states and cross-sectionally associated with reduced levels of nervousness (Swendsen et al., 2000).

The distinctions between positive and negative affect in the prediction of treatment outcomes have been demonstrated in several studies. Hodgins and colleagues (1995) showed that both positive and negative affect were associated with alcohol relapse; however, negative affect was associated with heavy drinking and positive affect was related to lighter drinking episodes. The authors concluded that negative affect may be more predictive of major relapses, while positive affect is more often predictive of lapses. Similarly, Borland (1990) found that lapses occurring in conjunction with a positive mood were more likely to lead to successful (abstinent) recovery. In experimental manipulations, positive and negative mood inductions are both related to increases in smoking urges (Taylor, Harris, Singleton, Moolchan, & Heishman, 2000) and alcohol cue reactivity (Cooney et al., 1997). Positive affect has also been associated with more positive treatment outcomes and lower relapse rates (McKay, Merikle, Mulvaney, Weiss, & Koppenhaver, 2001).

In opposition to the prominent view of negative affect as a strong predictor of substance use, Shiffman and colleagues (2002) have recently shown that daily changes in affect, as measured using EMA (Stone & Shiffman, 1994), were not significantly associated with *ad lib.* smoking in heavy smokers prior to a designated quit date. The only psychological states that were predictive of smoking behavior were urges to smoke and restlessness. Arousal, negative affect, and attention disturbance were unrelated to smoking. In a related study using EMA, Shiffman and Waters (2004) again demonstrated that negative affect in the days prior to a smoking lapse was not predictive of the lapse event, but negative affect steadily rises in the 6 hours prior to a smoking lapse. They also found that smoking lapses were often preceded by the combination of negative affect, stress, and arguing with another individual. In the author's discussion of their findings, they state: "An argument can easily spring up in minutes and lead quickly to a lapse, without any advance build-up or predictability" (p. 198).

A behavior analysis of drug addiction demonstrates that many drugs provide both negative reinforcement (e.g., the reduction of negative affect, referred to as "self-medication") and positive reinforcement (e.g., positive outcome expectancies, or the "problem of immediate gratification"). The self-medication hypothesis applies when the individual is using a substance as a means of coping with negative emotions, conflict, or stress. The problem of immediate gratification (PIG) applies when the person is focusing on the positive aspects and euphoria of using a substance, while ignoring the negative consequences (Marlatt, 1988). The biphasic sequence of immediate reductions in dysphoria and increases in euphoria provides the temporal contingencies required for maintaining drug use behavior. In addition, the negative consequences that may accompany drug use (e.g., hangovers, loss of employment, financial strain) are often delayed. As described earlier, from a behavioral economics perspective, the value of consequences decreases as the time between the behavior and the contigency increases (Bickel & Vuchinich, 2000). Unfortunately, some of the most negative consequences resulting from addictive behavior (e.g., HIV or hepatitis C infection, liver disease, lung cancer) often occur years after the instatement of the behavior. Therefore the probability of relapse is increased when negative consequences are delayed and/or alternative reinforcers are not available (Bickel, Madden, & Petry, 1998). Bickel has provided the example that an effective treatment may provide an immediate alternative reinforcer, but only when the treatment is desired by the individual client (Marlatt & Kilmer, 1998).

Craving

Craving is possibly the most widely studied and the most poorly understood concept in the study of drug addiction (Lowman, Hunt, Litten, & Drummond, 2000). Patients, clinicians, and researchers often describe craving as a formidable adversary in the recovery and persistence of addictive disorders. The history of alcohol-craving research dates back to Isbell (1955), who described both physical (indicated by withdrawal symptoms) and psychological (related to outcome expectancies and urge) types of craving. Later, Jellinek (1960) associated craving with both a *loss of control* and the inability to abstain from alcohol, emphasizing both acute physical withdrawal and an impulsive compulsion to drink. Edwards and Gross (1976) described an "alcohol dependence syndrome" characterized by a narrow drinking repertoire, the importance of drinking, tolerance, withdrawal, and "subjective awareness of the compulsion to drink." This last characteristic was associated with both craving, defined as an irrational desire to drink, and loss of control.

Empirical investigations, incorporating a placebo design, have provided evidence that disconfirms the *loss of control* hypothesis. In one study (Marlatt, Demming, & Reid, 1973), alcohol-dependent participants who consumed alcohol, even though they were told they would not be drinking alcohol, did not consume more alcohol in an *ad lib.* consumption period than social drinkers after both groups were given an initial (priming) dose of alcohol. When the participants thought they were drinking alcohol, although they were actually drinking a nonalcoholic placebo, they continued to "lose control" and drink more of the placebo than the social drinkers following a priming dose of alcohol. Bickel and colleagues (1998) proposed that the *loss of control* phenomenon can be explained within a behavioral economics framework, based on the discounting of delayed reinforcers. Essentially, substance abusers impulsively select smaller, more immediate reinforcers in place of larger, delayed reinforcers.

Siegel, Krank, and Hinson (1988) propose that both craving and symptoms of withdrawal may be acting as conditioned drug-compensatory responses, which are often in the opposite direction from the actual unconditioned drug effect. These responses are conditioned by several exposures to drug-related stimuli paired with physiological effects of the drug. Often referred to as tolerance, this process is explained by environmental drug cues eliciting a preparatory physiological response to prepare the individual for the drug effects (e.g., the elevation of blood glucose caused by nicotine over several occasions of smoking is preceded by an anticipatory hypoglycemic response in the presence of future nicotine cues). The preparatory response allows the individual to consume more of a desired substance while reducing the effects of the drug. Symptoms of withdrawal and craving may also be limited to situations in which prior learning of preparatory responses to drug effects has occurred, such as in reactions to the exposure to drug cues (Siegel, Baptista, Kim, McDonald, & Weise, 2000).

More recently, craving has been broadly defined by conditioned rein-forcement models (Li, 2000), incentive-sensitization models (Robinson & Berridge, 2000), dopamine system regulation (Grace, 1995), social learn-ing theory (Marlatt, 1985), and cognitive processing models (Tiffany, 1990). These recent models of craving have been thoroughly discussed in a 2000 supplement of the journal, *Addiction* (Volume 95, Supplement 2), de-voted to current research perspectives on alcohol craving. In addition to the problem of defining "craving" (Lowman et al., 2000), several research-ers discussed the larger problem of measuring this phenomenon (Sayette et al., 2000; Tiffany, Carter, & Singleton, 2000). Sayette and colleagues (2000) encourage a multidimensional and theory-driven approach to the definition and measurement of craving, while Tiffany and colleagues (2000) highlight the need for more sensitive measures of craving and the revisiting of basic measurement issues, such as the reliability and validity of craving measures.

One common finding of recent addiction research is the lack of a strong association between subjective reports of craving and relapse (e.g., Kassel & Shiffman, 1992; Tiffany, 1990). Drummond and colleagues (Drummond, Litten, Lowman, & Hunt, 2000) identified four possible explanations for this finding: (1) craving and relapse are unique and inde-pendent phenomena, (2) craving is predictive of relapse, but current mea-sures of craving are not sensitive enough to detect this relationship, (3) craving is only predictive of relapse in select conditions, and (4) "the subjective experience of craving is not predictive of relapse," but the corre-lates and underlying mechanisms of craving do predict relapse. Therefore, subjective reports of craving do not predict relapse (as they are currently measured), but other factors that cause craving (such as the opponent pro-cess of drug preparatory responses or incentive-sensitization models de-scribed earlier) may also be predictive of relapse (Sayette et al., 2000).

The fourth explanation of craving described by Drummond is most consistent with a cognitive social learning model of craving as it applies to relapse and RP. According to this model, cognitive expectations impact how an individual responds to conditioned substance-related stimuli and his or her ability to utilize effective coping mechanisms. Based on this model, Marlatt and colleagues (Larimer, Palmer, & Marlatt, 1999) distin-guish craving, or the subjective desire to experience an addictive substance, from an urge, the behavioral intention or impulse to consume alcohol or drugs. Using this conceptualization, cravings may be reduced or eliminated by focusing on client's subjective biases and outcome expectancies for a de-sired substance. The current state of knowledge regarding craving and re-lapse leads us to focus on the integration of physiological, learning, and cognitive theories of drug addiction. A transactional model, whereby physiological responses, tolerance, outcome expectancies, and/or self-efficacy moderate the relationship between subjective reports of "craving" and relapse to drug addiction should be tested in future research (Niaura, 2000).

Interpersonal Determinants: Social Support

In addition to the intrapersonal influences described earlier, social support plays a critical role as an interpersonal determinant of relapse. Positive social support is highly predictive of long-term abstinence rates across several addictive behaviors (Barber & Crisp, 1995; Beattie & Longabaugh, 1997, 1999; Dobkin, Civita, Paraherakis, & Gill, 2002; Gordon & Zrull, 1991; Havassy, Hall, & Wasserman, 1991; Humphreys, Moos, & Finney, 1996; McMahon, 2001; Noone, Dua, & Markham, 1999; Rosenberg, 1983). Similarly, negative social support in the form of interpersonal conflict (Cummings, Gordon, & Marlatt, 1980) and social pressure to use substances (Annis & Davis, 1988; Brown, Vik, & Craemer, 1989) has been related to an increased risk for relapse. Social pressure may be experienced directly, such as peers trying to convince a person to use, or indirectly through modeling (e.g., a friend ordering a drink at dinner) and/or cue exposure (e.g., friends with drug paraphernalia in the house). Social network size and the perceived quality of social support have also been shown to predict relapse (McMahon, 2001). Likewise, antisocial personality traits, which tend to preclude positive social relationships, are often associated with heightened relapse risk (Alterman & Cacciola, 1991; Fals-Stewart, 1992; Longabaugh, Rubin, Malloy, Beattie, Clifford, & Noel, 1994).

Beattie and Longabaugh (1997) demonstrated that functional social support is more predictive of drinking outcomes and psychological well-being than either quality or structural support. In a later study, the same authors found that alcohol-specific support (e.g., partner supporting the patient in abstinence goals) predicted more of the variance in short- (3 months) and long-term (15 months) posttreatment abstinence rates than general support (e.g., support from friends and extended family, which may include "drinking buddies"). Furthermore, alcohol-specific support mediated the relationship between general support and abstinence, suggesting that patients should be encouraged to seek out individuals who support them in their decisions to reduce drinking or remain abstinent following treatment (Beattie & Longabaugh, 1999). In support of these findings, behavioral marital therapy (Winters, Fals-Stewart, O'Farrell, Birchler, & Kelley, 2002), which incorporates partner support in treatment goals, has been described as one of the top three empirically supported treatment methods for alcohol problems (Finney & Monahan, 1996). (The community reinforcement approach, a skills training-based treatment that focuses on building a supportive social network, and RP were regarded as the other two supported methods for alcohol treatment.)

FUTURE DIRECTIONS IN THE DEFINITION, MEASUREMENT, AND TREATMENT OF RELAPSE

Two decades have elapsed since Marlatt and Gordon published the first edition of *Relapse Prevention*. During that time the term "relapse prevention" has been widely disseminated and tested, but it has also been misused, distorted, and embellished. Several authors have criticized RP, suggesting that it be modified to incorporate more complexity (Edwards, 1987), additional relapse determinants (e.g., craving; Longabaugh, et al., 1996), more information on the likelihood or timing of a relapse event (Stout, Longabaugh, & Rubin, 1996), and increased construct validity (Maisto, Connors, & Zwyiak, 1996). In addition to these critiques, there has been an accumulation of findings regarding the importance of self-efficacy (Greenfield et al., 2000), positive and negative affect (Hodgins et al., 1995), outcome expectancies (Jones et al., 2001), craving (Lowman et al., 2000), withdrawal symptomatology (Baker et al., 2004), coping (Morganstern & Longabaugh, 2000), motivation (Project MATCH Research Group, 1997), and social support (Beattie & Longabaugh, 1999) in the relapse process.

Reconceptualizing the Relapse Process

Synthesizing this accumulation of empirical findings into a unified theory requires a degree of complexity that has traditionally not been afforded to addictive behavior researchers. Unlike the simple path diagram of the cognitive-behavioral model presented in Figure 1.1, which centers on an individual's response in a high-risk situation, we propose that the determinants described herein are multidimensional and dynamic. The use of an effective coping response may not guarantee an increase in self-efficacy and continued abstinence, although in conjunction with functional social support, generalized positive affect, and negative outcome expectancies it may greatly improve the likelihood of maintenance.

Seemingly insignificant changes in one risk factor (e.g., an undetected reduction in self-efficacy) may kindle a downward spiral of increased craving, positive outcome expectancies, and intensified negative affect. These small changes may result in a major relapse, often initiated by a minor cue. The sheer disaster of a relapse crisis after an individual has been maintaining abstinence has bewildered patients, researchers, and clinicians for years. The symbolism of "falling from the wagon" provides an illustration of the sudden, devastating experience of the chronic return to previous levels of abuse. This experience is often followed by the harsh realization that getting back on the wagon will not be as effortless as the fall from it.

The picture of relapse painted here would most likely be described as unpredictable or chaotic. In fact, many researchers and clinicians have de-

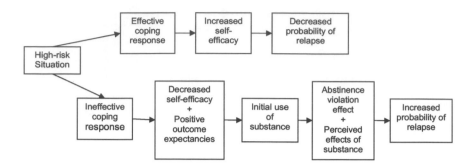

FIGURE 1.1. Cognitive-behavioral model of relapse (Marlatt & Gordon, 1985).

scribed relapse using these descriptors (Brownell et al., 1986; Donovan, 1996; Shiffman, 1989). The current reconceptualization of relapse acknowledges the complexity and dynamic nature of this process. Consider a simple example, an individual with a family history of alcoholism and low baseline self-efficacy who is likely to make more negative appraisals of perceived coping (e.g., "I can't do this. . . . Mom was always an alcoholic and I will be too"). This lowered coping-efficacy makes the person more susceptible to an ineffective coping response in a high-risk situation, and increased probability of a lapse. The lapse is followed by further reductions in self-efficacy, which combined with a higher likelihood for physical dependence (given the family history), leads to a full-blown relapse.

Focusing on the situation, we propose a dynamic interaction between several factors leading up to, and during, a high-risk situation. In every situation, an individual is faced with the challenge of balancing multiple cues and possible consequences. The individual's response can be described as a self-organizing system, incorporating distal risk factors (e.g., years of dependence, family history, social support, and comorbid psychopathology), cognitive processes (e.g., self-efficacy, outcome expectancies, craving, the AVE, motivation), and cognitive and behavioral coping skills. As shown in Figure 1.2, this dynamic model of relapse allows for several configurations of distal and proximal relapse risks (Witkiewitz & Marlatt, 2004). Dotted lines represent the proximal influences and solid lines represent distal influences. Connected boxes are hypothesized to be nonrecursive, that is, there is a reciprocal causation between them (e.g., coping skills influence drinking behavior and, in return, drinking influences coping). These *feedback loops* allow for the interaction between coping skills, cognitions, affect, and substance use behavior. As depicted by the large striped circle in Figure 1.2, situational cues (e.g., walking by the liquor store) play a prominent role in the relationship between risk factors and substance use behavior.

In order to test this new theory, future research will need to incorpo-

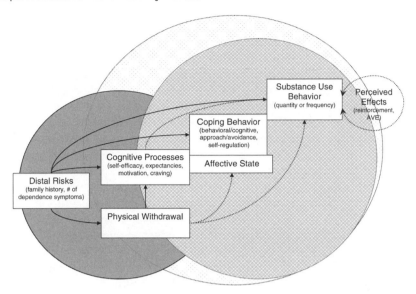

FIGURE 1.2. Dynamic model of relapse (Witkiewitz & Marlatt, 2004).

rate innovative data analytic strategies that will allow for complex and discontinuous relationships between variables. For example, Piasecki and colleagues (2000) have provided interesting findings on the withdrawal dynamics of smoking cessation, demonstrating that relapse vulnerability is indexed by the combination of severity, trajectory, and variability of withdrawal symptoms. Boker and Graham (1998) investigated dynamic instability and self-regulation in the development of adolescent substance abuse; they found that relatively small changes feedback into the system can lead to large changes over a relatively short period of time. Warren and colleagues (2003) successfully modeled an individual's daily alcohol intake using nonlinear time series analysis, which provided a data fit superior to that of a comparable linear model, and more accurately described the idiosyncrasies of drinking dynamics. Hawkins and Hawkins (1998) also present a case study of an individual's alcohol intake over a 6-year period of treatment. Based on more than 2,000 data points, analyses revealed a periodic cycle defined by bifurcations, in which lapses predicted discontinuous changes in the trajectory of the system.

The utility of nonlinear dynamical systems, such as models based on chaos and/or catastrophe theory, in the prediction and explanation of substance abuse has been described by several authors (Ehlers, 1992; Hawkins & Hawkins, 1998; Skinner, 1989; Warren et al., 2003). For example, catastrophe theory has been used to predict alcohol relapse (Hufford, Witkiewitz, Shields, Kodya, & Caruso, 2003; Witkiewitz, Hufford, Caruso, & Shields, 2002). Catastrophe models allow for the prediction of sudden discontinuous change in a measured behavior resulting from slight continuous changes in environmental and situational variables (Thom, 1975). Hufford and colleagues (Hufford, Witkiewitz, Shields, Kodya, & Caruso, 2003) evaluated a catastrophe model incorporating alcohol dependence, self-efficacy, depression, alcohol-use severity, family history, family conflict, and stress as predictors of 6-month alcohol consumption in small samples of individuals treated in both inpatient (more severe addiction) and outpatient (less severe addiction) treatment facilities. The catastrophe model provided a significantly better fit to the data in both samples, predicting 58% (inpatient) and 83% (outpatient) of the variance in posttreatment drinking, than the best-fitting linear models, which only predicted 19% (inpatient) and 14% (outpatient). Witkiewitz and colleagues (2002) replicated these initial findings using data from Project MATCH (Project MATCH Research Group, 1997), which showed alcohol risk, addiction severity, self-efficacy, depression, social support, and motivation for change predicted 77% of the variance in 12-month percentage of days abstinent (PDA) using a catastrophe model, and only 2% of the variance using a linear model. The striking amount of variance explained by the catastrophe models in these studies is posited to be a function of the underlying assumptions of catastrophe theory. Catastrophe modeling techniques allow for discontinuous functions and attempt to capture more of the data surrounding statistical modes. Oftentimes data (and behavior) is multimodal, yet linear functions will estimate a best fit line between two statistical modes. Catastrophe models seek to maximize the function near statistical modes, allowing for more data to be classified as unique variance, rather than error.

Assessing Relapse

Progress in the area of quantitative modeling procedures will only inform our understanding of the relapse process to the extent that we improve upon our operational definitions of relapse. Advancements in the assessment of lapses and relapse may provide the impetus for providing a more comprehensive definition of relapse and exhaustive understanding of this complex process (Haynes, 1995). A few of the recent developments that may increase our ability to accurately measure addictive behavior include EMA (Stone & Shiffman, 1994), interactive voice response technology (IVR; Mundt, Bohn, Drebus, & Hartley, 2001), physiological measures (Niaura, Shadel, Britt, & Abrams, 2002), and brain imaging techniques (Bauer, 2001). Many of these approaches are discussed at greater length in *Assessment of Addictive Behaviors* (Donovan & Marlatt, 2005).

EMA utilizes handheld computers to collect momentary, daily, and weekly assessments of self-reported behavior. Individuals carrying the palmtops are queried randomly, daily, and weekly. The individuals are also instructed to complete reports after an episode of use or strong temptation to use. The strength of EMA is its ability to collect data anonymously and in the moment, without the problems of retrospective recall (Shiffman et al., 1997). Using EMA, Shiffman and colleagues have been able to tease apart the differences between baseline differences and daily variation in relapse risk factors. For example, Shiffman and colleagues (2002) have recently demonstrated that daily reports of affect are not highly predictive of smoking behavior in heavy smoking adults, which is not consistent with the well-established association between affect and substance use described earlier. The weakness of EMA, like many other assessments of alcohol and drug use, is the reliance on self-reported information and the possibility of reactivity to the assessment device (e.g., participant noncompliance). IVR is very similar to EMA; however, the participants are instructed to make a telephone call to an automated telephone service, which feeds data directly from the participant's voice into a computer database. IVR is effective in that it also allows for immediate, anonymous reporting. The downfall of IVR is that it also relies on participant self-report and may result in reactivity and noncompliance (Mundt et al., 2001). Both EMA and IVR are time-consuming and more invasive than simple paper-and-pencil questionnaires, which may lead to higher rates of participant attrition and nonresponding.

Physiological measurements and brain-imaging techniques are unique to the study of relapse because they do not rely on self-report data. For example, Niaura and colleagues (2002) measured heart rate changes during a laboratory investigation of the effects of social anxiety on the prediction of relapse. The results demonstrated that an increase in social skills and a decrease in heart rate during the anxiety induction procedure predicted 3-month smoking abstinence rates. Imaging studies have also provided successful results. Using electroencephalography techniques, Bauer (2001) demonstrated that participants who relapsed during the first 6 months following treatment had enhanced high-frequency beta activity in regions of the frontal cortex, when compared to abstinent and non-drug-dependent participants. These results support the findings from previous imaging studies that showed functional deficits in the orbitofrontal cortex of relapse-prone patients, an area of the brain that has been shown to inhibit highly emotional responding (Bauer, 1994, 1997). Taken together these studies demonstrate that relapse may be assessed and predicted on an objective, physiological level.

White Bears and Mice

Gaining a better understanding of the relapse process will largely benefit from the incorporation of research on nonaddictive behavior and nonhuman animals. In this section we review social psychological models of self-control and thought suppression, and recent animal models of relapse.

With regard to addictive behaviors, the issue of self-regulation and "will-power" is commonly referenced as an explanation for success (Norcross & Vangarelli, 1989). Mischel and colleagues (Mischel, Shoda, & Mendoza-Denton, 1988) have identified self-regulation as a central feature of personality, which requires strength to maintain. For example, Wegner and Wheatley (1999) have demonstrated that self-control may be inhibited by the exercise of thought suppression. For example, when participants are told to not think about a white bear, they engage in more of the prohibited behavior than individuals who are instructed to think about white bears. These findings are highly relevant to the study of craving and the AVE. If an individual is told, either by treatment staff or family and friends, not to think about using cocaine and to avoid all cues associated with cocaine, they may be more likely to have intrusive thoughts about using cocaine and increased craving.

Recent work by Baumeister, Heatherton, and Tice (1994) has described self-control and self-regulation as a type of psychological muscle, which may be strengthened and may also become fatigued. The "fatigue" of self-regulation, which has also been called "ego-depletion," provides an explanation for why individuals are more likely to succumb to temptation (i.e., self-regulatory failure) when they are experiencing stress and/or negative affect. Coping with stressful life events and emotional distress are related to the deterioration of self-control (Muraven, Baumeister, & Tice, 1999). Fortunately, muscles that are deteriorating may be strengthened, and recent research from Baumeister's lab has demonstrated that the exertion of self-regulatory control can be strengthened over time. Therefore, exerting self-control leads to ego depletion over the short-term, but over time self-control becomes stronger with exercise. These findings have strong implications for the treatment of addiction. Individuals who are encouraged to exert willpower in the face of cravings, negative affect, and stressful events can be validated for how difficult it is to maintain treatment gains and reinforced for their efforts by describing the evidence of willpower as a muscle that needs to be continually strengthened and stretched.

Unlike models of self-control, certain hypothesized precipitants of relapse cannot be ethically demonstrated in an experimental setting. For example, researchers are unable to empirically show that environmental stress and low self-efficacy cause relapse in participants who are attempting to maintain abstinence. Alternatively, research may be conducted with animal models of human behavior; some aspects of stress, cue reactivity, and craving have been shown to predict "relapse" in animals (Littleton, 2000; Marlatt, 2002). Shaham, Erb, and Stewart (2000) have demonstrated that footshock stress causes reinstatement of heroin and cocaine seeking in rats. Roberts, Cole, and Koob (1996) verified that rats engage in significantly more ethanol seeking and consumption during withdrawal,

and several researchers have demonstrated environment-dependent tolerance and "place-preferences" for cages previously associated with alcohol
administration (e.g., Cole, Littleton, & Little, 1999; Kalant, 1998; Siegel et
al., 1988).

Unfortunately, animals do not truly experience "relapse," "craving,"
or "alcoholism," and models tested within the confines of a rat's cage do
not easily generalize to the high-risk situations and subsequent responses
experienced by humans (Littleton, 2000). Nevertheless, recent advances
using drug reinstatement, priming, and extinction models have demonstrated the effects of addictive substances on anticipation, postwithdrawal
consumption, and incentive motivation, and future work with animal
models may continue to provide more insight into human relapse (Li,
2000). Recently, Leri and Stewart (2002) trained rats to self-administer
heroin in the presence of a light stimulus. After extinction the rats experienced one of six different types of lapses (no heroin and no-light stimulus,
no heroin with light stimulus, self-administered heroin and no-light stimulus, self-administered heroin with light stimulus, investigator-administered
heroin yoked with self-administering rats with light stimulus). This design
is both innovative and informative because it is the first study of its kind to
measure the lapse–relapse process in animals (Baker & Curtin, 2002).
Further, Leri and Stewart (2002) provide data that asks whether a
self-administered lapse is associated with different relapse rates than an
investigator-administered lapse (called "priming"). The results from this
study demonstrated that self-initiated heroin use and heroin administration
paired with a heroin-related stimuli lead to heroin seeking during the relapse test. Mere exposure to heroin or heroin-related stimuli had little or
no effect on subsequent heroin-seeking behavior during the relapse test.
The robustness of their results is notable; however; animal models of relapse will never provide an analogue for the cognitive (e.g., abstinence violation effect) and environmental (e.g., peer pressure) precipitants of relapse
in humans (Baker & Curtin, 2002; Marlatt, 2002). Furthermore, rats cannot make a voluntary commitment to either abstinence or moderation
goals during the extinction phase, which has been shown to be a powerful
predictor of relapse in human substance users (Sobell, Sobell, Bogardis,
Leo, & Skinner, 1992).

Relapse Prevention Treatment in the 21st Century

Two recent, methodologically rigorous meta-analyses of treatment outcome studies for alcohol use disorders provided invaluable data on the
present state and proposed future direction of alcohol treatment. Moyer
and colleagues (Moyer, Finney, & Searingen, 2002) demonstrated that for
less severe cases, brief interventions are more effective than extensive interventions; for severe cases, brief interventions were found to be as effective

as extended interventions. This finding coincides with the results from Project MATCH (Project MATCH Research Group, 1997), in which the four-session motivational enhancement treatment was as successful as 12 sessions of either cognitive behavioral or 12-step facilitation therapies. Likewise, Miller and Wilbourne (2002) found brief interventions to be one of the most efficacious treatments. Other treatments with the strongest evidence of efficacy were social skills training (broadly defined as RP by McCrady, 2000), the community reinforcement approach, behavior contracting, behavioral marital therapy, and case management. Given the restrictive climate of health care and the time limitations imposed by managed care and health maintenance organizations, it is very encouraging that briefer interventions are at least as effective as more intensive, extended treatments. Furthermore, advertising a less intensive and more supportive intervention, rather than a traditional 28-day inpatient treatment program, may reduce the fears and stigma associated with seeking treatment for alcohol and drug problems (Marlatt & Witkiewitz, 2002).

We view RP as playing a role in the continuous development of brief interventions for alcohol and drug problems. Motivational interviewing (Miller & Rollnick, 2002), brief physician advice (Fleming, Barry, Manwell, Johnson, & London, 1997), and two-session assessment and feedback (Dimeff, Baer, Kivlahan, & Marlatt, 1999) are three examples of brief interventions that have demonstrated success in reducing alcohol and drug use in a variety of populations. Other studies have found that many participants are maintaining abstinence at 6 and 12 months following treatment. Incorporating the cognitive-behavioral model of relapse and RP techniques, either within the brief intervention or as a booster session of the initial intervention, will provide additional help for individuals who are attempting to abstain following treatment. In addition, RP techniques may be supplemented by other treatments for addictive behaviors, such as pharmacotherapy (Schmitz, Stotts, Rhoades, & Grabowski, 2001) or mindfulness meditation (Marlatt, 2002). Currently, a treatment is being developed that will integrate RP techniques with mindfulness training into a cohesive treatment package for addictive behaviors (see Witkiewitz, Marlatt, & Walker, in press, for an extensive introduction).

Adjunct Treatment Approaches: Medication and Meditation

Medication

Pharmacotherapy has often been the first line of defense in the fight against substance use disorders. With regard to alcohol use disorders, disulfiram (Antabuse) has been widely used as behavioral control agent designed to prevent an individual from drinking by bringing about an aversive response (sickness) to drinking alcohol. Compliance with disulfiram treatment is extremely low, and it has not been shown to be superior to placebo in double-blind studies (Schuckit, 1996). More recently, naltrexone (an opiate antagonist) and acamprosate (calcium acetyle homotaurine) have both been shown to be better than placebo at reducing cravings and increasing the percentage of days abstinent following treatment (Sass, Soyka, Mann, & Zieglgansberger, 1996; Volpicelli, Alterman, Hayashida, & O'Brien, 1992).

Smoking cessation has been successfully treated using nicotine replacement therapy (NRT; Hughes, 1993). Although the effectiveness of NRT varies widely (18–77%), more successful outcomes have been found when NRT is combined with a behavioral treatment (Fiore, Smith, Jorenby, & Baker, 1994). It appears that continuous exposure to low doses of nicotine, which decreases acute physical withdrawal symptoms, in combination with providing individuals with the skills to quit smoking (e.g., teaching effective coping strategies), is related to increased abstinence success, coping skills, and self-efficacy (Cinciriprini, Cinciriprini, Wallfisch, Haque, & Van Vunakis, 1996).

Opiate addiction has been primarily treated with a variety of opioid replacement agents, such as methadone, LAAM (levo-alpha-acetylmethadol), buprenorphine, and naltrexone (Hart, McCance-Katz, & Kosten, 2001). The efficacy of methadone in reducing relapse has been well demonstrated (Ling, Rawson, & Compton, 1994), although the higher doses required for better outcomes can be highly addictive (Caplehorn, Bell, Kleinbaum, & Gebski, 1993). LAAM is an opioid agonist with a longer duration of action than methadone, although higher doses of LAAM may have undesirable and/or unsafe side effects (Jones et al., 1998). Ling and colleagues (1994) demonstrated that buprenorphine may result in less physical dependence than methadone, although more large-scale research needs to be conducted on the efficacy and side-effects of buprenorphine (Hart et al., 2001). One new approach to opiate dependence that may be more desirable for clients and cost-effective for society is the implementation of methadone maintenance by primary care providers. A randomized controlled trial comparing a traditional narcotic treatment program with methadone delivered in the primary care office demonstrated that office-based methadone maintenance was as feasible and effective, and was significantly more satisfactory than the narcotic treatment program (Fiellin et al., 2001).

Cocaine has been treated within an RP framework using both acute treatment (drugs that work to suppress acute withdrawal from cocaine) and maintenance treatments (drugs that help patients maintain abstinence, albeit with limited sucess). Placebo-controlled trials with two acute treatments, bromocriptine and amantidine, have demonstrated mixed findings (Kosten, 1989; Kosten et al., 1992). Among the maintenance treatments, desipiramine has been shown to reduce cocaine use (Feingold, Oliveto, Schottenfeld, & Kosten, 2002). Naltrexone (50 mg) has also been shown to be effective in the reduction of cocaine use following treatment, but only if it is combined with RP therapy (Schmitz et al., 2001). This dosage of naltrexone may be ineffective for individuals with co-occurring cocaine and alcohol dependence (Hersh, Van Kirk, & Kranzler, 1998). Other studies have demonstrated that disulfiram is effective in the treatment of this polysubstance combination (Carroll et al., 1993; Higgins, Bundey, Bickel, Hughes, & Foerg, 1993), and is regularly prescribed within community reinforcement approaches (Budney & Higgins, 1998). Although multiple pharmacotherapies have been evaluated as treatments, or adjuncts to therapy for cocaine addiction, no medication has consistently demonstrated efficacy in comparison to placebo.

Meditation

Recently our laboratory, the Addictive Behaviors Research Center at the University of Washington, completed a pilot study on the use of meditation as a "treatment" for alcohol and drug problems. Inmates, many of whom were heavy substance abusers prior to incarceration, were recruited from a minimal security rehabilitation facility (North Rehabilitation Facility, Seattle) to participate in a 10-day Vipassana meditation course. Inmates who did not want to participate in the course were recruited to serve as case-matched, treatment as usual, control participants. Three months following their release from prison, Vipassana participants demonstrated significant decreases in alcohol and drug consumption, increased self-regulation, higher levels of optimism, and less recidivism, when compared to a case-matched control group (Marlatt, Witkiewitz, Dillworth, et al., 2004). Currently we are extending this study to include nonincarcerated individuals taking Vipassana courses in Washington, California, Massachusetts, and Illinois. Similarly, meditation-type interventions have been shown to be effective in the treatment of alcohol relapse (Taub, Steiner, Weingarten, & Walton, 1994), depression (Teasdale et al., 2002), personality disorders (Linehan, 1993), stress reduction (Bishop, 2002), and irritable bowel syndrome (Keefer & Blanchard, 2001).

CONCLUSIONS

Relapse is a formidable challenge in the treatment of all behavior disorders. Individuals working on behavior change are confronted with urges, cues, and automatic thoughts regarding the maladaptive behaviors they are attempting to change. Several authors have described relapse as complex, dynamic, and unpredictable (Buhringer, 2000; Donovan, 1996; Marlatt, 1996a; Shiffman, 1989), but previous conceptualizations have proposed static models of relapse risk factors (e.g., Marlatt & Gordon, 1985; Stout et al., 1996). The reconceptualization of relapse proposed in this chapter acknowledges the complexity and unpredictable nature of substance use behavior following the commitment to abstinence or a moderation goal. Future research should continue to focus on refining measurement devices and developing better data analytic strategies for assessing behavior change. Empirical testing of the postcessation response system and further refinements of this new model will add to our understanding of relapse and how to prevent it.

The chapters that follow in this volume focus on intervention strategies designed to both prevent and manage relapse in the treatment of addictive behaviors. Each chapter provides an overview of the treatment approach for specific problem areas, including both substance use and other addictive behaviors. This book is designed to be used with *Assessment of Addictive Behaviors* (Donovan & Marlatt, 2005). Taken together, these two books provide the foundation for an evidence-based assessment and a cognitive-behavioral intervention approach to relapse prevention.

REFERENCES

Allsop, S., & Saunders, B. (1989). Relapse and alcohol problems. In M. Gossop (Ed.), *Relapse and addictive behavior* (pp. 11–40). London: Routledge.

Alterman, A. I., & Cacciola, J. S. (1991). The antisocial personality disorder diagnosis in substance abusers: Problems and issues. *Journal of Nervous and Mental Disease, 179*, 401–409.

Annis, H. M. (1982a). *Inventory of Drinking Situations.* Toronto: Addiction Research Foundation.

Annis, H. M. (1982b). *Situational Confidence Questionnaire.* Toronto: Addiction Research Foundation.

Annis, H. M., & Davis, C. S. (1988). Assessment of expectancies. In D. M. Donovan & G. A. Marlatt (Eds.), *Assessment of addictive behaviors* (1st ed., pp. 84–111). New York: Guilford Press.

Baker, T. B., & Curtin, J. J. (2002). How will we know a lapse when we see one? Comment on Leri and Stewart experimental and clinical. *Psychopharmacology, 10*(4), 350–352.

Baker, T. B., Piper, M. E., McCarthy, D. E., Majeskie, M. R., & Fiore, M. C. (2004). Addiction motivation reformulated: An affective processing model of negative reinforcement. *Psychological Bulletin, 111*, 33–51.

Bandura, A. (1977). Self-efficacy: Toward a unifying theory of behavioral change. *Psychological Review, 84*, 191–215.

Barber, J. G., & Crisp, B. R. (1995). Social support and prevention of relapse following treatment for alcohol abuse. *Research on Social Work Practice, 5*(3), 283–296.

Bauer, L. O. (1994). Electroencephalographic and autonomic predictors of relapse in alcohol-dependent patients. *Alcoholism: Clinical and Experimental Research, 18*(3), 755–760.

Bauer, L. O. (1997). Frontal P300 decrements, childhood conduct disorder, family history and the prediction of relapse among abstinent cocaine abusers. *Drug and Alcohol Dependence, 44*(1), 1–10.

Bauer, L. O. (2001). Predicting relapse to alcohol and drug abuse via quantitative electroencephalography. *Neuropsychopharmacology, 25*(3), 332–340.

Baumeister, R. F., Heatherton, T. F., & Tice, D. M. (1994). *Losing control: How and why people fail at self-regulation.* San Diego, CA: Academic Press.

Beattie, M. C., & Longabaugh, R. (1997). Interpersonal factors and post-treatment drinking and subjective well-being. *Addiction, 92,* 1507–1521.

Beattie, M. C., & Longabaugh, R. (1999). General and alcohol-specific social support following treatment. *Addictive Behaviors, 24*(5), 593–606.

Bickel, W. K., Madden, G. J., & Petry, N. M. (1998). The price of change: Behavioral economics of drug dependence. *Behavior Therapy, 29,* 545–565.

Bickel, W. K., & Vuchinich, R. E. (2000). *Reframing health behavior change with behavioral economics.* Mahwah, NJ: Erlbaum.

Bien, T. H., Miller, W. R., & Boroughs, J. M. (1993). Motivational interviewing with alcohol outpatients. *Behavioral and Cognitive Psychotherapy, 21,* 347–356.

Bishop, S. R. (2002). What do we really know about mindfulness-based stress reduction? *Psychosomatic Medicine, 64*(1), 71–83.

Boker, S. M., & Graham, J. (1998). A dynamical systems analysis of adolescent substance abuse. *Multivariate Behavioral Research, 33*(4), 479–507.

Bolles, R. (1972). Reinforcement, expectancy, and learning. *Psychological Review, 79,* 394–409.

Borland, R. (1990). Slip-ups and relapse in attempts to quit smoking. *Addictive Behaviors, 15,* 235–245.

Brandon, T. H., Tiffany, S. T., Obremski, K. M., & Baker, T. B. (1990). Postcessation cigarette use: The process of relapse. *Addictive Behaviors, 15,* 105–114.

Brown, S. A., Goldman, M. S., & Christiansen, B. A. (1985). Do alcohol expectancies mediate drinking patterns of adults? *Journal of Consulting and Clinical Psychology, 53,* 512–519.

Brown, S. A., Vik, P. W., & Craemer, V. A. (1989). Characteristics of relapse following adolescent substance abuse treatment. *Addictive Behaviors, 14,* 291–300.

Brownell, K. D., Marlatt, G. A., Lichtenstein, E., & Wilson, G. T. (1986). Understanding and preventing relapse. *American Psychologist, 41,* 765–782.

Brownell, K. D., & Wadden, T. A. (1992). Etiology and treatment of obesity: Understanding a serious, prevalent, and refractory disorder. *Journal of Consulting and Clinical Psychology, 60*(4), 505–517.

Bruce, T. J., Spiegel, D., & Hegel, M. (1999). Cognitive-behavioral therapy helps prevent relapse and recurrence of panic disorder following alprazolam discontinuation: A long-term follow-up of the Peoria and Dartmouth studies. *Journal of Consulting and Clinical Psychology, 67*(1), 151–156.

Budney, A., & Higgins, S. T. (1998). *A community reinforcement plus vouchers approach: Treating cocaine addiction* (Manual 3, Therapy Manuals for Drug Addiction). Rockville, MD: National Institute on Drug Abuse.

Budney, A. J., Higgins, S. T., Radonovich, K. J., & Novy, P. L. (2000). Adding voucher-based incentives to coping skills and motivational enhancement improves outcomes during treatment for marijuana dependence. *Journal of Consulting and Clinical Psychology, 68*(6), 1051–1061.

Buhringer, G. (2000). Testing CBT mechanisms of action: Humans behave in a more complex way than our treatment studies would predict. *Addiction, 95*(11), 1715–1716.

Burke, B. L., Arkowitz, H., & Menchola, M. (2003). The efficacy of motivational interviewing: A meta-analysis of controlled clinical trials. *Journal of Consulting and Clinical Psychology, 71*(5), 843–861.

Burling, T. A., Reilly, P. M., Molten, J. O., & Ziff, D. C. (1989). Self-efficacy and relapse among inpatient drug and alcohol abusers: A predictor of outcome. *Journal of Studies on Alcohol, 50*(4), 354–360.

Butler, C., Rollnick, S., Cohen, D., Russell, I., Bachmann, M., & Stott, N. (1999). Motivational consulting versus brief advice for smokers in general practice: A randomized trial. *British Journal of General Practice, 49*, 611–616.

Caplehorn, J. R., Bell, J., Kleinbaum, D. G., & Gebski, V. J. (1993). Methadone dose and heroin use during maintenance treatment. *Addiction, 88*, 119–124.

Carey, M. P., Braaten, L. S., Maisto, S. A., Gleason, J. R., Forsyth, A. D., Durant, L. E., & Jaoworski, B. C. (2000). Using information, motivational enhancement, and skills training to reduce the risk of HIV infection for low-income urban women: A second randomized clinical trial. *Health Psychology, 19*, 3–11.

Carroll, K. M. (1996). Relapse prevention as a psychosocial treatment: A review of controlled clinical trials. *Experimental and Clinical Psychopharmacology, 4*, 46–54.

Carroll, K. M., Rounsaville, B. J., & Gawin, F. H. (1991). A comparative trial of psychotherapies for ambulatory cocaine abusers: Relapse prevention and interpersonal psychotherapy. *American Journal of Drug and Alcohol Abuse, 17*(3), 229–247.

Carroll, K. M., Rounsaville, B. J., Nich, C., & Gordon, L. T. (1994). One-year follow-up of psychotherapy and pharmacotherapy for cocaine dependence: Delayed emergence of psychotherapy effects. *Archives of General Psychiatry, 51*(12), 989–997.

Carroll, K. M., Ziedonis, D., O'Malley, S., McCance-Katz, E., Gordon, L., & Rounsaville, B. (1993). Pharmacological interventions for abusers of alcohol and cocaine: Disulfiram versus naltrexone. *American Journal of Addictions, 2*, 77–79.

Carter, B. L., & Tiffany, S. T. (1999). Meta-analysis of cue-reactivity in addiction research. *Addiction, 94*(3), 327–340.

Chamberlain, L. L., & Butz, M. R. (1998). *Clinical chaos: A therapist's guide to nonlinear dynamics and therapeutic change.* Philadelphia: Brunner/Mazel.

Chaney, E. R., O'Leary, M. R., & Marlatt, G. A. (1978). Skill training with alcoholics. *Journal of Consulting and Clinical Psychology, 46*, 1092–1104.

Chung, T., Langenbucher, J., Labouvie, E., Pandina, R. J., & Moos, R. H. (2001). Changes in alcoholic patients' coping responses predict 12-month treatment outcomes. *Journal of Consulting and Clinical Psychology, 69*(1), 92–100.

Cinciriprini, P. M., Cinciriprini, L. G., Wallfisch, A., Hague, W., & Van Vunakis, H. (1996). Behavior therapy and the transdermal nicotine patch: Effects on cessation outcome, affect, and coping. *Journal of Consulting and Clinical Psychology, 64*, 314–323.

Cinciriprini, P. M., Wetter, D. W., Fouladi, R. T., Blalock, J. A., Carter, B. L., Cinciriprini, L. G., et al. (2003). The effects of depressed mood on smoking cessation: Mediation by postcessation self-efficacy. *Journal of Consulting and Clinical Psychology, 71*(2), 292–301.

Cole, J. C., Littleton, J. M., & Little, H. J. (1999). Effects of repeated ethanol administration in the plus maze: A simple model for conditioned abstinence behavior. *Psychopharmacology, 142,* 270–279.

Collins, L. R., & Lapp, W. M. (1991). Restraint and attributions: Evidence of the abstinence violation effect in alcohol consumption. *Cognitive Therapy and Research, 15*(1), 69–84.

Connors, G. J., Maisto, S. A., & Zywiak, W. H. (1996). Extensions of relapse predictors beyond high-risk situations: Understanding relapse in the broader context of post-treatment functioning. *Addiction, 91*(Suppl.), 173–189.

Connors, G. J., Tarbox, A. R., & Faillace, L. A. (1993). Changes in alcohol expectancies and drinking behavior among treated problem drinkers. *Journal of Studies on Alcohol, 54,* 676–683.

Cooney, N. L., Litt, M. D., Morse, P. A., Bauer, L. O., & Gaupp, L. (1997). Alcohol cue reactivity, negative-mood reactivity, and relapse in treated alcoholic men. *Journal of Abnormal Psychology, 106,* 243–250.

Cox, W. M., & Klinger, E. (1988). A motivational model of alcohol use. *Journal of Abnormal Psychology, 97,* 165–180.

Cummings, C., Gordon, J. R., & Marlatt, G. A. (1980). Relapse: Strategies of prevention and prediction. In W. R. Miller (Ed.), *The addictive behaviors* (pp. 291–321). Oxford, UK: Pergamon Press.

Curry, S., Marlatt, G. A., & Gordon, J. R. (1987). Abstinence violation effect: Validation of an attributional construct with smoking cessation. *Journal of Consulting and Clinical Psychology, 55,* 145–149.

Daley, D. C., & Marlatt, G. A. (2005). Relapse prevention. In J. H. Lowinson, P. Ruiz, R. B. Millman, & J. G. Langrod (Eds.), *Substance abuse: A comprehensive textbook* (4th ed., pp. 772–785). Philadelphia: Lippincott, Williams, & Wilkins.

Daley, D. C., Marlatt, G. A., & Spotts, C. E. (2003). Relapse prevention: Clinical models and intervention strategies. In A. W. Graham et al. (Eds.), *Principles of addiction medicine* (3rd ed., pp. 467–485). Chevy Chase, MD: American Society of Addiction Medicine.

Davis, J. R., & Glaros, A. G. (1986). Relapse prevention and smoking cessation. *Addictive Behaviors, 11*(2), 105–114.

DiClemente, C. C., Carbonari, J. P., Montgomery, R. P. G., & Hughes, S. O. (1994). The Alcohol Abstinence Self-Efficacy Scale. *Journal of Studies on Alcohol, 55*(2), 141–148.

DiClemente, C. C., & Hughes, S. O. (1990). Stages of change profiles in outpatient alcoholism treatment. *Journal of Substance Abuse, 2,* 217–235.

Dimeff, L. A., Baer, J. S., Kivlahan, D. R., & Marlatt, G. A. (1999). *Brief Alcohol Screening and Intervention for College Students (BASICS): A harm reduction approach.* New York: Guilford Press.

Dimeff, L. A., & Marlatt, G. A. (1998). Preventing relapse and maintaining change in addictive behaviors. *Clinical Psychology: Science and Practice, 5*(4), 513–525.

Dobkin, P. L., Civita, M., Paraherakis, A., & Gill, K. (2002). The role of functional social support in treatment retention and outcomes among outpatient adult substance abusers. *Addiction, 97*(3), 347–356.

Donovan, D. M. (1996). Marlatt's classification of relapse precipitants: Is the emperor still wearing clothes? *Addiction, 91*(Suppl.), 131–137.

Donovan, D. M., & Marlatt, G. A. (Eds.). (2005). *Assessment of addictive behaviors* (2nd ed.). New York: Guilford Press.

Drummond, D. C., Litten, R. Z., Lowman, C., & Hunt, W. A. (2000). Craving research: Future directions. *Addiction, 95*(Suppl. 2), 247–255.

Edwards, G. (1987). [Book review of *Relapse Prevention*, edited by G. A. Marlatt and J. R. Gordon.] *British Journal of Addiction, 82,* 319–323.

Edwards, G., & Gross, M. M. (1976). Alcohol dependence: Provisional description of a clinical syndrome. *British Medical Journal, 1,* 1058–1061.

Ehlers, C. L. (1992). The new physics of chaos: Can it help us understand the effects of alcohol? *Alcohol Health and Research World, 16*(4), 169–176.

Fals-Stewart, W. (1992). Personality characteristics of substance abusers: An MCMI cluster typology of recreational drug users treated in a therapeutic community and its relationship to length of stay and outcome. *Journal of Personality Assessment, 59*(3), 515–527.

Feingold, A., Oliveto, A., Schottenfeld, R., & Kosten, T. R. (2002). Utility of crossover designs in clinical trials: Efficacy of desipramine vs. placebo in opioid-dependent cocaine abusers. *American Journal of Addictions, 11*(2), 111–123.

Fiellin, D. A., O'Connor, P. G., Chawarski, M., Pakes, J. P., Pantalon, M. V., & Schottenfeld, R. S. (2001). Methadone maintenance in primary care: A randomized controlled trial. *Journal of the American Medical Association, 286*(14), 1724–1731.

Finney, J. W., & Monahan, S. C. (1996). The cost-effectiveness of treatment for alcoholism: A second approximation. *Journal of Studies on Alcohol, 52,* 517–540.

Fiore, M. D., Smith, S. S., Jorenby, D. E., & Baker, T. B. (1994). The effectiveness of the nicotine patch for smoking cessation: A meta-analysis. *Journal of the American Medical Association, 271,* 1940–1947.

Fleming, M. F., Barry, K. L., Manwell, L. B., Johnson, K., & London, R. (1997). Brief physician advice for problem alcohol drinkers: A randomized controlled trial in community-based primary care practices. *Journal of the American Medical Association, 277*(13), 1039–1045.

Goldman, M. S., Brown, S. A., Christiansen, B. A., & Smith, G. T. (1991). Alcoholism etiology and memory: Broadening the scope of alcohol expectancy research. *Psychological Bulletin, 110,* 137–146.

Goldstein, M. G., Niaura, R., Follick, M. J., & Abrahms, D. B. (1989). Effects of behavioral skills training and schedule of nicotine gum administration on smoking cessation. *American Journal of Psychiatry, 146*(1), 56–60.

Gordon, A. J., & Zrull, M. (1991). Social networks and recovery: One year after inpatient treatment. *Journal of Substance Abuse Treatment, 8*(3), 143–152.

Grace, A. A. (1995). The tonic/phasic model of dopamine system regulation: Its relevance for understanding how stimulant abuse can alter basal ganglia function. *Drug and Alcohol Dependence, 37,* 111–129.

Greenfield, S., Hufford, M., Vagge, L., Muenz, L., Costello, M., & Weiss, R. (2000). The relationship of self-efficacy expectancies to relapse among alcohol dependent men and women: A prospective study. *Journal of Studies on Alcohol, 61,* 345–351.

Groves, P., & Farmer, R. (1994). Buddhism and addictions. *Addictions Research*, 2, 183–194.

Gwaltney, C. J., Shiffman, S., Paty, J. A., Liu, K. S., Kassel, J. D., Gnys, M., et al. (2002). Using self-efficacy judgments to predict characteristics of lapses to smoking. *Journal of Consulting and Clinical Psychology*, 70, 1140–1149.

Hart, C., McCance-Katz, E. F., & Kosten, T. R. (2001). Pharmacotherapies used in common substance use disorders. In F. M. Tims, C. G. Leukefeld, & J. J. Platt (Eds.), *Relapse and recovery in addictions* (pp. 303–333). New Haven, CT: Yale University Press.

Havassy, B. E., Hall, S. M., & Wasserman, D. A. (1991). Social support and relapse: Commonalities among alcoholics, opiate users, and cigarette smokers. *Addictive Behaviors*, 16, 253–246.

Hawkins, J. D., Catalano, R. F., Gillmore, M. R., & Wells, E. A. (1989). Skills training for drug abusers: Generalization, maintenance, and effects on drug use. *Journal of Consulting and Clinical Psychology*, 75(4), 559–563.

Hawkins, R. C., & Hawkins, C. A. (1998). Dynamics of substance abuse: Implications of chaos theory for clinical research. In L. Chamberlain & M. Butz (Eds.), *Clinical chaos*. NY: Taylor & Francis.

Haynes, S. N. (1995). Introduction to the special section on chaos theory and psychological assessment. *Psychological Assessment*, 7(1), 3–4.

Heather, N., & Stallard, A. (1989). Does the Marlatt model underestimate the importance of conditioned craving in the relapse process? In M. Gossop (Ed.), *Relapse and addictive behavior* (pp. 180–208). London: Routledge.

Hersh, D., Van Kirk, J. R., & Kranzler, H. R. (1998). Naltrexone treatment of comorbid alcohol and cocaine use disorders. *Psychopharmacology*, 139, 44–52.

Herz, M. I., Lamberti, J. S., Mintz, J., Scott, R., O'Dell, S., McCartan, L., et al. (2000). A program for relapse prevention in schizophrenia: A controlled study. *Archives of General Psychiatry*, 57, 277–283.

Higgins, S. T., Budney, A. J., Bickel, N. K., Hughes, J. R., & Foerg, F. (1993). Disulfiram therapy in patients abusing cocaine and alcohol. *American Journal of Psychiatry*, 150, 576–676.

Hiss, H., Foa, E., & Kozak, M. J. (1994). Relapse prevention for treatment of obsessive–compulsive disorder. *Journal of Consulting and Clinical Psychology*, 62(4), 801–808.

Hodgins, D. C., el Guebaly, N., & Armstrong, S. (1995). Prospective and retrospective reports of mood states before relapse to substance use. *Journal of Consulting and Clinical Psychology*, 63, 400–407.

Hufford, M. H., Witkiewitz, K., Shields, A. L., Kodya, S., & Caruso, J. C. (2003). Applying nonlinear dynamics to the prediction of alcohol use disorder treatment outcomes. *Journal of Abnormal Psychology*, 112(2), 219–227.

Hughes, J. R. (1993). Pharmacotherapy for smoking cessation: Unvalidated assumptions, anomalies, and suggestions for future research. *Journal of Consulting and Clinical Psychology*, 61, 751–760.

Humphreys, K., Moos, R. H., & Finney, J. W. (1996). Life domains, Alcoholics Anonymous, and role incumbency in the 3-year course of problem drinking. *Journal of Nervous and Mental Disease*, 184(8), 475–481.

Hunt, W. A., Barnett, L. W., & Branch, L. G. (1971). Relapse rates in addiction programs. *Journal of Clinical Psychology, 27,* 455–456.

Irvin, J. E., Bowers, C. A., Dunn, M. E., & Wang, M. C. (1999). Efficacy of relapse prevention: A meta-analytic review. *Journal of Consulting and Clinical Psychology, 67*(4), 563–570.

Isbell, H. (1955). Craving for alcohol. *Quarterly Journal of Studies on Alcohol, 16,* 38–42.

Jellinek, E. M. (1960). *The disease concept of alcoholism.* Highland Park, NJ: Hillhouse Press.

Jones, B. T., Corbin, W., & Fromme, K. (2001). A review of expectancy theory and alcohol consumption. *Addiction, 96,* 57–72.

Jones, B. T., & McMahon, J. (1996). A comparison of positive and negative alcohol expectancy value and their multiplicative composite as predictors of post-treatment abstinence survivorship. *Addiction, 91,* 89–99.

Jones, H. E., Strain, E. C., Bigelow, G. E., Walsh, S. L., Stitzer, M. L., Eissenberg, T., et al. (1998). Induction with levomethadyl acetate: Safety and efficacy. *Archives of General Psychiatry, 55*(8), 729–736.

Kadden, R. (1996). Is Marlatt's taxonomy reliable or valid? *Addiction, 91*(Suppl.), 139–146.

Kalant, H. (1998). Research on tolerance: What can we learn from history? *Alcoholism: Clinical and Experimental Research, 22,* 67–76.

Kassel, J. D., & Shiffman, S. (1992). What can hunger tell us about drug craving? A comparative analysis of the two constructs. *Advances in Behaviour Therapy and Research, 14,* 141–167.

Katon, W., Rutter, C., Ludman, E. J., Von Korff, M., Lin, E., Simon, G., et al. (2001). A randomized trial of relapse prevention of depression in primary care. *Archives of General Psychiatry, 58,* 241–247.

Keefer, L., & Blanchard, E. B. (2001). The effects of relaxation response meditation on the symptoms of irritable bowel syndrome: Results of a controlled treatment study. *Behaviour Research and Therapy, 39*(7), 801–811.

Kelly, A. B., & Witkiewitz, K. (2003). Accessibility of alcohol-related attitudes: A cross-lag panel model with young adults. *Alcoholism: Clinical and Experimental Research, 27*(8), 1241–1250.

Khantzian, E. J. (1974). Opiate addiction: A critique of theory and some implications for treatment. *American Journal of Psychotherapy, 28*(1), 59–70.

Kosten, T. R. (1989). Pharmacotherapeutic interventions for cocaine abuse: Matching patients to treatments. *Journal of Nervous and Mental Disease, 177,* 379–389.

Kosten, T. R., Silverman, D. G., Fleming, J., Kosten, T. A., Gawin, F. H., Compton, M., Jatlow, P., & Byck, R. (1992). Intravenous cocaine challenges during naltrexone maintenance: A preliminary study. *Biological Psychiatry, 32,* 543–548.

Lam, D. H., Watkins, E., Hayward, P., Bight, J., Wright, K., Kerr, N., Parr-Davis, G., & Sham, P. (2003). A randomised controlled study of cognitive therapy of relapse prevention for bipolar affective disorder—Outcome of the first year. *Archives of General Psychiatry, 60,* 145–152.

Larimer, M. E., Palmer, R. S., & Marlatt, G. A. (1999). Relapse prevention: An overview of Marlatt's cognitive-behavioral model. *Alcohol Research and Health,* 23(2), 151–160.

Laws, D. R. (1995). Central elements in relapse prevention procedures with sex offenders. *Psychology, Crime and Law,* 2(1), 41–53.

Laws, D. R., Hudson, S. M., & Ward, T. (Eds.). (2000). *Remaking relapse prevention with sex offenders: A sourcebook.* Thousand Oaks, CA: Sage.

Lazarus, R. S. (1966). *Psychological stress and the coping process.* New York: McGraw-Hill.

Lazarus, R. S., & Folkman, S. (1984). *Stress, appraisal, and coping.* New York: Springer.

Leigh, B. C., & Stacy, A. W. (1991). On the scope of alcohol expectancy research: Remaining issues of measurement and meaning. *Psychological Bulletin, 110,* 147–154.

Leri, F., & Stewart, J. (2002). The consequences of different "lapses" on relapse to heroin seeking in rats. *Experimental and Clinical Psychopharmacology, 10*(4), 339–349.

Li, T. K. (2000). Clinical perspectives for the study of craving and relapse in animal models. *Addiction, 95*(Suppl. 2), 55–60.

Linehan, M. M. (1993). *Cognitive-behavioral treatment of borderline personality disorder.* New York: Guilford Press.

Ling, W. L., Rawson, R. A., & Compton, M. A. (1994). Substitution pharmacotherapies for opioid addiction: From methadone to LAAM to buprenorphine. *Journal of Psychoactive Drugs, 26,* 119–128.

Litman, G. (1984). The relationship between coping behaviors, their effectiveness and alcoholism relapse and survival. *British Journal of Addiction, 79*(3), 283–291.

Litman, G., Stapleton, J., Oppenheim, A. N., & Peleg, M. (1983). An instrument for measuring coping behaviors in hospitalized alcoholics: Implications for relapse prevention treatment. *British Journal of Addiction, 78*(3), 269–276.

Litman, G., Stapleton, J., Oppenheim, A. N., Peleg, M., & Jackson, P. (1983). Situations related to alcoholism relapse. *British Journal of Addiction, 78,* 381–389.

Litt, M. D., Cooney, N. L., Kadden, R. M., & Gaupp, L. (1990). Reactivity to alcohol cues and induced moods in alcoholics. *Addictive Behaviors, 15,* 137–146.

Litt, M. D., Cooney, N. L., & Morse, P. (2000). Reactivity to alcohol-related stimuli in the laboratory and in the field: Predictors of craving in treated alcoholics. *Addiction, 95,* 889–900.

Litt, M. D., Kadden, R. M., Cooney, N. L., & Kabela, E. (2003). Coping skills and treatment outcomes in cognitive-behavioral and interactional group therapy for alcoholism. *Journal of Consulting and Clinical Psychology, 71*(1), 118–128.

Littleton, J. (2000). Can craving be modeled in animals? The relapse prevention perspective. *Addiction, 95,* 83–90.

Longabaugh, R., Rubin, A., Malloy, P., Beattie, M., Clifford, P. R., & Noel, N. (1994). Drinking outcomes of alcohol abusers diagnosed as antisocial personality disorder. *Alcoholism: Clinical and Experimental Research, 18*(4), 778–785.

Longabaugh, R., Rubin, A., Stout, R. L., Zywiak, W. H., & Lowman, C. (1996). The reliability of Marlatt's taxonomy for classifying relapses. *Addiction, 91*(Suppl.), 73–88.

Lowman, C., Allen, J., Stout, R. L., & the Relapse Research Group. (1996). Replication and extension of Marlatt's taxonomy of relapse precipitants: Overview of procedures and results. *Addiction, 91*(Suppl.), 51–71.

Lowman, C., Hunt, W. A., Litten, R. Z., & Drummond, D. C. (2000). Research perspectives on alcohol craving: An overview. *Addiction, 95*(Suppl. 2), 45–54.

Maisto, S. A., Connors, G. J., & Zwyiak, W. H. (1996). Construct validation analyses on the Marlatt typology of relapse precipitants. *Addiction, 91*(Suppl.), 89–98.

Marlatt, G. A. (1978). Craving for alcohol, loss of control, and relapse: A cognitive-behavioral analysis. In P. E. Nathan, G. A. Marlatt, & T. Loberg (Eds.), *New directions in behavioral research and treatment* (pp. 271–314). New Brunswick, NJ: Rutgers Center of Alcohol Studies.

Marlatt, G. A. (1985). Relapse prevention: Theoretical rationale and overview of the model. In G. A. Marlatt & J. R. Gordon (Eds.), *Relapse prevention* (1st ed., pp. 280–250). New York: Guilford Press.

Marlatt, G. A. (1988). Research on behavioral strategies for the prevention of alcohol problems. *Contemporary Drug Problems, 15,* 31–45.

Marlatt, G. A. (1998). *Harm reduction: Pragmatic strategies for managing high-risk situations.* New York: Guilford Press.

Marlatt, G. A. (1996a). Lest taxonomy become taxidermy: A comment on the relapse replication and extension project. *Addiction, 91*(Suppl.), 147–153.

Marlatt, G. A. (1996b). Taxonomy of high-risk situations for alcohol relapse: Evolution and development of a cognitive-behavioral model of relapse. *Addiction, 91*(Suppl.), 37–50.

Marlatt, G. A. (2002). Buddhist philosophy and the treatment of addictive behavior. *Cognitive and Behavioral Practice, 9,* 44–49.

Marlatt, G. A., Baer, J. S., & Quigley, L. A. (1995). Self-efficacy and addictive behaviour. In A. Bandura (Ed.), *Self-efficacy in changing societies* (pp. 289–315). New York: Cambridge University Press.

Marlatt, G. A., & George, W. H. (1984). Relapse prevention: Introduction and overview of the model. *British Journal of Addiction, 79,* 261–273.

Marlatt, G. A., & Gordon, J. R. (1980). Determinants of relapse: Implications for the maintenance of behavior change. In P. O. Davidson & S. M. Davidson (Eds.), *Behavior medicine: Changing health lifestyles* (pp. 410–452). New York: Brunner/Mazel.

Marlatt, G. A., & Gordon, J. R. (Eds.). (1985). *Relapse prevention: Maintenance strategies in the treatment of addictive behaviors* (1st ed.). New York: Guilford Press.

Marlatt, G. A., & Kilmer, J. R. (1998). Consumer choice: Implications of behavioral economics for drug use and treatment. *Behavior Therapy, 29*(4), 567–576.

Marlatt, G. A., & Kristeller, J. (1999). Mindfulness and meditation. In W. R. Miller (Ed.), *Integrating spirituality in treatment: Resources for practitioners* (pp. 67–84). Washington, DC: American Psychological Association Books.

Marlatt, G. A., Pagano, R. R., Rose, R. M., & Marques, J. K. (1984). Effects of meditation and relaxation training upon alcohol use in male social drinkers. In D. H. Shapiro & R. N. Walsh (Eds.), *Meditation: Classic and contemporary perspectives* (pp. 105–120). New York: Aldine.

Marlatt, G. A., & Witkiewitz, K. (2002). Harm reduction approaches to alcohol use: Health promotion, prevention, and treatment. *Addictive Behaviors, 901,* 1–20.

Marlatt, G. A., Witkiewitz, K., Dillworth, T., Bowen, S. W., Parks, G., Macpherson,

L. M., et al. (2004). Vipassana meditation as a treatment for alcohol and drug use disorders. In S. C. Hayes, V. M. Follette, & M. M. Linehan (Eds.), *Mindfulness and acceptance: Expanding the cognitive-behavioral tradition* (pp. 261–287). New York: Guilford Press.

McCrady, B. S. (2000). Alcohol use disorders and the Division 12 Task Force of the American Psychological Association. *Psychology of Addictive Behaviors, 14,* 267–276.

McKay, J. R., Merikle, E., Mulvaney, F. D., Weiss, R. V., & Koppenhaver, J. M. (2001). Factors accounting for cocaine use two years following initiation of continuing care. *Addiction, 96,* 213–225.

McKay, J. R., Rutherford, M. J., Alterman, A. I., Cacciola, J. S., & Kaplan, M. R. (1995). An examination of the cocaine relapse process. *Drug and Alcohol Dependence, 38,* 35–43.

McMahon, R. C. (2001). Personality, stress, and social support in cocaine relapse prediction. *Journal of Substance Abuse Treatment, 21,* 77–87.

Miller, W. R., Benefield, R. G., & Tonigan, S. O. (1993). Enhancing motivation for change in problem drinking: A controlled comparison of two therapist styles. *Journal of Consulting and Clinical Psychology, 61*(3), 455–461.

Miller, W. R., & Rollnick, S. (1991b). *Motivational interviewing: Preparing people to change addictive behavior* (1st ed.). New York: Guilford Press.

Miller, W. R., & Rollnick, S. (2002). *Motivational interviewing: Preparing people for change* (2nd ed.). New York: Guilford Press.

Miller, W. R., Westerberg, V. S., Harris, R. J., & Tonigan, J. S. (1996). What predicts relapse? Prospective testing of antecedent models. *Addiction, 91*(Suppl.), 155–171.

Miller, W. R., & Wilbourne, P. L. (2002). Mesa Grande: A methodological analysis of clinical trials of treatments for alcohol use disorders. *Addiction, 97,* 265–277.

Mischel, W., Shoda, Y., & Mendoza-Denton, R. (1988). Situation-behavior profiles as a locus of consistency in personality. *Current Directions in Psychological Science, 11*(2), 50–54.

Monti, P. M., Rohsenow, D. J., Abrams, D. B., Zwick, W. R., Binkoff, J. A., Munroe, S. M., et al. (1993). Development of a behavior analytically derived alcohol-specific role-play assessment instrument. *Journal of Studies on Alcohol, 54,* 710–721.

Mooney, J. P., Burling, T. A., Hartman, W. M., & Brenner-Liss, D. (1992). The abstinence violation effect and very low calorie diet success. *Addictive Behaviors, 17*(4), 319–324.

Moos, R. H. (1993). *Coping Responses Inventory.* Odessa, FL: Psychological Assessment Resources.

Morganstern, J., & Longabaugh, R. (2000). Cognitive-behavioral treatment for alcohol dependence: A review of evidence for its hypothesized mechanisms of action. *Addiction, 95*(10), 1475–1490.

Moyer, A., Finney, J. W., & Swearingen, C. E. (2002). Methodological characteristics and quality of alcohol treatment outcome studies, 1970–98: An expanded evaluation. *Addiction, 97,* 253–263.

Mundt, J. C., Bohn, M. J., Drebus, D. W., & Hartley, M. T. (2001). Development and validation of interactive voice response (IVR) alcohol use assessment instruments. *Alcoholism: Clinical and Experimntal Research, 25*(5, Suppl.), 248.

Muraven, M., Baumeister, R. F., & Tice, D. M. (1999). Longitudinal improvement of self-regulation through practice: Building self-control strength through repeated exercise. *Journal of Social Psychology, 139*(4), 446–457.

Niaura, R. (2000). Cognitive social learning and related perspectives on drug craving. *Addiction, 95,* 155–163.

Niaura, R., Shadel, W. G., Britt, D. M., & Abrams, D. B. (2002). Response to social stress, urge to smoke, and smoking cessation. *Addictive Behaviors, 27*(2), 241–250.

Noone, M., Dua, J., & Markham, R. (1999). Stress, cognitive factors, and coping resources as predictors of relapse in alcoholics. *Addictive Behaviors, 24,* 687–693.

Norcross, J. C., & Vangarelli, D. J. (1989). The resolution solution: Longitudinal examination of New Year's change attempts. *Journal of Substance Abuse, 1*(2), 127–134.

O'Malley, S. S., Jaffe, A. J., Chang, G., Rode, S., Schottenfeld, R., Meyer, R., et al. (1996). Six-month follow-up of naltrexone and psychotherapy for alcohol dependence. *Archives of General Psychiatry, 53,* 217–224.

Ostafin, B. D., Palfai, T. P., & Wechsler, C. E. (2003). The accessibility of motivational tendencies toward alcohol: Approach, avoidance, and disinhibited drinking. *Experimental and Clinical Psychopharmacology, 11*(4), 294–301.

Palfai, T. P., & Ostafin, B. D. (2003). Alcohol-related motivational tendencies in hazardous drinkers: Assessing implicit response tendencies using the modified-IAT. *Behaviour Research and Therapy, 41*(10), 1149–1162.

Perri, M. G., Nezu, A. M., McKelvey, W. F., Shermer, R. L., Renjilian, D. A., & Viegener, B. J. (2001). Relapse prevention training and problem-solving therapy in the long-term management of obesity. *Journal of Consulting and Clinical Psychology, 69*(4), 722–726.

Piasecki, T. M., Niaura, R., Shadel, W. G., Abrams, D., Goldstein, M., Fiore, M. C., & Baker, T. B. (2000). Smoking withdrawal dynamics in unaided quitters. *Journal of Abnormal Psychology, 109,* 74–86.

Polivy, J., & Herman, C. P. (2002). If at first you don't succeed: False hopes of self-change. *American Psychologist, 57*(9), 677–689.

Prochaska, J. O., & DiClemente, C. C. (1984). *The transtheoretical approach: Crossing the traditional boundaries of therapy.* Malabar, FL: Krieger.

Project MATCH Research Group. (1997). Matching alcoholism treatment to client heterogeneity: Post-treatment drinking outcomes. *Journal of Studies on Alcohol, 58,* 7–29.

Project MATCH Research Group. (1998). Matching alcoholism treatments to client heterogeneity: Project MATCH three-year drinking outcomes. *Alcoholism: Clinical and Experimental Research, 22*(6), 1300–1311.

Raimo, E. B., & Schuckit, M. A. (1998). Alcohol dependence and mood disorders. *Addictive Behaviors, 23*(6), 933–946.

Rawson, R. A., McCann, M., Flammino, F., Shoptaw, S., Miotto, K., Reiber, C., et al. (2002). A comparison of contingency management and cognitive-behavioral approaches for cocaine- and methamphetamine-dependent individuals. *Archives of General Psychiatry, 59,* 817–824.

Roberts, A. J., Cole, M., & Koob, G. F. (1996). Intra-amygdala muscimol decreases operant ethanol self-administration in dependent rats. *Alcoholism: Clinical and Experimental Research, 20,* 1289–1298.

Robinson, T. E., & Berridge, K. C. (2000). The psychology and neurobiology of addiction: An incentive-sensitization view. *Addiction, 95*(Suppl. 2), 91–118.

Roffman, R. A., Stephens, R. S., Simpson, E. E., & Whitaker, D. L. (1990). Treatment of marijuana dependence: Preliminary results. *Journal of Psychoactive Drugs, 20*(1), 129–137.

Rosenberg, H. (1983). Relapsed versus non-relapsed alcohol abusers: Coping skills, life events, and social support. *Addictive Behaviors, 8*(2), 183–186.

Rychtarik, R. G., Prue, D. M., Rapp, S. R., & King, A. C. (1992). Self-efficacy, aftercare and relapse in a treatment program for alcoholics. *Journal of Studies on Alcohol, 53*(5), 435–440.

Sass, H., Soyka, M., Mann, K., & Zieglgansberger, W. (1996). Relapse prevention by acamprosate. *Archives of General Psychiatry, 53,* 673–680.

Sayette, M. A., Shiffman, S., Tiffany, S. T., Niaura, R. S., Martin, C. S., & Shadel, W. G. (2000). The measurement of drug craving. *Addiction, 95*(Suppl. 2), 189–210.

Schmitz, J. M., Stotts, A. L., Rhoades, H. M., & Grabowski, J. (2001). Naltrexone and relapse prevention treatment for cocaine-dependent patients. *Addictive Behaviors, 26*(2), 167–180.

Schuckit, M. A. (1996). Recent developments in the pharmacotherapy of alcohol dependence. *Journal of Consulting and Clinical Psychology, 64,* 669–676.

Segal, Z., Williams, J. M. G., & Teasdale, J. D. (2002). *Mindfulness-based cognitive therapy for depression: A new approach to preventing relapse.* New York: Guilford Press.

Shaham, Y., Erb, S., & Stewart, J. (2000). Stress-induced relapse to heroin and cocaine seeking in rats: A review. *Brain Research Reviews, 33,* 13–33.

Shiffman, S. (1984). Coping with temptations to smoke. *Journal of Consulting and Clinical Psychology, 52*(2), 261–267.

Shiffman, S. (1989). Conceptual issues in the study of relapse. In M. Gossop (Ed.), *Relapse and addictive behavior* (pp. 149–179). London: Routledge.

Shiffman, S., Balabanis, M., Paty, J., Engberg, J., Gwaltney, C., Liu, K., et al. (2000). Dynamic effects of self-efficacy on smoking lapse and relapse. *Health Psychology, 19,* 315–323.

Shiffman, S., Dresler, C. M., Hajek, P., Gilburt, S. J., Targett, D. A., & Strahs, K. R. (2002). Efficacy of a cotinine lozenge for smoking cessation. *Archives of Internal Medicine, 162,* 1267–1276.

Shiffman, S., Engberg, J. B., Paty, J. A., Perz, W. G., Gnys, M., Kassel, J. D., & Hickcox, M. (1997). A day at a time: Predicting smoking lapse from daily urge. *Journal of Abnormal Psychology, 106,* 104–116.

Shiffman, S., Paty, J. A., Gnys, M., Kassel, J. D., & Hickcox, M. (1996). First lapses to smoking: Within subjects analysis of real time reports. *Journal of Consulting and Clinical Psychology, 2,* 366–379.

Shiffman, S., & Waters, A. J. (2004). Negative affect and smoking lapses: A prospective analysis. *Journal of Consulting and Clinical Psychology, 72,* 192–201.

Siegel, S., Baptista, M. A. S., Kim, J. A., McDonald, R. V., & Weise, K. L. (2000). Pavlovian psychopharmacology: The associate basis of tolerance. *Experimental and Clinical Psychopharmacology, 8*(3), 276–293.

Siegel, S., Krank, M. D., & Hinson, R. E. (1988). Anticipation of pharmacological and nonpharmacological events: Classical conditioning and addictive behavior. In S. Peele (Ed.), *Visions of addiction: Major contemporary perspectives on addiction and alcoholism* (pp. 85–116). Washington, DC: Lexington Books.

Skinner, H. A. (1989). Butterfly wings flapping: Do we need more "chaos" in understanding addictions? *British Journal of Addiction, 84,* 353–356.

Sobell, M. B., Sobell, L. C., Bogardis, J., Leo, G., & Skinner, W. (1992). Problem drinkers' perceptions of whether treatment goals should be self-selected or therapist selected. *Behavior Therapy, 23,* 43–52.

Solomon, K. E., & Annis, H. M. (1990). Outcome and efficacy expectancy in the prediction of post-treatment drinking behavior. *British Journal of Addiction, 85*(5), 659–665.

Stacy, A. W., Ames, S. L., & Leigh, B. C. (2004). An implicit cognition assessment approach to relapse, secondary prevention, and media effects. *Cognitive and Behavioral Practice, 11*(2), 139–148.

Stacy, A. W., Widaman, K. F., & Marlatt, G. A. (1990). Expectancy models of alcohol use. *Journal of Personality and Social Psychology, 58*(5), 918–928.

Stephens, R. S., Curtin, L., & Roffman, R. A. (1994). Testing the abstinence violation effect construct with marijuana cessation. *Addictive Behaviors, 19,* 23–32.

Stephens, R. S., Roffman, R. A., & Curtin, L. (2000). Comparison of extended versus brief treatments for marijuana use. *Journal of Consulting and Clinical Psychology, 68*(5), 898–908.

Stone, A. A., & Shiffman, S. (1994). Ecological momentary assessment (EMA) in behavioral medicine. *Annals of Behavioral Medicine, 16*(3), 199–202.

Stout, R. L., Longabaugh, R., & Rubin, A. (1996). Predictive validity of Marlatt's taxonomy versus a more general relapse code. *Addiction, 91*(Suppl.), 99–110.

Supnick, J. A., & Colletti, G. (1984). Relapse coping and problem solving training following treatment for smoking. *Addictive Behaviors, 9*(4), 401–404.

Sutton, S. R. (1979). Interpreting relapse curves. *Journal of Consulting and Clinical Psychology, 47,* 96–98.

Swendsen, J., Tennen, H., Carney, M. A., Affleck, G., Willard, A., & Hromi, A. (2000). Mood and alcohol consumption: An experience sampling test of the self-medication hypothesis. *Journal of Abnormal Psychology, 109,* 198–204.

Taub, E., Steiner, S. S., Weingarten, E., & Walton, K. G. (1994). Effectiveness of broad spectrum approaches to relapse prevention in severe alcoholism: A long-term, randomized, controlled trial of transcendental meditation, EMG biofeedback and electronic neurotherapy. *Alcoholism Treatment Quarterly, 11,* 187–220.

Taylor, R. C., Harris, N. A., Singleton, E. G., Moolchan, E. T., & Heishman, S. J. (2000). Tobacco craving: Intensity-related effects of imagery scripts in drug abusers. *Experimental and Clinical Psychopharmacology, 8,* 75–87.

Teasdale, J. D., Moore, R. G., Hayhurst, H., Pope, M., Williams, S., & Segal, Z. V. (2002). Metacognitive awareness and prevention of relapse in depression: Empirical evidence. *Journal of Consulting and Clinical Psychology, 70*(2), 275–287.

Thom, R. (1975). *Structural stability and morphogenesis: An outline of a general theory of models.* Reading, MA: Benjamin-Cummings.

Tiffany, S. T. (1990). A cognitive model of drug urges and drug use behavior: Role of automatic and non-automatic processes. *Psychological Review, 97,* 147–168.

Tiffany, S. T., Carter, B. L., & Singleton, E. G. (2000). Challenges in the manipulation, assessment and interpretation of craving relevant variables. *Addiction, 95*(Suppl. 2), 177–187.

Volpicelli, J. R., Alterman, A. I., Hayashida, M., & O'Brien, C. P. (1992). Naltrexone in the treatment of alcohol dependence. *Archives of General Psychiatry, 48,* 876–880.

Vuchinich, R. E., & Tucker, J. A. (1996). Life events, alcoholic relapse, and behavioral theories of choice: A prospective analysis. *Experimental and Clinical Psychopharmacology, 4,* 19–28.

Walton, M. A., Castro, F. G., & Barrington, E. H. (1994). The role of attribution in abstinence, lapse, and relapse following substance abuse treatment. *Addictive Behaviors, 19*(3), 319–331.

Warren, K., Hawkins, R. C., & Sprott, J. C. (2003). Substance abuse as a dynamical disease: Evidence and clinical implications of nonlinearity in a time series of daily alcohol consumption. *Addictive Behaviors, 28,* 369–374.

Wegner, D. M., & Wheatley, T. (1999). Apparent mental causation: Sources of the experience of will. *American Psychologist, 54*(7), 480–492.

Weiner, B. (1974). *Achievement motivation and attribution theory.* Morristown, NJ: General Learning Press.

Wilson, P. H. (1992). Relapse prevention: Conceptual and methodological issues. In P. H. Wilson (Ed.), *Principles and practice of relapse prevention.* New York: Guilford Press.

Winters, J., Fals-Stewart, W., O'Farrell, T. J., Birchler, G. R., & Kelley, M. L. (2002). Behavioral couples therapy for female substance-abusing patients: Effects on substance use and relationship adjustment. *Journal of Consulting and Clinical Psychology, 70*(2), 344–355.

Witkiewitz, K., Hufford, M. R., Caruso, J. C., & Shields, A. S. (2002, November). *Increasing the prediction of alcohol relapse using catastrophe theory: Findings from Project MATCH.* Poster session presented at the annual meeting of the Association for Advancement of Behavior Therapy, Reno, NV.

Witkiewitz, K., & Marlatt, G. A. (2004). Relapse prevention for alcohol and drug problems: That was zen, this is tao. *American Psychologist, 59,* 224–235.

Witkiewitz, K., Marlatt, G. A., & Walker, D. D. (in press). Mindfulness-based relapse prevention: The meditative tortoise wins the race. *Journal of Cognitive Psychotherapy.*

CHAPTER 2

Relapse Prevention among Diverse Populations

Arthur W. Blume
Berenice García de la Cruz

Ethnic-minority groups in the United States experience disproportionately high numbers of health problems related to substance abuse and are typically underserved when it come to treatment services. For instance, alcohol-related deaths tend to be much higher for some ethnic-minority populations than for whites, with deaths from cirrhosis, alcohol-related injuries, violence, and suicide being significant problems for some ethnic-minority communities (National Center for Injury Prevention and Control, 2004). Interestingly, the research suggests that treatment may be as effective for ethnic-minority patients as for those who are white Americans. However, there are identified disparities in accessing treatment services among ethnic-minority clients, especially African American and Hispanic/Latinos, suggesting that certain nonmajority groups may be significantly underrepresented in substance abuse treatment (National Institute on Alcohol Abuse and Alcoholism [NIAAA], 2001). Economic disparities caused by lack of insurance or lower income have been identified as a reason why nonmajority clients may not be able to access treatment services. However, it also is possible that treatment may not be appealing to ethnic minorities. Since treatment modalities often are developed within majority culture, the models may not be relevant to the needs of potential clients from nonmajority cultures.

One of the shortcomings of research concerning many empirically developed and supported interventions has been testing whether those interventions work effectively in nonmajority populations. Historically, behavioral intervention strategies have been tested in more "representative" samples in order to assess their efficacy for the general population. However, there is no guarantee that interventions developed for the general population will work with more specific populations, such as those from nonmajority cultures.

Interventions developed and tested among "representative" samples are generally developed with majority-culture norms and reflect majority culture's worldview. However, many ethnic-minority groups have different norms and worldviews than the larger majority culture. Assumptions used to develop a more generalized model in the majority populations may not fit well with cultures that have different assumptions about life, the world, and social behavior. In the following section, we discuss potential differences in worldviews among ethnic-minority communities that may influence the efficacy of therapeutic interventions developed within majority culture.

CULTURAL DIFFERENCES THAT MAY INFLUENCE TREATMENT

Although it is difficult to generalize due to differences in acculturation, the worldviews held among certain ethnic-minority groups can differ vastly from the prevailing worldview of the majority culture. For instance, in the United States, the majority worldview tends to be very individualistic, with a strong emphasis on constructs such as "self" and "autonomy." Majority culture also tends to view time and history as linear and progressive. These majority culture ideas can influence how we conceptualize therapy, health, and behavior change, as well as human relationships.

However, some ethnic-minority subcultures within the United States do not subscribe to this type of individualistic worldview. Instead, collectivism may be more valued than individualism and interdependency and relationships may be more important than autonomy and self (Gaines et al., 1997; Sue & Sue, 2003a). In addition, gender roles may be much different than majority culture and may be highly prescribed within certain ethnic-minority cultures. These roles may vary according to birth order within a family, and birth order may prescribe very specific expectations for children within the family structures (Gushue & Sciarra, 1995; McGoldrick, Pearce, & Giordano, 1982; Sue & Sue, 2003b, 2003c). Since family life tends to be at the center of many ethnic-minority cultures, familial roles and relationships can be much more powerful influences on individuals than one would expect by majority-culture standards.

Ethnic-minority cultures often have different value systems than those emphasized by majority culture. For instance, generally speaking, among collectivistic cultures relationships are highly valued. Since relationships are highly valued, social values, such as honor, respect, and role in the community, are often very important and develop in the context of service to others rather than as a result of individual achievement. "Self" often is defined by a person's relationship or role in the community, and autonomy is often a foreign construct since interdependence rather than independence is valued (Sue & Sue, 2003a).

Many ethnic-minority communities have a different view of time and history than majority culture (e.g., Sue & Sue, 2003c). Whereas white Western culture tends to think of history as linear and progressive, many people from nonmajority cultures see time and history as cyclical and potentially repetitive. Personal growth might be defined much differently in the context of this worldview than it is for majority culture. Many ethnic-minority communities also place great importance on oral traditions, so that stories and shared histories take on great meaning, and the cadence of life may be much slower than is often witnessed in majority culture.

Ethnic-minority clients also may experience discrimination, prejudice, and racism. Epidemiological research has suggested that racism can be a contributing factor to increased psychopathology, including substance abuse (Carter, 1994; Wingo, 2001). Prejudice and racism also tend to cluster with financial disadvantage, which can be a risk factor for relapse (e.g., Brewer, Catalano, Haggerty, Gainey, & Fleming, 1998; Ellis & McClure, 1992). Unfortunately, traditional substance abuse therapy does not typically address the relationship between racism and substance abuse in clients, which may cause therapists to overlook a potentially noxious stressor (Rhodes & Johnson, 1997). Furthermore, little research has been conducted to examine how prejudice and racism may be addressed in therapy to aid clients from ethnic-minority groups.

The differences between majority and minority cultures can be vast enough to cause concern about whether therapy models developed for use in the general population will be efficacious for ethnic-minority clients. Because substance abuse is of great concern among ethnic-minority communities, it is imperative that existing treatment models be tested for efficacy among these populations. Cultural enhancements should be considered to make these models more appealing to potential clients and more effective for those who do seek help. Relapse prevention (RP) has been beneficial in enhancing treatment success for many clients. However, as noted in the following section, RP, like so many other empirically validated therapies, has not been widely tested among ethnic-minority communities.

RESEARCH ON RELAPSE DETERMINANTS AND RELAPSE PREVENTION

Marlatt and colleagues reported finding several types of overt determinants of relapse that cluster in two broad areas: intrapersonal determinants and interpersonal determinants (Larimer, Palmer, & Marlatt, 1999; Mackay & Marlatt, 1990; Marlatt, 1985d, 1996; Marlatt & Gordon, 1980). Intrapersonal or environmental determinants include within-person or contextual variables (such as cognitive factors), and interpersonal determinants include relationship or social variables (such as coping with marital or couple conflict). Other researchers also have found intrapersonal and interpersonal determinants to be predictive of relapse after alcohol treatment (Maisto, O'Farrell, McKay, Connors, & Pelcovits, 1988; Schonfeld, Rohrer, Dupree, & Thomas, 1989; Smith & Frawley, 1993; Strowig, 2000; Vuchinich & Tucker, 1996).

In Marlatt's (1985d) early research, intrapersonal determinants may be more commonly linked to actual relapse than interpersonal determinants. In addition, a subsequent study found no gender differences in overt relapse determinants (Rubin, Stout, & Longabaugh, 1996). However, little is known about what kinds of determinants will predict relapse in some ethnic-minority cultures, which have remarkably different worldviews, values, and family and social organizational structures. For instance, it is possible that a person who holds a collectivistic worldview may be more sensitive to interpersonal determinants of relapse than intrapersonal determinants.

Marlatt and others have identified covert determinants of relapse, including use of inappropriate coping responses in high-risk drinking situations after treatment (Chaney, O'Leary, & Marlatt, 1978; Connors, Maisto, & Zywiak, 1996; Miller, Westerberg, Harris, & Tonigan, 1996; Monti, Gulliver, & Myers, 1994; Walton, Blow, & Booth, 2000), low self-efficacy for the ability to cope effectively with high-risk relapse situations (Alsop, Saunders, & Phillips, 2000; Greenfield et al., 2000; Marlatt, 1985c, 1996; Marlatt & Barrett, 1994; Miller, McCrady, Abrams, & Labouvie, 1994), and increased positive expectancies that place the person at high risk for relapse (Brown, 1985; Marlatt, 1985a, 1985b; Rather & Sherman, 1989). However, many of these constructs have been conceptualized in the context of valuing autonomy and individuality. There is no guarantee that these constructs will be identical in cultures where "self," "coping," and "skills" may have different meanings than they do in majority culture.

CULTURAL DIFFERENCES AND COPING SKILLS

Teaching and rehearsal of coping skills has been used effectively in prevention programs that target addictive behaviors in ethnic-minority youth. For instance, successful prevention programs have taught coping skills to prevent alcohol- and smoking-related problems among Hispanic-migrant adolescents (Litrownik et al., 2000), to prevent both alcohol and drug abuse among both African Americans and Hispanics (Botvin & Kantor, 2000; Botvin, Schinke, Epstein, Diaz, & Botvin, 1995), and to prevent smoking problems among American Indians (Schinke, Tepavac, & Cole, 2000).

However, research is quite limited on whether teaching skills are effective among ethnic-minority clients for the prevention of relapse. One small study found possible cultural differences in perceptions concerning skill level and in self-efficacy to use skills. In this particular study, African American clients reported significantly greater coping skills and higher self-efficacy to use those skills than whites, in spite of reporting they had fewer resources to support them after discharge from a substance abuse treatment unit (Walton, Blow, & Booth, 2001). These results are not conclusive and should be viewed with caution, but the study does highlight how little is known about the use of coping skills for RP among clients from nonmajority cultures.

Ethnic-minority clients live in two (or possibly more than two) cultures. In order for the person to cope effectively, it would follow that ethnic-minority clients must be competent in the skills of both cultures in which they interact. This hypothesized model for coping has been referred to as bicultural competence, and the model suggests that a person may need different skills to successfully negotiate the different cultures (LaFromboise & Rowe, 1983). Many intervention programs developed for use within ethnic-minority communities have attempted to culturally enhance skills training in order to promote bicultural competence. On the surface, teaching bicultural competence to ethnic-minority clients has intuitive appeal. These skills could be potentially valuable for preventing relapse in clients, since these competencies theoretically would allow a client to succeed and fit in with both the ethnic-minority and majority cultures. An example might include a person who actively participates in traditional healing practices to purify the body and mind and to restore harmony and balance of self with nature while learning new drink-refusal skills in therapy, both actions completed with the goal of preventing relapse. However, no research has been conducted to test the relationship between bicultural competence and RP.

Before training in bicultural-competence skills, a therapist would want to know the client's level of acculturation into majority culture, or the level of enculturation in his or her traditional culture. Acculturation in this case can be thought of as how much an ethnic-minority client has adopted the majority culture, whereas enculturation is identification with the ethnic-minority culture. Researchers who have studied acculturation and its impact upon therapy have suggested that treatment matching to level of acculturation may be important for success. For instance, if an ethnic-minority client is not highly acculturated, interventions that assume a high level of acculturation (meaning a high level of familiarity with and skills in negotiating majority culture) may not be very effective. Ideally, acculturation levels should be matched between client and therapist, as well as between client and content of therapy (Atkinson & Lowe, 1995; Sue & Sue, 2003b).

However, knowing the acculturation level alone is not sufficient to assess a person's ethnic identity. It is possible that a client may strongly (or weakly) identify with both majority and minority culture. Ethnic identity has been postulated to be orthogonal, so that identification with one culture is not dependent upon the level of identification with the other culture (Oetting & Beauvais, 1991). Therefore, the level of identification with both cultures should be assessed, since acculturation alone will not provide adequate information to determine treatment and therapist matches.

Little is known about the effectiveness of traditional RP skills with someone who is low in acculturation and high in enculturation. Although the research suggests that skills training can be effectively done for prevention of certain addictive behaviors among some ethnic-minority groups, little is known about how acculturation/enculturation levels may mediate or moderate the learning of these skills. Intuitively, matching skills to acculturation/enculturation levels would seem warranted, but a great deal of research needs to be done in order to understand how to match with confidence.

CULTURAL DIFFERENCES AND SELF-EFFICACY

Another important factor in preventing relapse is developing higher self-efficacy in clients for successfully mastering and negotiating high-risk relapse situations. There are indications that self-efficacy may be an important predictor of successful behavior change for at least some ethnic-minority clients as well. For instance, in one study investigating drinking behavior among college students, increased numbers of drinking expectancies in conjunction with lowered levels of self-efficacy predicted greater numbers of drinking-related problems for both whites and Mexican American students (Kercher, 2000). However, one would presume that Mexican American college students would have a higher acculturation level than Mexican Americans not in college, so there may have been sample bias for a group more versed in majority-culture values. Indeed, in another study regarding prevention of smoking, an inverse relationship was found between level of acculturation and reported self-efficacy among Hispanic study participants (Sabogal, Otero-Sabogal, Perez-Stable, Marin, & Marin, 1989).

Research in other domains suggests that the construct of self-efficacy may be different among people from ethnic-minority populations than it is for whites. In one study, participants from a collectivistic culture were more able to process group-efficacy feedback rather than self-efficacy feedback (Earley, Gibson, & Chen, 1999), and another study found that people who had collectivistic worldviews had increased self-efficacy for completing tasks when exposed to group training sessions rather than when exposed to individual training sessions (Earley, 1994). Although none of these studies examined the relationship of self-efficacy with addictive behaviors, they do suggest that self-efficacy may develop differently among people who hold collectivistic worldviews.

Indeed, collective efficacy may be a more appropriate construct to consider regarding successful behavior change among people from collectivistic societies than self-efficacy. Collective efficacy can be thought of as the shared belief by a group of people in their ability to successfully organize and complete particular tasks in order to achieve specified goals (Bandura, 1997). From the perspective of collectivistic culture, social institutions such as the family or the community are the principle reference groups for normative behavior. Therefore, it would follow that efficacy in terms of successful action and behavior change would be interpreted through these referent social groups. One particular study examined the constructs of self-efficacy and collective efficacy to predict mental health symptoms and job satisfaction across American (individualistic) culture and Chinese (collectivistic) culture. The researchers found that for American workers, increased self-efficacy predicted better mental health and job satisfaction, whereas for Chinese workers, increased collective efficacy predicted better mental health and job satisfaction (Schaubroeck, Lam, & Xie, 2000).

Collective efficacy does not have a place per se in the traditional relapse model, but it may be that high collective efficacy may be equally or perhaps more important than high self-efficacy to prevent relapse for some clients from collectivistic communities. If such a hypothesis were to be supported, then RP for people from collectivistic worldviews might be enhanced by the inclusion of community-oriented strategies to skills training to enhance mastery in high-risk situations, and by development of competence and confidence in abilities within cultural reference groups. However, this hypothesis needs to be tested.

Given that collective efficacy may be an important consideration for some minority groups, it would beg the question of whether relapse prevention should be conducted within groups for certain populations. Evidence exists that some ethnic groups that value interdependence may be good candidates for group therapy, such as African Americans and Hispanic/Latino groups. However, in other cultural groups, such as American Indians, Alaska Natives, and Asian origin populations, competing cultural values, such as concern for protecting honor and avoiding shame, may preclude sharing among a gathering of relative strangers (Merta, 1995). The issue of whether to conduct RP in group settings with some ethnic-minority clients is complex and requires further evaluation.

In addition, there is evidence that some ethnic-minority groups are highly underrepresented in the membership of Alcoholics Anonymous (Alcoholics Anonymous World Services, 2004). Although the reason for the low membership numbers of minorities in Alcoholics Anonymous is unknown, it may be in part due to clash of cultural values with the group format or even with 12-step philosophy. For some ethnic-minority clients, sharing about substance use amongst strangers would be considered potentially dishonorable and shameful. Care should taken to consider the client's cultural values when deciding upon a referral to a support group as part of an RP plan.

CULTURAL DIFFERENCES AND EXPECTANCIES

Another important predictor of relapse in the Marlatt taxonomy is expectancies. Although expectancies are likely to be a factor among ethnic-minority clients as well as whites, there is evidence that expectancies may vary across cultures (Daisy, 1989). For example, one research study found that alcohol expectancies for enhanced mood and for improved celebration among Japanese college students were significantly lower than for American college students (Nagoshi, Nakata, Sasano, & Wood, 1994). Another study found that Irish adolescents had significantly lower alcohol expectancies for physical, sexual, and cognitive enhancement but significantly greater alcohol-related expectancies for aggressiveness than American adolescents (Christiansen & Teahan, 1987). An interesting but small cross-cultural study examined the "motives" for drinking in both American and Nigerian adults to examine differences between "individualistic" and "collectivistic" cultures. The researchers found that the American participants used drinking as a coping strategy, whereas the Nigerian participants reported drinking for socialization (Gire, 2002), again suggesting there may be the potential for vast cultural differences for reasons to drink and expected outcomes for drinking behavior.

Even within the United States cultural differences have been found in alcohol expectancies. One study investigated expectancy differences between native Puerto Ricans and college students in the United States and found that expectancy responses for the Puerto Rican participants were significantly associated with increased sociability, whereas this was not true for American college students (Velez-Blasini, 1997). In another study investigating smoking, significant differences were found between Hispanic and non-Hispanic white smoking expectancies. Hispanic participants expected smoking to be significantly less relaxing than whites and were significantly more concerned about the effects of secondhand smoke and the effects of modeling smoking behavior on their children. In addition, similar to findings concerning self-efficacy, acculturation level for Hispanics moderated differences in expectancies; the smoking expectancies of highly acculturated Hispanics tended to be very similar to smoking expectancies of non-Hispanic whites (Marin, Marin, Perez-Stable, Sabogal, & Otero-Sabogal, 1990).

Interestingly, some researchers have found implied relationships between cultural norms for behavior in general and for alcohol expectancies. One study (n = 1,008) that investigated differences in alcohol expectancies in college students in eight countries found significant national differences in expected aggressiveness after drinking that were independent of alcohol consumption patterns or rates. These alcohol-expectancy patterns in fact closely mirrored norms about aggressive behavior in the countries being assessed, the authors argued, so that aggressive countries had similarly aggressive expectations related to drinking behavior (Lindman & Lang, 1994). Another more recent study examined differences in alcohol expectancies between Puerto Ricans and Irish Americans and found that expected loss of control predicted greater numbers of alcohol problems among Irish American participants but predicted fewer alcohol problems among Puerto Rican participants. The authors suggest that different cultural expectations shape beliefs about alcohol outcome expectancies: Loss of control is not a socially acceptable outcome in Puerto Rican culture (Johnson & Glassman, 1999).

Expectancies also may change from generation to generation. In one particular epidemiological study, the investigators found that expectancies changed over time among different ethnic-minority groups (Caetano & Clark, 2002). Such findings remind researchers and therapists that not only are there may be possible variance of psychological constructs across cultures, but that many of these constructs may be subject to intergenerational changes within cultures.

Since very little research has been conducted to assess differences of alcohol expectancies across cultures, it is difficult to speculate what potential cultural differences may mean for RP strategies. The RP model anticipates a wide range of different kinds of substance use expectancies (Marlatt, 1985a) and appears to have the flexibility to adjust to cultural differences. However, it would be helpful to identify culturally relevant ways to assess expectancies and challenge expectancies.

OTHER UNKNOWNS ABOUT RELAPSE BEHAVIOR IN ETHNIC-MINORITY CLIENTS

One important unknown among ethnic-minority clients is whether lapses and relapses are the same across cultures. For instance, there are some cultures where binge substance abuse is the norm rather than a regular use pattern. In this type of cultural context, lapse and relapse behavior may be somewhat different than what was described in the original Marlatt model. Furthermore, abstinence violation effects (AVE) may be different across cultures. Whereas in majority culture guilt may be the principle emotion experienced when a lapse has occurred and the violation of abstinence may be attributed to the self (Marlatt, 1985c; Marlatt & Gordon, 1980), there may be differences in ethnic-minority cultures. In some cultures, community-based shame may be much more powerful in shaping behavior after a lapse than individual feelings of guilt, and attributions made to fate or destiny may be more common for violations than attributions to self. We simply do not know whether there are cultural differences regarding this part of the relapse process since no research has examined potential cultural differences for lapse and relapse patterns or for the AVE.

RELAPSE PREVENTION RESEARCH AMONG ETHNIC MINORITIES

Although relapse prevention has substantial empirical support as an efficacious treatment in the general population, especially for alcohol abuse (Carroll, 1996; Irvin, Bowers, Dunn, & Wang, 1999), there have been very few studies on the efficacy of RP strategies and therapy in homogeneous samples of ethnic-minority participants who abuse substances. In one such study, the investigator found that African Americans with schizophrenia were more likely to have a cocaine relapse if they did not have a case manager assigned to them and did not complete the inpatient treatment provided. Among those who completed the program, those who used alcohol to relieve their schizophrenic symptoms were more likely to relapse (Rosa, 1996). In another study, homeless African American mothers who abuse cocaine were treated with a promising RP program that included intensive support from congregational members of a community church (Stahler et al., 1997).

Among American Indian adolescents, a successful RP program was developed using mentorship to provide social support for maintaining sobriety (Lefler, 1997). Providing mentorship as part of program is an excellent example of culturally enhancing traditional RP since it incorporates the traditional cultural model of eldership into the scientifically efficacious model of RP. Another excellent example of culturally enhancing RP strategies is the Journey of the Circle project that targeted Native Alaskan and American Indian adolescent substance users (Marlatt et al., 2003). In this project, participants received culturally relevant skills training in conjunction with involvement in traditional cultural activities that were lead by community elders.

Some limited research has been conducted among Hispanic and Latino groups as well. A study with a small sample ($n = 18$) of Hispanic/Latino abusers of heroin found qualitative evidence that use of effective coping skills, focusing on negative expectancies, and changes in peer associations were effective for prevention of relapse (Jorquez, 1984). Among participants who abuse methamphetamine, other researchers found that the Hispanic participants tended to relapse more quickly than non-Hispanic whites (Brecht, von Mayrhauser, & Anglin, 2000). Finally, in a study of adolescents, Stewart (1999) found that rates of relapse 6 months after treatment were similar among Hispanics and non-Hispanic whites. However, the relapses experienced by Hispanic participants resulted in significantly greater numbers of negative consequences and risks. Stewart also found that Hispanic adolescents who were more acculturated were less likely to relapse after treatment.

THE MARLATT MODEL AND APPEAL TO NONMAJORITY CULTURES

Although the RP model has not been widely empirically tested within nonmajority populations, especially among clients who are low in acculturation, aspects of the model seem to match well with a collectivistic worldview. First, the model provides for specific interventions for overt relapse determinants, such as interpersonal determinants and environmental determinants. Intuitively, substance-abusing clients from cultures with a strong emphasis on community structures, leadership, and institutions and on family ties, roles, and structure may benefit from the interventions that address interpersonal and environmental determinants, even if there is little empirical data about the effectiveness of such approaches among nonmajority clients. An RP therapist may wish to focus more upon plans to reduce the risk of interpersonal and environmental triggers for relapse than for within-person triggers when conducting therapy with highly enculturated clients from collectivistic cultural groups.

Second, the emphasis of the model on lifestyle balance (Marlatt, 1985b) may be highly appealing to groups that believe in living in harmony and balance with nature, such as many indigenous communities and Asian American cultures (Sue & Sue, 2003b). Using RP strategies that focus upon restoration of lifestyle balance and upon oneness and harmony with the web of life may be culturally relevant and personally appealing to clients who come from a culture that subscribes to an interdependent worldview. Using lapse or relapse management (Larimer & Marlatt, 1990; Larimer et al., 1999), which offers moderation as one of its possible range of goals, also might be quite appealing to certain communities that strive for lifestyle balance. The use of harm reduction strategies as part of relapse management may be compatible with certain cultural perspectives that emphasize moderation and in which abstinence may not be culturally appropriate (Blume, Anderson, Fader, & Marlatt, 2001). The sanctioned use of specific substances for religious or spiritual purposes in some cultures may contribute to complete abstinence being a culturally incompatible goal for some clients.

Third, the RP model places an emphasis on the use of positive addictions (or habits) as a substitute for detrimental addictive behaviors (Marlatt, 1985c). These activities take on a new and profound twist within many ethnic-minority communities because substituting new positive habits has become synonymous with reclaiming traditional cultural practices through what has been termed "alternative activities." Many alternative activities involve participation in the cultural and religious/spiritual heritage of the ethnic-minority community. Examples include use of folk medicine, community-building experiences, traditional forms of recreation, religious, and spiritual practices, storytelling, dances, and the arts.

Alternative activities in ethnic-minority communities also may include skills building experiences that aid in developing majority-culture competence (such as educational and vocational training). However, since there is research suggesting that greater acculturation into majority culture is a risk factor for substance abuse among some ethnic minority groups (e.g., Caetano, 1987; Vega et al., 1998), there is some controversy as to whether greater acculturation into majority culture is ultimately useful for ethnic minority communities. Certainly those who believe in the value of bicultural competence would argue that learning these skills may be potentially useful for reducing other risk factors for substance abuse such as unemployment and poverty, but that they should be balanced with competence in traditional culture.

The use of these alternative activities could theoretically be very helpful in preventing relapse among ethnic-minority clients for several reasons. First, the alternative activities provide structured time in which substance use is not allowed or sanctioned. Second, engagement in traditional activities related to the community would likely have the effect of promoting greater collective efficacy among the members of that community. Third, the alternative activities allow the person to develop bicultural or multicultural competence by engagement in activities that develop skills in both traditional and majority cultures. However, these hypothetical assertions about the possible positive effects of alternative activities should be empirically tested in order to fully understand the value of these activities.

There are some constructs within the Marlatt relapse model that may not hold in nonmajority cultures, and certainly much more research on the model in specific ethnic-minority populations is warranted. However, possible shortcomings of using traditional RP with nonmajority cultures may be overcome with cultural enhancements. The relapse model seems to allow for within-construct flexibility. For example, therapists may wish to enhance self-efficacy *and* collective efficacy, and they may wish to address/challenge individual substance use expectancies *and* community and/or familial expectancies related to substance use. In the following section, we suggest possible cultural enhancements that may be useful for RP among people from ethnic-minority cultures and that seem highly compatible with Marlatt's model.

CULTURALLY ENHANCING RELAPSE PREVENTION

A first step to developing RP that is successfully matched to the needs of an ethnic-minority client is to assess acculturation/enculturation and to what degree he or she identifies with the minority culture and the majority culture. In the case of multiracial clients, it would be important to assess how much that person would identify with all relevant cultural traditions. Intuitively, more highly acculturated clients will likely require fewer cultural enhancements to an existing relapse program.

If a person is not highly acculturated or is distressed about being alienated from the traditional culture of his or her family, then cultural enhancements may be quite helpful and should be considered. The first enhancement may be to simply conduct the RP training and intervention in the client's first language (which cannot be assumed to be English even if he or she is speaking English). An assessment of English language skills also would be part of this process. Furthermore, since English words do not always translate into other languages, it would be very important for the therapist to understand the differences between the nuances of word meaning across both languages to avoid misunderstandings.

As previously described, bicultural competence may be very important for treatment success for an ethnic-minority client, and a determination of a client's skills to cope well in both majority and minority culture is recommended. In order to do so, a behavioral analysis of the time spent interacting in the different cultures (majority and nonmajority), as well as of the context of those interactions, should be made. This analysis should provide useful information of what type of skills may be needed in order to negotiate more efficiently in both majority and nonmajority culture. A bicultural behavior analysis will help therapists determine if there are skills deficits related to successfully interacting in either culture, as well as provide direction of what kinds of bicultural skills training should take place in order to aid the client in preventing relapse.

After determining deficits, the therapist would want to incorporate alternative activities that match the needs of the client into RP therapy, with the goal of developing competence in areas that are in need of enhancement within his or her traditional and majority culture. In creating a bicultural skills training program, it is important to have community collaboration. The community should be consulted in order to effectively develop the skills training program because they can provide insight into what would be culturally relevant and appropriate programs. In addition, the bicultural skills training program should be open to the entire community since collectivistic societies believe in sharing of resources (Daisy, Thomas, & Worley, 1998). Other relapse management strategies can be practiced communitywide as well and linked with the use of alternative activities that are culturally relevant for the community (Groth-Marnat, Leslie, & Renneker, 1996). Involvement of the extended family in these activities is strongly suggested if the client and the family remain on good terms.

Community leaders should be involved in both developing and implementing these activities if they are to succeed. In many ethnic-minority communities, leaders are highly respected and often entrusted with a tremendous amount of authority for developing and implementing community policy and activities. Many cultures have a greatly esteemed place for elders, who serve as highly respected role models for appropriate lifestyle practices. Within these communities, elders can be highly effective as mentors for alternative activities and as role models and leaders of community-based treatment services, including RP. Using the eldership model as a guide, mentorship programs can provide a strong and culturally relevant community support system for preventing relapse (Lefler, 1997).

Many ethnic-minority cultures place great value in oral tradition and the value of storytelling in the exchange of ideas and the intergenerational transmission of cultural identity (Woods, 1998). RP, as a cognitive-behavioral intervention, can be conducted in a very linear fashion if the therapist focuses solely on the science of behavior change. With some ethnic-minority clients, it also would be very important to conduct cognitive-behavioral therapy in a relational fashion, by illustrating the science of behavior change with very allegorical and relational examples. Stories that illustrate risky behavior, how the strategies work, or even how some activities are related to others may illustrate RP lessons more clearly among ethnic-minority clients than traditional cognitive-behavioral protocols. The ability to engage in the oral tradition with a client requires listening and storytelling skills on the part of the therapist. It would be even more helpful if the therapist is able to use traditional stories from the culture of the client to illustrate the lessons about relapse and its prevention.

Storytelling can be an especially effective technique to address cognitions related to destiny and fatalism if clients come from such a worldview. If clients believe it is destiny to be addicted or destined to relapse, then encouraging them to retell their stories with different outcomes (using imagery or other in-session means) could allow patients to believe in a more positive destiny. Retelling of these stories with different outcomes also could be particularly powerful for clients who have felt alienated from the community. The stories can provide examples of how to become positively reengaged in the community and also can reaffirm the person's place in the context of the larger web of life.

In addition, it is important to acknowledge the importance that traditional healing practices may play in the process of successfully overcoming substance abuse problems in particular communities. A successful RP program in some ethnic-minority communities would include traditional healing practices and folk medicine. Collaborative efforts between some treatment programs in ethnic-minority communities with traditional religious leaders and healers have been established and can work well (e.g., Mail & Shelton, 2002). This form of bicultural treatment also has the added benefit of enhancing the therapeutic alliance between an ethnic-minority client and the RP specialist by validating the client's cultural needs. Again, in order to determine the appropriate match of traditional practices with client, acculturation and ethnic identity are important to assess.

CONCLUSIONS

Many traditional practices have been used in substance abuse treatment of ethnic-minority clients, but it is unclear whether any of these approaches have empirical support for preventing relapse. Therefore, one of the great challenges for behavioral scientists interested in RP is to test the efficacy of culturally enhanced relapse prevention among ethnic-minority communities, as well as to test the relevance of specific relapse model constructs within different cultures. Future relapse research conducted in homogeneous ethnic-minority samples is sorely needed. However, in the absence of such research, it is recommended that therapists pay close attention to cultural differences when working with ethnic-minority clients. In the meantime, therapists will have to creatively use available knowledge and resources to tailor RP programs that will meet both the clinical and cultural needs of their ethnic-minority clients.

REFERENCES

Alcoholics Anonymous World Services. (2004). *Alcoholics Anonymous 2001 membership survey.* Available at www.alcoholics-anonymous.com/English/E_FactFile/P-48_02survey.html.

Alsop, S., Saunders, B., & Phillips, M. (2000). The process of relapse in severely dependent male problem drinkers. *Addictions, 95,* 95–106.

Atkinson, D. R., & Lowe, S. M. (1995). The role of ethnicity, cultural knowledge, and conventional techniques in counseling and psychotherapy. In J. G. Ponterotto, J. M. Casas, L. A. Suzuki, & C. M. Alexander (Eds.), *Handbook of multicultural counseling* (pp. 387–414). Thousand Oaks, CA: Sage.

Bandura, A. (1997). Collective efficacy. In *Self-efficacy: The exercise of control* (pp. 477–525). New York: Freeman.

Blume, A. W., Anderson, B. K., Fader, J. S., & Marlatt, G. A. (2001). Harm reduction programs: Progress rather than perfection. In R. H. Coombs (Ed.), *Addiction recovery tools: A practical handbook* (pp. 367–382). Thousand Oaks, CA: Sage.

Botvin, G. J., & Kantor, L. W. (2000). Preventing alcohol and tobacco use through life skills training. *Alcohol Health and Research World, 24,* 250–257.

Botvin, G. J., Schinke, S. P., Epstein, J. A., Diaz, T., & Botvin, E. M. (1995). Effectiveness of culturally focused and generic skills training approaches to alcohol and drug abuse prevention among minority adolescents: Two-year follow-up results. *Psychology of Addictive Behaviors, 9,* 183–194.

Brecht, M. L., von Mayrhauser, C., & Anglin, M. D. (2000). Predictors of relapse after treatment for methamphetamine use. *Journal of Psychoactive Drugs, 32,* 211–220.

Brewer, D. D., Catalano, R. F., Haggerty, K., Gainey, R. R., & Fleming, C. B. (1998). A meta-analysis of predictors of continued drug use during and after treatment for opiate addiction. *Addiction, 93,* 73–92.

Brown, S. A. (1985). Reinforcement expectancies and alcoholism treatment outcome after a one-year follow-up. *Journal of Studies on Alcohol, 46,* 304–308.

Caetano, R. (1987). Acculturation and drinking patterns among U.S. Hispanics. *British Journal of Addictions, 82,* 789–799.

Caetano, R., & Clark, C. L. (2002). Acculturation, alcohol consumption, smoking, and drug use among Hispanics. In K. M. Chun, P. B. Organista, & G. Marín (Eds.), *Acculturation: Advances in theory, measurement, and applied research* (pp. 223–239). Washington, DC: American Psychological Association.

Carroll, K. M. (1996). Relapse prevention as a psychosocial treatment: A review of controlled trials. *Experimental and Clinical Psychopharmacology, 4,* 46–54.

Carter, J. H. (1994). Racism's impact on mental health. *Journal of the American Medical Association, 86,* 543–547.

Chaney, E. F., O'Leary, M. R., & Marlatt, G. A. (1978). Skills training with alcoholics. *Journal of Clinical and Consulting Psychology, 46,* 1092–1104.

Christiansen, B. A., & Teahan, J. E. (1987). Cross-cultural comparisons of Irish and American adolescent drinking practices and beliefs. *Journal of Studies on Alcohol, 48,* 558–562.

Connors, G. J., Maisto, S. A., & Zywiak, W. H. (1996). Understanding relapse in the broader context of post-treatment functioning. *Addictions, 91*(Suppl.), S173–S189.

Daisy, F. (1989). *Ethnic differences in alcohol outcome expectancies and drinking patterns.* Unpublished dissertation, University of Washington, Seattle.

Daisy, F., Thomas, L. R., & Worley, C. (1998). Alcohol use and harm reduction within the Native community. In G. A. Marlatt (Ed.), *Harm reduction: Pragmatic strategies for managing high risk behaviors* (pp. 327–350). New York: Guilford Press.

Earley, P. C. (1994). Self or group? Cultural effects of training on self-efficacy and performance. *Administrative Science Quarterly, 39,* 89–117.

Earley, P. C., Gibson, C. B., & Chen, C. C. (1999). "How did I do?" versus "how did we do?" Cultural contrasts of performance feedback use and self-efficacy. *Journal of Cross-Cultural Psychology, 30,* 594–619.

Ellis, D., & McClure, J. (1992). In-patient treatment of alcohol problems—Predicting and preventing relapse. *Alcohol and Alcoholism, 27,* 449–456.

Gaines, S. O., Jr., Marelich, W. D., Bledsoe, K. L., Steers, W. N., Henderson, M. C.,

Granrose, C. S., Barajas, L., Hicks, D., Lyde, M., Takahashi, Y., Yum, N., Rios, D. I., Garcia, B. F., Farris, K. R., & Page, M. S. (1997). Links between race/ethnicity and cultural values as mediated by racial/ethnic identity and moderated by gender. *Journal of Personality and Social Psychology, 72*, 1460–1476.

Gire, J. T. (2002). A cross-national study of motives for drinking alcohol. *Substance Use and Misuse, 37*, 215–223.

Greenfield, S. F., Hufford, M. R., Vagge, L. M., Muenz, L. R., Costello, M. E., & Weiss, R. D. (2000). The relationship of self-efficacy expectancies to relapse among alcohol dependent men and women: A prospective study. *Journal of Studies on Alcohol, 61*, 345–351.

Groth-Marnat, G., Leslie, S., & Renneker, M. (1996). Tobacco control in a traditional Fijian village: Indigenous methods of smoking cessation and relapse prevention. *Social Science and Medicine, 43*, 473–477.

Gushue, G. V., & Sciarra, D. T. (1995). Culture and families: A multidimensional approach. In J. G. Ponterotto, J. M. Casas, L. A. Suzuki, & C. M. Alexander (Eds.), *Handbook of multicultural counseling* (pp. 586–606). Thousand Oaks, CA: Sage.

Irvin, J. E., Bowers, C. A., Dunn, M. E., & Wang, M. C. (1999). Efficacy of relapse prevention: A meta-analytic review. *Journal of Consulting and Clinical Psychology, 67*, 563–570.

Johnson, P. B., & Glassman, M. (1999). The moderating effects of gender and ethnicity on the relationship between effect expectancies and alcohol problems. *Journal of Studies on Alcohol, 60*, 64–69.

Jorquez, J. S. (1984). Heroin use in the barrio: Solving the problem of relapse or keeping the tecato gusano asleep. *American Journal of Drug and Alcohol Abuse, 10*, 63–75.

Kercher, L. S. (2000). *Alcohol expectancies, coping responses, and self-efficacy judgments: Predictors of alcohol use and alcohol-related problems for Anglo-American and Mexican-American college students.* Unpublished doctoral dissertation, California School of Professional Psychology, San Diego.

LaFromboise, T. D., & Rowe, W. (1983). Skills training for bicultural competence: Rationale and application. *Journal of Counseling Psychology, 30*, 589–595.

Larimer, M. E., & Marlatt, G. A. (1990). Application of relapse prevention with moderation goals. *Journal of Psychoactive Drugs, 22*, 189–195.

Larimer, M. E., Palmer, R. S., & Marlatt, G. A. (1999). Relapse prevention: An overview of Marlatt's cognitive-behavioral model. *Alcohol Health and Research World, 23*, 151–160.

Lefler, L. J. (1997). *Mentorship as an intervention strategy in relapse reduction among Native American youth.* Unpublished dissertation, North Dakota State University, Fargo.

Lindman, R. E., & Lang, A. R. (1994). The alcohol-aggression stereotype: A cross-cultural comparison of beliefs. *International Journal of the Addictions, 29*, 1–13.

Litrownik, A. J., Elder, J. P., Campbell, N. R., Ayala, G. X., Slymen, D. J., Parra-Medina, D., Zavala, F. B., & Lovato, C. Y. (2000). Evaluation of a tobacco and alcohol use prevention program for Hispanic migrant adolescents: Promoting the protective factor of parent–child communication. *Preventive Medicine, 31*, 124–133.

Mackay, P. W., & Marlatt, G. A. (1990). Maintaining sobriety: Stopping is starting. *International Journal of the Addictions, 25*, 1257–1276.

Mail, P. D., & Shelton, C. (2002). Treating Indian alcoholics. In P. D. Martin, S. Heurtin-Roberts, S. E. Martin, & J. Howard (Eds.), *Alcohol use among American Indians and Alaska Natives: Multiple perspectives on a complex problem* (National Institute on Alcohol Abuse and Alcoholism [NIAAA] Research Monograph No. 37.) Bethesda, MD: NIAAA.

Maisto, S. A., O'Farrell, T. J., McKay, J. R., Connors, G. J., & Pelcovits, M. (1988). Alcoholic and spouse concordance on attributions about relapse to drinking. *Journal of Substance Abuse Treatment, 5*, 179–181.

Marin, G., Marin, B. V., Perez-Stable, E. J., Sabogal, F., & Otero-Sabogal, R. (1990). Cultural differences in attitudes and expectancies between Hispanic and non-Hispanic White smokers. *Hispanic Journal of Behavioral Sciences, 12*, 422–436.

Marlatt, G. A. (1985a). Cognitive factors in the relapse process. In G. A. Marlatt & J. R. Gordon (Eds.), *Relapse prevention: Maintenance strategies in the treatment of addictive behaviors* (1st ed., pp. 128–200). New York: Guilford Press.

Marlatt, G. A. (1985b). Lifestyle modification. In G. A. Marlatt & J. R. Gordon (Eds.), *Relapse prevention: Maintenance strategies in the treatment of addictive behaviors* (1st ed., pp. 280–348). New York: Guilford Press.

Marlatt, G. A. (1985c). Relapse prevention: Theoretical rationale and overview of the model. In G. A. Marlatt & J. R. Gordon (Eds.), *Relapse prevention: Maintenance strategies in the treatment of addictive behaviors* (1st ed., pp. 3–70). New York: Guilford Press.

Marlatt, G. A. (1985d). Situational determinants of relapse and skills-training interventions. In G. A. Marlatt & J. R. Gordon (Eds.), *Relapse prevention: Maintenance strategies in the treatment of addictive behaviors* (1st ed., pp. 71–127). New York: Guilford Press.

Marlatt, G. A. (1996). Taxonomy of high-risk situations for alcohol relapse: Evolution and development of a cognitive-behavioral model. *Addictions, 91*(Suppl.), S37–S49.

Marlatt, G. A., & Barrett, K. (1994). Relapse prevention. In M. Galanter & H. D. Kleber (Eds.), *The textbook of substance abuse treatment* (pp. 285–299). Washington, DC: American Psychiatric Press.

Marlatt, G. A., & Gordon, J. R. (1980). Determinants of relapse: Implications for the maintenance of behavior change. In P. O. Davidson & S. M. Davidson (Eds.), *Behavioral medicine: Changing health lifestyles* (pp. 410–445). New York: Brunner/Mazel.

Marlatt, G. A., Larimer, M. E., Mail, P. D., Hawkins, E. H., Cummins, L. H., Blume, A. W., Lonczak, H. S., Burns, K. M., Chan, K. K., Cronce, J. M., LaMarr, J., Radin, S., Forquera, R., Gonzales, R., Tetrick, C., & Gallion, S. (2003). Journeys of the circle: A culturally congruent life skills intervention for adolescent Indian drinking. *Alcoholism: Clinical and Experimental Research, 27*, 1327–1329.

McGoldrick, M., Pearce, J. K., & Giordano, J. (Eds.). (1982). *Ethnicity and family therapy*. New York: Guilford Press.

Merta, R. J. (1995). Group work. In J. G. Ponterotto, J. M. Casas, L. A. Suzuki, & C. M. Alexander (Eds.), *Handbook of multicultural counseling* (pp. 567–585). Thousand Oaks, CA: Sage.

Miller, K. J., McCrady, B. S., Abrams, D. B., & Labouvie, E. W. (1994). Taking an individualized approach to the assessment of self-efficacy and the prediction of alcoholic relapse. *Journal of Psychopathology and Behavioral Assessment, 16,* 111–120.

Miller, W. R., Westerberg, V. S., Harris, R. J., & Tonigan, J. S. (1996). What predicts relapse? Prospective testing of antecedent models. *Addiction, 91*(Suppl.), S155–S172.

Monti, P. M., Gulliver, S. B., & Myers, M. G. (1994). Social skills training for alcoholics: Assessment and treatment. *Alcohol and Alcoholism, 29,* 627–637.

Nagoshi, C. T., Nakata, T., Sasano, K., & Wood, M. D. (1994). Alcohol norms, expectancies and reasons for drinking and alcohol use in a U. S. versus a Japanese college sample. *Alcoholism: Clinical and Experimental Research, 18,* 671–678.

National Center for Injury Prevention and Control. (2004). *10 leading causes of death, United States.* http://webapp.cdc.gov/sasweb/ncipc/leadcaus10.html

National Institute on Alcohol Abuse and Alcoholism. (2001). *Forecast for the future: Strategic plan to address health disparities.* Bethesda, MD: Author.

Oetting, E. R., & Beauvais, F. (1991). Orthogonal cultural identification theory: The cultural identification of minority adolescents. *International Journal of the Addictions, 25,* 655–685.

Rather, B. C., & Sherman, M. F. (1989). Relationship between alcohol expectancies and length of abstinence among Alcoholics Anonymous members. *Addictive Behaviors, 14,* 531–536.

Rhodes, R., & Johnson, A. (1997). A feminist approach to treating alcohol and drug addicted African-American women. *Women and Therapy, 20,* 23–37.

Rosa, M. E. (1996). *Cognitive-behavioral processes that affect substance-dependent schizophrenic African-American males' completion of inpatient treatment.* Unpublished dissertation, University of California at Los Angeles.

Rubin, A., Stout, R. L., & Longabaugh, R. (1996). Gender differences in relapse situations. *Addiction, 91,* 111–120.

Sabogal, F., Otero-Sabogal, R., Perez-Stable, E. J., Marin, B. V., & Marin, G. (1989). Perceived self-efficacy to avoid cigarette smoking and addiction: Differences between Hispanics and non-Hispanic Whites. *Hispanic Journal of Behavioral Sciences, 11,* 136–147.

Schaubroeck, J., Lam, S. S. K., & Xie, J. L. (2000). Collective efficacy versus self-efficacy in coping responses to stressors and control: A cross-cultural study. *Journal of Applied Psychology, 85,* 512–525.

Schinke, S. P., Tepavac, L., & Cole, K. C. (2000). Preventing substance abuse among Native American youth: Three year results. *Addictive Behaviors, 25,* 387–397.

Schonfeld, L., Rohrer, G. E., Dupree, L. W., & Thomas, M. (1989). Antecedents of relapse and recent substance use. *Community Mental Health Journal, 25,* 245–249.

Smith, J. W., & Frawley, P. J. (1993). Treatment outcome of 600 chemically dependent patients treated in a multimodal inpatient program including aversion therapy and pentothal interviews. *Journal of Substance Abuse Treatment, 10,* 359–369.

Stahler, G. J., Godboldte, C., Shipley, T. E., Shandler, I. W., Ijoy, L., Weinberg, A., Harrison-Horn, N., Nichols, C., Simons, L., & Koszowski, L. (1997). Preventing relapse among crack-using homeless women with children: Building bridges to the community. *Journal of Prevention and Intervention in the Community, 15,* 53–66.

Stewart, D. G. (1999). *Differences in substance abuse treatment outcome in Hispanic and non-Hispanic Caucasian adolescents: The role of delinquency, acculturation, and cultural stress.* Unpublished dissertation, University of California at San Diego and San Diego State University.

Strowig, A. B. (2000). Relapse determinants reported by men treated for alcohol addiction: The prominence of depressed mood. *Journal of Substance Abuse Treatment, 19,* 469–474.

Sue, D. W., & Sue, D. (2003a). Barriers to effective multicultural counseling/therapy. In D. W. Sue & D. Sue, *Counseling the culturally diverse: Theory and practice* (pp. 95–121). New York: Wiley.

Sue, D. W., & Sue, D. (2003b). Counseling and therapy with racial/ethnic-minority populations. In D. W. Sue & D. Sue, *Counseling the culturally diverse: Theory and practice* (pp. 291–376). New York: Wiley.

Sue, D. W., & Sue, D. (2003c). Multicultural family counseling and therapy. In D. W. Sue & D. Sue, *Counseling the culturally diverse: Theory and practice* (pp. 151–176). New York: Wiley.

Vega, W. A., Kolody, B., Aguilar-Gaxiola, S., Aldrete, E., Catalano, R., & Caraveo-Anduaga, J. (1998). Lifetime prevalence of DSM-III-R psychiatric disorders among urban and rural Mexican Americans in California. *Archives of General Psychiatry, 55,* 771–778.

Velez-Blasini, C. J. (1997). A cross-cultural comparison of alcohol expectancies in Puerto Rico and the United States. *Psychology of Addictive Behaviors, 11,* 124–141.

Vuchinich, R. E., & Tucker, J. A. (1996). Alcoholic relapse, life events, and behavioral theories of choice: A prospective analysis. *Experimental and Clinical Psychopharmacology, 4,* 19–28.

Walton, M. A., Blow, F. C., & Booth, B. M. (2000). A comparison of substance abuse patients' and counselors' perceptions of relapse risk: Relationship to actual relapse. *Journal of Substance Abuse Treatment, 19,* 161–169.

Walton, M. A., Blow, F. C., & Booth, B. M. (2001). Diversity in relapse prevention needs: Gender and race comparisons among substance abuse treatment patients. *American Journal of Drug and Alcohol Abuse, 27,* 225–240.

Wingo, L. K. (2001). Substance abuse in African American women. *Journal of Cultural Diversity, 20,* 23–37.

Woods, I. P. (1998). Bringing harm reduction to the black community: There's a fire in my house and you're telling me to rearrange my furniture? In G. A. Marlatt (Ed.), *Harm reduction: Pragmatic strategies for managing high risk behaviors* (pp. 301–326). New York: Guilford Press.

CHAPTER 3

Treating Alcohol Problems

Ronald M. Kadden
Ned L. Cooney

From the perspective of cognitive-behavioral theory, alcohol dependence is viewed as a set of learned behaviors that are acquired through experience. If alcohol provides certain desired effects (e.g., good feelings, reduced tension, etc.) on repeated occasions, it may become the preferred way of achieving those effects, particularly in the absence of other ways of achieving them. From the relapse prevention (RP) perspective, the primary tasks of treatment are to (1) identify as many as possible of the needs that are being met by alcohol use, and (2) develop coping skills that provide alternative ways of meeting those needs, thereby reducing the likelihood of relapsing to drinking as a way of meeting them.

Both of the major types of learning that have been identified in behavior laboratories, learning by association ("Pavlovian" or "classical" conditioning) and learning by consequences ("operant" conditioning), may be involved. In learning by association, originally neutral stimuli become triggers for cravings or drinking as a result of repeated associations of those stimuli with alcohol use. Triggers may be external to the individual (e.g., settings, specific objects, or the people one drinks with regularly) or internal (e.g., thoughts, emotions, or physiological changes). Associations between these various objects/occurrences and alcohol use are gradually strengthened if they repeatedly occur in close temporal proximity. Through this associative process, a growing array of stimuli that were previously neutral become capable of triggering alcohol cravings.

In the operant conditioning model, drinking behavior is strengthened by the consequences that follow. If after drinking a person feels euphoric, more comfortable in social situations, or less tense, the likelihood of future drinking is increased. The negative consequences of drinking, such as withdrawal symptoms, depression, and anxiety, which would be expected to reduce the likelihood of future alcohol use, occur so long after drinking that they have little if any impact, and are therefore no match for the more immediate reinforcing consequences.

The coping skills training approach to RP seeks to identify ways of avoiding triggers, or failing that, to train alternative responses to them. The alternative responses are intended to give a person additional ways of coping with the occurrence of trigger situations, and of obtaining the outcomes that were sought by means of drinking. With sufficient practice of alternative coping skills, it becomes increasingly likely that they will be utilized in trigger situations, in place of drinking. The RP approach provides a systematic way (1) of assessing the full range of antecedents and consequences of drinking that may influence an individual's relapse potential, and (2) of selecting interventions that will help clients to avoid or deal with risky situations in ways that are likely to reduce the probability of a relapse.

ASSOCIATION OF COPING SKILLS WITH DRINKING

A basic assumption of this overall model is that the development of problems with drinking, and recovery from them, are both related to a person's coping ability. The present section reviews evidence for such a connection. Abrams et al. (1991) found that alcoholics differ from nonalcoholics in skills for coping with alcohol-related high-risk situations. Litman et al. (Litman, Stapleton, Oppenheim, Peleg, & Jackson, 1984) used the Coping Behavior Inventory (CBI) to assess coping strategies and found that alcoholics' ratings of the Positive Thinking and Avoidance categories discriminated abstainers from relapsers (see also Miller, Westerberg, Harris, & Tonigan, 1996). Maisto, Connors, and Zywiak (2000) found that changes in the total score on the CBI from baseline to 6 months following treatment predicted drinking at 12 months. Cronkite and Moos (1980) found a strong association between coping at posttreatment and drinking outcomes 2 years later. Moser and Annis (1996) found that maintaining abstinence after a relapse crisis was related to the number of coping strategies utilized, and to the use of active rather than avoidant strategies. Wunschel, Rohsenow, Norcross, and Monti (1993) reported that clients drank less if they engaged in substitute activities as a way of coping with urges to drink. Chung et al. (Chung, Langenbucher, Labouvie, Pandira, & Moos, 2001) found that cognitive approach coping was a significant factor throughout a 12-month posttreatment follow-up period, whereas behavioral approach coping only showed significant effects between months 6 and 12. Schutte,

Byrne, Brennan, and Moos (2001) also found that the use of approach coping was associated with reductions in drinking and alcohol-related problems.

Jones and Lanyon (1981) and Moggi, Ouimette, Moos, and Finney (1999) found that both alcohol-specific and general coping skills were correlated with drinking outcome. In contrast, Wells, Catalano, Plotnick, Hawkins, and Brattesani (1989) and Monti et al. (1990) found that skills for handling drug-related situations were associated with less alcohol use among substance abusers following treatment, whereas general coping skills (e.g., assertiveness, problem solving) were not. Rohsenow et al. (2001) found that less drinking during a 12-month follow-up was related to the use of alcohol-specific skills, including delay, thinking about consequences, substitute behavior, substitute consumption, and escape/avoidance of high-risk situations, but not to the use of more general skills such as relaxation, imagery, mastery messages, or distraction. Complete abstinence was associated with thinking about positive or negative consequences and escape/avoidance.

In summary, studies of coping skills in alcoholics suggest that abstinence is more likely with utilization of a greater number of coping skills and with alcohol-specific skills as opposed to general coping skills, that it is more advantageous to use active than avoidant coping strategies, and that both cognitive and behavioral strategies are beneficial.

IMPACT OF COPING SKILLS TRAINING

A number of studies have examined the efficacy of cognitive-behavioral treatment for alcoholic clients. In early work, Hedberg and Campbell (1974) found that rehearsal of communication and assertiveness skills in the context of behavioral family counseling was more effective than other behavioral interventions, such as desensitization, covert sensitization, and aversion therapy in reducing alcohol intake over a 6-month period. Chaney, O'Leary, and Marlatt (1978) found that RP training (e.g., drink refusal, coping with negative moods, and coping with interpersonal conflict) led to reductions in days of drinking, amount drunk, and length of drinking episodes, compared to a discussion control group or to no additional treatment. Those who received the skills training responded more rapidly in role-played high-risk situations, which was also associated with less subsequent drinking. Freedberg and Johnston (1978) found that adding assertiveness training to inpatient treatment significantly improved treatment outcome.

Oei and Jackson (1980, 1982) reported that social skills training and cognitive restructuring, whether provided as individual or group therapy for alcoholics, were superior to supportive therapy, and that cognitive restructuring fostered better maintenance of treatment gains. Eriksen, Björnstad, and Götestam (1986) found better drinking outcomes (less drinking, more sober days, and more continuous abstinence, as well as more working days) 1 year after social skills training, as compared to a discussion control group. The duration of effects in this study was particularly encouraging. Similarly, Ferrell and Galassi (1981) found, at a 2-year follow-up, that clients who had received social skills (assertiveness) training as a treatment adjunct maintained sobriety significantly longer than those who had received human relations training. Monti et al. (1990) compared two elements of skills training and found that inpatient alcoholics who received communication skills training, with or without family involvement, consumed less alcohol and obtained higher skill ratings than those who received cognitive-behavioral mood management training.

Not all studies have demonstrated superior outcomes from cognitive-behavioral skills training. Jones, Kanfer, and Lanyon (1982) found that the Chaney et al. (1978) package of skills training was not superior to simply discussing means of handling high-risk situations. This raises the question of whether actual practice of skills is required, or whether simply identifying high-risk situations and becoming aware of how to cope with them might be sufficient. Comparisons between the two studies are complicated by the fact that the Chaney et al. sample was more impaired than the relatively high-functioning alcoholics studied by Jones et al.

There have been other negative studies as well. Sanchez-Craig and Walker (1982) provided residents of an alcoholism halfway house with coping skills training (goal setting, problem solving, and cognitive coping with urges to drink) and found no differences from control procedures (covert sensitization or discussions of goals and problem solving) on any outcome variables out to an 18-month follow-up. Sjoberg and Samsonowitz (1985) found no differences between outpatient skills training and traditional counseling, and Ito, Donovan, and Hall (1988) found that in an aftercare setting, skills training was not different from interpersonal-process groups. Finney, Noyes, Coutts, and Moos (1998) found that clients enrolled in either 12-step-oriented or cognitive-behavioral-oriented treatment programs showed outcomes that had been anticipated to be specific to cognitive-behavioral treatment.

Project MATCH was a multisite alcoholism treatment trial that compared the effects of 12 sessions of cognitive-behavioral therapy (CBT), 12 sessions of 12-step facilitation (TSF), and 4 sessions of motivational enhancement therapy (MET), delivered either as outpatient treatment or as aftercare following inpatient or intensive outpatient treatment. In general, there were no outcome differences among the three treatments in the Aftercare arm. In the Outpatient arm, CBT and TSF clients drank less often (an average of 15 out of 90 days) during treatment than MET clients (20 days). More than 40% of CBT and TSF clients were classified as either abstinent or drinking moderately without problems, compared with 28% of MET clients (Project MATCH Research Group, 1998). Treatment differences faded among Outpatients in the year after treatment so that no enduring clinically significant differences were found among treatments on measures of frequency of drinking, intensity of drinking or negative consequences (Project MATCH Research Group, 1997). Thus, Project MATCH found that cognitive-behavioral coping skills treatment was roughly equivalent to other credible, manual-guided active treatment approaches when provided either as the sole outpatient treatment or as aftercare following a more intensive program.

Longabaugh and Morgenstern (1999) examined controlled clinical trials of CBT for alcohol dependence to determine whether coping behaviors were more likely following CBT treatment and whether coping behaviors covaried with drinking outcomes. Nine studies met scientific criteria for inclusion in their review. Longabaugh and Morgenstern found that some studies provided evidence for an increase in coping behaviors with CBT treatment, and that other studies provided evidence for drinking outcomes covarying with level of coping. However, only one of the nine studies provided evidence that a measure of coping differentially changed in the CBT condition *and* covaried with drinking outcome. Many of the studies were unable to provide tests of the complete mediational model because of methodological reasons. Longabaugh and Morgenstern concluded that research has yet to establish precisely why CBT may be effective for treating alcohol dependence.

Interventions that focus specifically on RP have been found beneficial for sustaining the effects of treatment during follow-up and for reducing the severity of relapse episodes that do occur (Carroll, 1996). However, there are a number of reports in which these benefits have been found to decrease with increasing time since treatment completion (e.g., Allsop, Saunders, Phillips, & Carr, 1997). Another finding of clinical relevance from RP treatment outcome studies is that among the various categories of risk for relapse specified by Marlatt and Gordon (1985), negative emotions have been consistently identified as a major relapse precipitant (Longabaugh, Rubin, Stout, Zywiak, & Lowman, 1996). Based on that, coupled with findings that coping ability is related to treatment outcome (Connors, Maisto, & Zywiak, 1996; Miller et al., 1996), it has been recommended that skills training to foster improved coping with negative emotions be provided as a means of reducing relapse risk (Connors, Longabaugh, & Miller, 1996).

TREATMENT MATCHING STUDIES

Some support for the CBT approach has also been provided by treatment matching studies. Coping skills training was more effective than a comparison treatment for alcoholics who had high scores on measures of socio-pathy and/or psychiatric severity (Cooney, Kadden, Litt, & Getter, 1991; Kadden, Cooney, Getter, & Litt, 1989; Longabaugh et al., 1994). How-ever, neither Kadden, Litt, Cooney, Kabela, and Getter (2001) in a close replication of their earlier procedures, nor Kalman, Longabaugh, Clifford, Beattie & Maisto (2000) in a replication of Longabaugh et al., were able to reproduce their earlier matching findings. Another matching study (Rohsenow et al., 1991) found that training in intrapersonal coping skills was selectively effective for patients with higher education, lower anxiety, or lower urges to drink, while interpersonal skills training was effective re-gardless of individual differences.

Project MATCH found only 4 treatment matching interactions, out of 21 that were tested, and those interactions involved only small improve-ments in drinking outcomes. TSF and MET were more effective in all but one of the successful matches, and CBT was more effective for aftercare clients low in alcohol dependence. Thus, treatment matching studies over-all have not provided strong support for the efficacy of CBT for specific cli-ent needs.

META-ANALYSES OF ALCOHOLISM TREATMENT OUTCOME STUDIES

Meta-analyses comparing the outcomes of various approaches to alcohol-ism treatment have ranked coping skills training interventions either first (Holder, Longabaugh, Miller, & Rubonis, 1991) or second (Finney & Monahan, 1996; Miller et al., 1995) among alcoholism treatments, based on evidence of effectiveness. Morgenstern and Longabaugh (2000) con-ducted a box-score analysis of CBT skills training studies and found that, when added to another treatment, CBT did enhance treatment effective-ness, but that as a stand-alone treatment or as aftercare, it was not superior to alternative treatments. CBT was superior to no-treatment controls and to some treatments, but was not more effective than robust comparison treatments.

A meta-analysis by Irvin, Bowers, Dunn, and Wang (1999) indicated that RP has its primary impact on psychosocial functioning, with less effect on substance use outcomes. Carroll's (1996) review of RP-oriented studies found that RP demonstrated efficacy, for substance use outcomes, when compared to no-treatment controls or to some alternative treatments (such as sobriety education or supportive therapy), but when compared to other alternative treatments (such as problem-solving training), it was compara-ble in effects. The review also concluded that RP is effective for sustaining the effects of treatment and reducing the severity of subsequent relapses, but these benefits diminish with increasing time after treatment.

Although a number of important issues have yet to be resolved, the coping skills training approach has strong theoretical grounding, and the supporting evidence for it and for RP indicates that they are at least equal to, and in some cases superior to, other treatment approaches that are currently available.

COPING SKILLS TRAINING

The RP approach to treatment utilizes coping skills training to develop a number of alternative responses to situations that are high risk for relapse. The most obvious strategy for preventing relapse is to avoid high-risk situations altogether. Therefore, one element of skills training involves helping clients to anticipate and avoid decision paths that could lead them into a high-risk situation. Another strategy for avoiding high-risk situations is to review a client's lifestyle, identifying those activities that tend to place him or her at risk for drinking, and fostering development of alternative activities that are incompatible with drinking.

If a high-risk situation was not avoided, whether because of lack of trying or despite one's best efforts, it must be coped with adequately if drinking is to be prevented. The first step is recognition that a risky situation is at hand. This requires developing clients' awareness of what their high-risk situations generally tend to be, paying attention to the situations in which they find themselves, and monitoring their thoughts and feelings, all for the purpose of detecting warning signs of risk as early as possible. Risky situations detected early are usually more easily controlled than situations that are ignored until they become intense. Once clients are in a high-risk situation, deficits in coping skills become a major risk factor due to the tendency among alcoholics to rely on drinking in the absence of adequate coping skills. Therefore, within the RP model, coping skills training is essential, to enable clients to manage high-risk situations without relapsing (Marlatt & Gordon, 1985).

The central role of coping skills training may be conceptualized in terms of psychological dependence (Miller & Pechacek, 1987). Heavy drinkers often use alcohol to cope with certain (or, in some cases, most) of the problems in their lives. Through repeated experience of the apparent short-term benefits of alcohol, drinking may become the preferred way of coping, especially in the absence of other coping skills. If alcohol is the *only* way a person has to cope with certain things, then he or she has become psychologically dependent upon it. Such a person has no choice; he or she must drink if those needs are to be met. To the extent that this is true for a person, coping skills deficits are a major obstacle to his or her recovery from alcohol dependence. On the other hand, if a person has several ways of meeting a need, then he or she has a *choice* about whether or not to drink when that need arises. Thus, providing coping skills training is of major importance since it develops alternative ways of meeting needs, thereby reducing psychological dependence on alcohol.

Determining the skills for which training is required necessitates a functional analysis to identify the antecedents to a person's use of alcohol and the functional relationship of drinking to the consequences that follow. This assessment may be in the form of structured interviews or question-naires, or it may take the form of a less structured clinical interview that seeks to identify the situations in which drinking or drug use are likely to occur, and the outcomes that are sought. A useful assessment instrument for identifying drinking antecedents is the Inventory of Drinking Situations (Annis, 1984), and an instrument for identifying consequences is the Drinker Inventory of Consequences (Miller, Tonigan, & Longabaugh, 1995). The Global Appraisal of Individual Needs (Dennis, Titus, White, Unsicker, & Hodgkins, 2003) assesses a wide range of factors that might be related to an individual's use of alcohol and/or drugs.

When searching for clients' antecedents to cravings and drinking, a range of domains should be explored, including social, situational, emo-tional, cognitive, and physiological antecedents (Miller & Mastria, 1977). For each antecedent factor identified, the client should be asked to specify what he or she expected to gain from drinking in that circumstance. To minimize clients' discomfort identifying positive expectations from drink-ing, they should be given the message that, by and large, what they sought from alcohol is not unreasonable or abnormal. If, for example, they were depressed and sought relief from it, or were socially inhibited and sought to feel more comfortable in social situations, those are very reasonable de-sires. The only problem is their use of alcohol to meet those needs. An im-portant goal, then, is to identify needs that are likely to trigger a desire to use alcohol, and, having done so, to develop alternative ways of meeting those needs. The process of identifying the outcomes that were being sought through the use of alcohol, and alternative ways of achieving those results, can be organized and facilitated using the scheme proposed by Miller and Pechacek (1987).

Coping skills deficits are viewed as a major risk factor because of the likelihood of substituting a reliance on alcohol as the default coping strat-egy. If a person never developed appropriate coping skills, or having once learned them can no longer apply them due to lack of recent practice or the presence of some inhibiting factor, he or she will need skills training to overcome the deficit or the factor preventing their use. Skills training can be used to teach coping behaviors not currently in a client's repertoire, to refresh or enhance deficient behaviors, and to identify and reduce inhibit-ing factors. In all cases, adequate practice of skills, during sessions and as homework, is essential, so that clients become "fluent" in the skills and are able to apply them fairly easily when the necessity arises, without having to do a lot of thinking about what has to be done.

Motivational Interviewing

Before proceeding on to a description of specific coping skills training elements, the issue of readiness to change and its impact on the timing of a skills training intervention must first be considered. Poor motivation for change is a particular problem in the field of alcoholism, where client ambivalence has been especially troublesome. A systematic approach, called "motivational interviewing," has been developed to address client motivation. Based upon principles of motivational psychology and the client-centered approach of Carl Rogers, its primary goals are to help clients resolve ambivalence and reach a commitment to change (Miller & Rollnick, 2002).

Motivational interviewing starts with the therapist's exploration and acceptance of client ambivalence. Proceeding through what may be characterized as a gradual shaping process, this approach attempts to move clients toward acknowledging current problems, developing a desire to change them, and identifying strategies that will enable this change. The basic therapist interventions involve discussion of problems that the client has perceived or concerns that others have voiced, and providing empathic feedback that communicates understanding and acceptance of the client. These aim at establishing trust in the therapist and a climate in which the client feels safe enough to explore areas of dissatisfaction with his or her life. The therapist assumes a reflective stance that allows exploration of both sides of the client's ambivalence without arousing defensiveness. By providing frequent summaries of what the client has said, the therapist focuses the client's attention on the problems that are being revealed and on motivational statements the client makes during the course of the discussion.

Through a gradual application of this process, the client is made more aware of problems, their ramifications, and their relationship to his or her drinking. The process is moved forward by the application of behavioral shaping to reinforce client verbalizations that indicate increased awareness of problems and of the need to change. The goal is for the client to move toward accepting the need for change and formulating a strategy for making behavior changes. Baer, Kivlahan, and Donovan (1999) stress the importance of adequate client motivation in order for skills training to be successful, and Annis, Schober, and Kelly (1996) provide a detailed plan for apportioning therapeutic strategies based on client readiness for change (Prochaska & DiClemente, 1984). For those who do not yet recognize the need to change, or who are not ready to commit to making any changes, the intervention strategy should be one of continued motivational interviewing built around feedback regarding the impact of drinking on various aspects of the client's life. As clients accept the need to change, the strategy shifts toward identifying and rehearsing behaviors that can be used to cope with the clients' most common and most potent high-risk situations. As changes in drinking occur, the strategy shifts further, to include practice of coping skills in real-life high-risk situations, fading the use of external aids to performance, and promoting self-attribution of control (Annis et al., 1996).

Coping Skills Modules

A number of coping skills training manuals are available. The one by Monti, Kadden, Rohsenow, Cooney, and Abrams (2002) provides session-by-session explanations, in considerable detail, of the rationale, skill components, and practice methods for 17 skills related to problem areas that are common among alcoholic clients. In the following sections of this chapter, synopses of the rationale and training guidelines for the skills taught in a number of key sessions are provided. The skills are organized according to two broad categories: intrapersonal and interpersonal skills. Further details on the implementation of each of the coping skills training sessions, as well as information on additional skills not reviewed here, and on other topics related to skills training, can be found in Monti et al. (2002).

Intrapersonal Skills

Managing Urges to Drink

Urges can range from thoughts about drinking, without any intention to actually drink, all the way to craving. Urges to resume using are common among people recovering from substance use disorders, and therefore this training module is generally used with all clients. They are taught a number of skills for managing urges, including challenging them, recalling unpleasant experiences that resulted from drinking, anticipating the benefits of not drinking, distracting oneself, delaying the decision about whether or not to drink, leaving the situation, and seeking support. Clients are given a 3 × 5 card on which to record the unpleasant effects of past use and the anticipated benefits of not drinking, and are instructed to carry it with them and refer to it whenever they think of using. They are also asked to imagine various high-risk situations, and to practice coping with the urges that might accompany them.

Anger Management

Anger is a very common antecedent to drinking. Clients are taught about the warning signs of anger, both external and internal signs, so they can identify them early and begin to manage them before anger grows strong and becomes difficult to control. Skills for anger management include using calm-down phrases, identifying the elements of the situation that are provoking anger, and considering options that might help to resolve the situation. These skills can be modeled by the therapist and then role-played by the client. For homework, clients are asked to record their handling of the next anger situation they encounter.

Negative Thinking

Since negative thoughts can be high-risk for drinking, clients are taught to recognize various types of negative thinking habits that may occur automatically. Skills for managing negative thoughts include thought stopping, substituting positive thoughts or feelings, and positive self-talk. Exercises give clients practice identifying their negative thoughts and negative self-talk, and provide an opportunity for them to prepare alternative, substitute responses for use when they occur. A related common problem is negative moods and/or depression. Guidelines for skills training to manage them can be found in Kadden et al. (1992).

Pleasant Activities

Clients may discover a void in their lives as free time becomes available once they are no longer so occupied with drinking and recovering from its effects. They may also find that they are leading an unbalanced lifestyle in which they fulfill numerous obligations, with little if any time devoted to recreation or self-fulfillment. A session on developing a pleasant activities plan is intended to help clients prepare enjoyable, low-risk ways of filling the free time that will be opened up, and achieve a better balance between their obligations and more enjoyable or self-fulfilling activities. A number of strategies for selecting and engaging in these activities are identified.

Decision Making

Sometimes clients end up relapsing after a series of incremental steps that gradually led them ever closer to craving and then to actually drinking. Decision-making training can help clients think ahead to the possible consequences of all the decisions they make, even the ones that are seemingly irrelevant to drinking, to increase the likelihood that they will anticipate potential risks associated with various decision options. They are offered a variety of practice scenarios and are assisted in thinking them through, to identify possible risks and to select a decision option that is likely to minimize the probability of drinking.

Problem Solving

This is a "generic" skill, not necessarily related to avoiding or coping with high-risk situations. Nevertheless, it is recommended to include it among the skills being trained, to provide a flexible coping repertoire in difficult situations for which clients have no apparent coping response immediately available. The steps in the problem-solving model include problem recognition, identification of the problem's component elements as precisely as possible, brainstorming potential solutions, selecting the most promising approach, trying it out, assessing its adequacy, and refining the plan if necessary. With this skill, clients are provided a way of coping with unanticipated problems that might otherwise stump them and put them at high risk for resorting to drinking.

Planning for Emergencies

This is in some ways similar to problem solving, inasmuch as it attempts to provide clients a way of coping with situations that were not specifically anticipated in their skills training, and for which no solution is immediately apparent. The difference here is that the precipitating events are so overwhelming, and so likely to precipitate drinking, that there may not be enough time to initiate the problem-solving process. In anticipation of such "emergency" situations, clients are provided with suggestions to assist them in setting up an emergency plan for use when strong cravings develop and drinking becomes imminent, or actually occurs.

Interpersonal Skills

These skills are taught for coping with situations in which other people are an important factor or are actually part of the problem.

Drink Refusal

Knowing how to cope with offers to drink is an important skill for the majority of clients because such offers are fairly common. Clients are taught to say "no" convincingly without giving a double message, to then suggest an alternative activity that does not involve alcohol, to change the subject to a different topic of conversation, and if the other person persists, to ask him or her not to offer alcohol any more. With considerable practice of this skill, clients should be able to respond quickly and convincingly when these situations arise. Role playing of refusal scenes progress from ones that are easy to handle, building to more persistent offers that are difficult to refuse. Homework involves planning how to respond in a variety of different situations in which alcohol may be offered.

Handling Criticism

Criticism, whether giving it or receiving it, can be high risk since it is often accompanied by feelings of anger. This is even more the case when receiving criticism about drinking. When giving criticism, clients are taught to calm down first, state the criticism in terms of their own feelings, use a firm and clear tone of voice but not an angry one, criticize specific behaviors, request a behavior change, and be willing to work out a compromise. When receiving criticism they are taught not to get defensive or to counterattack, but rather to ask the other person to clarify the purpose and content of the criticism, and to try to find something in the criticism to agree with, so that the parties can work together toward formulating a compromise. In this way, criticism may be transformed into a potentially constructive communication that could produce positive results for both parties involved. Clients practice using the skills in various situations, including those that specifically involve criticisms about drinking.

Relationship Problems

Some clients may experience difficulty expressing their feelings or communicating effectively and sensitively, particularly in intimate relationships, when there is conflict and tension as a result of drinking. This can be a bar to intimacy, both emotional and sexual. Clients are taught about self-disclosing their emotions, sharing their positive feelings, and expressing negative feelings in an appropriate way, to prevent tension from building up. They may also be taught listening skills, which are an essential component of an intimate relationship. Clients practice these skills in simulated situations drawn from their recent past in which they felt angry, anxious, or sad with loved ones. Homework involves planning how to handle one such situation, and then actually trying out the skills in the situation.

Enhancing Social Support Network

Support from others often makes people feel more confident about their ability to cope with problems. Given the number of life problems caused or exacerbated by alcoholism, a good social support network can enhance the chances of coping effectively. However, as their drinking increased, clients may have alienated potential supporters and will have to work to rebuild their support network. They are asked to consider the various types of support that might be helpful to them, who might be helpful in providing the support they need, and how to go about developing that support. They are also taught about the importance of reciprocity, that is, lending support to others as part of the process of building one's support network. They are provided opportunities to practice asking for support, and offering to support others.

General Social Skills

A number of additional social skills may also be taught to help clients better handle social situations that might otherwise put them at risk for drinking. Various communications skills (e.g., conversation skills, use of nonverbal behavior) may be taught to help clients cope with deficits in communications that could leave them feeling socially inadequate or isolated, and therefore at greater risk for relapsing. Assertiveness training may be offered to enable clients to express their emotions and opinions clearly and directly, in a manner that leaves them satisfied that their views were heard, but without doing so in a way that alienates or antagonizes others.

Coping Skills Training with Significant Others

Problems within an intimate relationship, such as maladaptive communication patterns, lack of intimacy, and control struggles, can be precipitants of drinking. Therefore, having a significant other participate in skills-oriented treatment can enhance treatment outcome. Issues to be dealt with in a session with a significant other include deciding whether or not to keep alcohol in the house, identifying how the sober partner can most effectively support and reinforce the alcoholic's efforts to change, fostering more positive communication within the relationship, and learning how to solve problems together. During the session, the couple may be assisted in practicing the problem-solving process as it applies to a current problem they are facing, and discussing how they might apply other skills taught in this program to their daily lives. Homework, designed with their collaboration, can be used to further the implementation of coping skills in their daily lives. O'Farrell (1995) provides descriptions of CBT-oriented marital and family interventions, including assessment, goal setting, fostering changes in drinking and in the relationship, dealing with obstacles that may be encountered, and maintenance of effects.

Skills Training Methods

Clients should be active participants in the skills training process. The more passive they are, the less likely they will be to develop sufficient motivation to follow through with the practice that is required to become fluent in implementing new skills. Clients who actively engage in the processes of skills acquisition and cognitive restructuring are more likely to accept responsibility for making changes. To enhance client involvement and participation, the selection of skills to be taught should match client needs, based on functional analyses of their drinking and related problems.

Regarding the sequence in which skills are taught, it would be good pedagogy to begin by training those skills that are the simplest and easiest to implement, and then adding skills in order of increasing complexity and difficulty. Nevertheless, in the interests of promoting sobriety and enhancing client involvement in what is being taught, it probably makes the most sense to begin skills training with topics that meet clients' most pressing immediate needs, returning at a later time, if possible, to more basic skills that might support implementation of the more complex ones.

At the beginning of each skills training session, the client's current status and recent problems should be assessed, and an opportunity provided to consider how the use of problem solving and other skills already taught could be incorporated in a plan for coping with them. Following this initial discussion, the therapist should review the skill(s) taught in the prior session, praise attempts at homework completion, and explore obstacles that may have interfered with doing the assignment.

A new coping skill is introduced by first providing a rationale for it, as it relates in general to achieving/maintaining sobriety, and specifically in terms of its usefulness for dealing with issues that the client has been facing. This is followed by a description of the steps involved in implementing the new skill, and modeling of them by the therapist. Then the client role-plays the skill with the therapist, or with a peer if it is a group setting, and is provided constructive feedback and an opportunity to try the skill again. At the end of each session, clients are given a written reminder of the steps for implementing the skill(s) they just learned, and a homework exercise to practice them. Strategies to increase the likelihood of doing the homework include placing reminder notes in strategic locations and associating the new behavior with already-established daily routines. As the final agenda item in each session, clients are asked to anticipate high-risk situations that might arise prior to the next session, and ways to avoid them or cope with them.

As with any newly acquired behaviors, coping skills are not likely to be retained or utilized if their acquisition is limited to a single session and one homework assignment. Considerable practice is needed to develop a sense of mastery of each skill and to increase the likelihood of its being used in real-life situations. Therefore, previously learned skills should be reviewed occasionally, be suggested as ways of coping with current problems in the discussions at the outset of sessions, and suggested as ways of handling anticipated high-risk situations, at the end of sessions.

The intensity and duration of treatment will be determined by a number of factors, most notably clinical need and what a third-party payer is willing to cover. Decisions regarding the most appropriate level of care can be made with the aid of the American Society of Addiction Medicine

(ASAM) Patient Placement Criteria (Mee-Lee, Shulman, Fishman, Gast-friend, & Griffith, 2001). With regard to treatment duration, in this era of emphasis on brief treatment and relentless attention to cost-containment, a lengthy course of treatment is not likely to be reimbursed. In many clinical studies it has been found that approximately half of clients drop out of treatment by about the sixth session, and six sessions may be about as much as most managed care organizations are willing to approve, at least initially. Topics that might be covered in a brief time frame include managing urges to drink, problem solving, drink refusal, planning for emergencies, anger management, and decision making, although the actual selection and sequencing of topics should be determined by a functional analysis and client preference. In addition, one or more "booster" follow-up sessions may be scheduled, at 1-month or 6-week intervals, to monitor progress and augment skills as needed to cope with new or persisting problem situations.

An additional consideration involves the relative advantages of skills training in group versus individual treatment. In a group format, peers are natural partners for role playing, group members' life experiences offer a host of examples to illustrate the applicability of skills and provide scenarios for role-playing them, and group members working together facilitate the brainstorming of strategies that is part of the problem-solving process. Peers sometimes trust one another more, or at least sooner, than they trust their therapist, so that peer support can be a very important asset in treatment. Despite these advantages of the group therapy setting, the coping skills training described here can nevertheless be successfully implemented in an individual treatment context, even though the opportunities for role playing are more limited and clients may feel more "on the spot" than in a group setting, where responsibilities can be shared. Trust issues with the treatment provider become more central, but if the therapist is able to adopt an empathic style (Miller & Rollnick, 2002), client trust and openness may emerge fairly rapidly. Thus, although individual treatment does present some challenges, they are not insurmountable, and that format can be effectively utilized with this treatment approach.

In the event that a person's coping in an actual high-risk situation was not adequate and he or she relapsed to substance use, the RP model offers recommendations for handling that eventuality. Slips should be viewed as a learning experience, an opportunity to identify trigger situations and the expectancies the client might have had regarding possible benefits of substance use in the circumstance. Clients should be encouraged to identify what they actually did in the high-risk situation, what turned out to have been helpful, and what was not helpful. Based on that review, they should formulate plans to strengthen the actions that worked and to compensate for those that did not, so that they will be likely to cope more effectively with similar trigger situations when they arise in the future. There should also be an exploration of feelings of guilt and self-blame that clients may experience in response to a relapse, and they should be cautioned that surrendering to those emotions places them at high risk for continuing to drink (Marlatt & Gordon, 1985).

Treatment Goal: Abstinence or Moderation?

Some clients will come to treatment with strong opinions about whether or not they can drink any longer. Some will believe that abstinence is a necessity, whereas others will hope that they can continue to drink at reduced levels (Pattison, 1985). At the outset of a self-help guide for controlled drinking, Miller and Muñoz (1982) provide guidelines indicating that moderation is appropriate for problem drinkers who have experienced some negative consequences of their drinking (but not major life crises), do not consider themselves alcoholic, have no alcoholic close relatives, and have not been physically addicted. Abstinence should be pursued if there are medical complications, such as liver disease, gastrointestinal problems, heart disease, or other physical problems that could be exacerbated by even moderate drinking, if a female is pregnant, if one is taking prescribed medications that could interact with alcohol, or if one experiences a loss of control when alcohol is consumed. Some clients for whom abstinence is recommended may nevertheless insist upon a goal of moderation. For them, a trial in which they are permitted to drink a substantially reduced amount of alcohol will determine whether such a limit can be adhered to. The National Institute on Alcohol Abuse and Alcoholism (1995) recommends limits of 14 drinks per week and no more than 4 drinks per occasion for men, and 7 drinks per week and no more than 3 per occasion for women and for both sexes over the age of 65. The "harm reduction" approach, which has become increasingly popular over the last decade, may be helpful with clients who refuse an abstinence goal, because of its focus on minimizing the harmful consequences of drinking rather than on the amount consumed (Marlatt, 1998). Some clients who initially choose a goal of controlled drinking may revert to abstinence at a later time (Hodgins, Leigh, Milne, & Gerrish, 1997).

RELATED TREATMENT APPROACHES

Several other behavioral and cognitive-behavioral approaches to treatment have demonstrated effectiveness and are compatible with the coping skills approach described here. Any one of them, or a combination of them, could be implemented together with a coping skills training intervention.

Contingency Management

The contingency management approach to treatment is based in operant conditioning theory and is primarily concerned with the events that follow behavior. From this perspective, drinking behavior is maintained by the reinforcing effects of alcohol and by social reinforcement. The treatment of excessive drinking involves eliminating or weakening naturally occurring reinforcements for drinking, and providing reinforcement for abstinence by means of tangible reinforcers, such as vouchers for goods or services (Higgins & Petry, 1999). There was a spate of research on this approach in the alcoholism literature of the 1970s (Liebson, Tommasello, & Bigelow, 1978; Miller, 1975; Miller, Hersen, Eisler, & Watt, 1974). Subsequently, however, interest in the use of this approach has centered primarily on drug dependence, and contingency management for alcoholism fell into disuse until recently. When applied to drug problems, the contingency management approach has been more efficacious than comparison treatments for reducing substance use and retaining clients in treatment (see Higgins & Silverman, 1999).

Iguchi et al. (Iguchi, Belding, Morral, Lamb, & Husband, 1997) demonstrated that reinforcement for completion of tasks specified in a treatment plan resulted in better attendance and a significant improvement in abstinence rates, which were maintained even after explicit reinforcement was discontinued. The finding of sustained maintenance suggests the possibility that this strategy brought participants into contact with naturally occurring reinforcers in their environments that continued to maintain behavior change after removal of the therapist-controlled contingencies.

In a study with alcohol dependent outpatients, Petry, Martin, Cooney, and Kranzler (2000) demonstrated that contingency management added to standard treatment improved both attendance and time to relapse. The use of other drugs was also reduced, although use of them was not specifically targeted by the contingency management intervention. Reinforcement was contingent upon negative breathalyzer readings and completion of steps related to clients' treatment goals, with bonuses for continuing compliance. Reinforcers were provided according to a variable ratio schedule that was effective, acceptable to clients, and less expensive to implement than the more usual voucher system.

Community Reinforcement

Although it too arose from the operant tradition, the Community Reinforcement Approach (CRA) employs a fairly eclectic array of interventions (Meyers & Smith, 1995; Smith & Meyers, 2000). Despite extremely promising early reports (Azrin, 1976; Azrin, Sisson, Meyers, & Godley, 1982), there was a long hiatus during which CRA was not widely utilized clinically and there was virtually no research outside of Azrin's circle. In the late 1990s, Smith, Meyers, and Delaney (1998) reported a trial with homeless alcoholics in which CRA outperformed standard treatment at all follow-up assessments, although drinking gradually increased during the follow-up interval. A subset of CRA participants drank heavily throughout, leading the authors to recommend a search for client variables that predict success versus failure with this approach. Budney and Higgins (1998) combined the two operant-oriented methods, community reinforcement and contingency management, for the treatment of cocaine dependence, with some treatment success, but the combined intervention has yet to be tested with alcoholics.

Behavioral Marital Therapy

The inclusion of a client's spouse/partner in treatment can be helpful to identify relationship problems that might trigger or reinforce substance use, and provide an opportunity to educate the partner about effective support for the client's recovery efforts (McCrady & Epstein, 1996). The behavioral marital approach to alcoholism treatment seeks to identify relationship conflicts that trigger drinking, improve communications in strained relationships, and develop reinforcing consequences for abstinence (Epstein & McCrady, 1998). Behavioral marital therapy has been shown to be associated with reduced domestic violence (O'Farrell, Van Hutton, & Murphy, 1999), reduced treatment attrition, improvements in marital functioning, and reduced alcohol consumption, although relapse to alcohol use is common (McCrady, Epstein, & Hirsch, 1999; McKay, Longabaugh, Beattie, Maisto, & Noel, 1993). Longabaugh, Wirtz, Beattie, and Noel (1995) found that the addition of a small amount of relationship enhancement to CBT was helpful for those who had nonproblematic relationships, but that a more extended intervention was necessary for those with problematic relationships. Fals-Stewart, O'Farrell, and Birchler (1997) report that behavioral couple therapy was both more effective and more cost-effective than individual therapy for reducing substance use, sustaining abstinence, and reducing legal, family, and social problems.

TREATMENT CONSIDERATIONS FOR DUAL-DIAGNOSIS CLIENTS

It is estimated that as many as 37% of those with alcohol abuse/dependence also have a psychiatric disorder, usually an affective, anxiety, psychotic, or personality disorder (Rosenthal & Westreich, 1999). Conversely, among psychiatric patients, 20–50% also have alcohol or drug use disorders. There are various possible etiologies of co-occurring psychiatric and substance use disorders: They might have independent etiologies, one of them may be secondary to the other, or both may be secondary to a common third factor (Meyer, 1986). Regardless of their etiology, each may influence the course of, and recovery from, the other, so that treatment programs focused primarily on either type of disorder must consider the possibility of the other in its clients. Routine screening is therefore recommended to detect psychiatric problems among clients who present in substance abuse settings, and to detect substance abuse problems among clients in psychiatric settings.

The processes of detection and diagnosis are complicated by the difficulty in discriminating between alcohol-induced psychiatric symptoms and symptoms of an independent psychiatric disorder (e.g., Schuckit et al., 1997). Information collected early in treatment is likely to be unreliable because of the lingering effects of alcohol and withdrawal, but nevertheless treatment decisions must be made. Drake et al. (1990) recommend utilizing a consensus approach combining self-report and interview data, collateral reports, and longitudinal data accumulated over time.

With respect to treatment for co-occurring alcoholism and psychiatric disorders, a number of psychosocial interventions can benefit both types of disorder. Since negative moods or anger may be concomitants of psychiatric disorders and may also be triggers for relapse to drinking, interventions that enhance clients' ability to identify and manage negative moods and/or anger will likely contribute to improvements in both the psychiatric and substance use disorders. Lack of social support may be an obstacle to recovery from both types of disorder, and here again both are likely to be improved by providing training in social skills, effective communication, and development of a social support network. Other skills training interventions that may be beneficial for both types of disorder include problem solving, stress management, increasing pleasant activities, and vocational rehabilitation.

The manner of delivery of interventions for co-occurring disorders must be adapted for these challenging clients. Providing a high degree of structure and clear ground rules can help to compensate for poorer internal controls seen among some dual-diagnosis clients. Possible cognitive limitations can be compensated for by providing simple explanations of new skills, breaking them down into small steps, and providing considerable practice. Therapists who adopt a "coaching" style, in which they avoid direct confrontations and work with clients toward mutually agreed-upon goals, are more likely to retain clients in treatment. Greater tolerance for relapses is often necessary, using them as opportunities to teach clients about drinking triggers and how to avoid or cope with them. Accordingly, Carey (1996) has advocated employing a harm reduction philosophy with dual-diagnosis clients, and has developed a 5-point program for implementing it. Since both psychiatric and chemical dependence problems may disrupt clients' functioning, initial treatment efforts must often be directed toward reducing or eliminating both the substance use and the most disruptive psychiatric symptoms.

CONCLUSIONS

A cognitive-behavioral conceptualization of addictive behavior has been described in which abusive drinking is considered to be a form of learned behavior that is acquired through the processes of Pavlovian and/or operant conditioning. As such, excessive drinking can be modified by the application of learning-based interventions. The coping skills approach to RP treatment was outlined in detail, providing examples of how it can be employed to deal with both the intrapersonal and interpersonal situations that tend to support substance use. While there is considerable evidence to support the efficacy of these interventions, it is not clear that they are superior to other interventions. Further clinical research is needed to assess the impact of coping skills training on treatment outcome, ascertain the relative effectiveness of the various skills training components, determine how each of the components can best be matched to particular client needs, and determine how much actual practice of skills is required for them to be useful in coping with high-risk situations.

REFERENCES

Abrams, D. B., Binkoff, J. A., Zwick, W. R., Liepman, M. R., Nirenberg, T. D., Munroe, S. M., & Monti, P. M. (1991). Alcohol abusers' and social drinkers' responses to alcohol-relevant and general situations. *Journal of Studies on Alcohol, 52*, 409–414.

Allsop, S., Saunders, B., Phillips, M., & Carr, A. (1997). A trial of relapse prevention with severely dependent male problem drinkers. *Addiction, 92*, 61–74.

Annis, H. M. (1984). *Inventory of Drinking Situations.* Toronto: Addiction Research Foundation.

Annis, H. M., Schober, R., & Kelly, E. (1996). Matching addiction outpatient counseling to client readiness for change: The role of structured relapse prevention counseling. *Experimental and Clinical Psychopharmacology, 4*, 37–45.

Azrin, N. H. (1976). Improvements in the community reinforcement approach to alcoholism. *Behavior Research and Therapy, 14*, 339–348.

Azrin, N. H., Sisson, W., Meyers, R. J., & Godley, M. (1982). Alcoholism treatment by disulfiram and community reinforcement therapy. *Journal of Behavior Therapy and Experimental Psychiatry, 13*, 105–112.

Baer, J. S., Kivlahan, D. R., & Donovan, D. M. (1999). Integrating skills training and motivational therapies: Implications for the treatment of substance dependence. *Journal of Substance Abuse Treatment, 17*, 15–23.

Budney, A. J., & Higgins, S. T. (1998). *A community reinforcement plus vouchers ap-*

proach: Treating cocaine addiction (National Institute on Drug Abuse Publication No. 98-4309). Rockville, MD: National Institute on Drug Abuse.

Carey, K. B. (1996). Substance use reduction in the context of outpatient psychiatric treatment: A collaborative, motivational, harm reduction approach. *Community Mental Health Journal, 32,* 291–306.

Carroll, K. M. (1996). Relapse prevention as a psychosocial treatment: A review of controlled clinical trials. *Experimental and Clinical Psychopharmacology, 4,* 46–54.

Chaney, E. F., O'Leary, M. R., & Marlatt, G. A. (1978). Skill training with alcoholics. *Journal of Consulting and Clinical Psychology, 46,* 1092–1104.

Chung, T., Langenbucher, J., Labouvie, E., Pandina, R. J., & Moos, R. H. (2001). Changes in alcoholic patients' coping responses predict 12-month treatment outcomes. *Journal of Consulting and Clinical Psychology, 69,* 92–100.

Connors, G. J., Longabaugh, R., & Miller, W. R. (1996). Looking forward and back to relapse: Implications for research and practice. *Addiction, 91*(Suppl.), S191–S196.

Connors, G. J., Maisto, S. A., & Zywiak, W. H. (1996). Understanding relapse in the broader context of post-treatment functioning. *Addiction, 91*(Suppl.), S173–S189.

Cooney, N. L., Kadden, R. M., Litt, M. D., & Getter, H. (1991). Matching alcoholics to coping skills or interactional therapies: Two-year follow-up results. *Journal of Consulting and Clinical Psychology, 59,* 598–601.

Cronkite, R. C., & Moos, R. H. (1980). Determinants of the posttreatment functioning of alcoholic patients: A conceptual framework. *Journal of Consulting and Clinical Psychology, 48,* 305–316.

Dennis, M. L., Titus, J. C., White, M., Unsicker, J., & Hodgkins, D. (2003). *Global Appraisal of Individual Needs (GAIN): Administration guide for the GAIN and related measures.* Bloomington, IL: Chestnut Health Systems. Web site: www.chestnut.org/li/gain

Drake, R. E., Osher, F. C., Noordsy, D. L., Hurlbut, S. C., Teague, G. B., & Beaudette, M. S. (1990). Diagnosis of alcohol use disorders in schizophrenia. *Schizophrenia Bulletin, 16,* 57–67.

Epstein, E. E., & McCrady, B. S. (1998). Behavioral couples treatment of alcohol and drug use disorders: Current status and innovations. *Clinical Psychology Review, 18,* 689–711.

Eriksen, L., Björnstad, S., & Götestam, K. G. (1986). Social skills training in groups for alcoholics: One-year treatment outcome for groups and individuals. *Addictive Behaviors, 11,* 309–329.

Fals-Stewart, W., O'Farrell, T. J., & Birchler, G. R. (1997). Behavioral couples therapy for male substance-abusing patients: A cost outcomes analysis. *Journal of Consulting and Clinical Psychology, 65*(5), 789–802.

Ferrell, W. L., & Galassi, J. P. (1981). Assertion training and human relations training in the treatment of chronic alcoholics. *International Journal of the Addictions, 16,* 959–968.

Finney, J. W., & Monahan, S. C. (1996). The cost-effectiveness of treatment for alcoholism: A second approximation. *Journal of Studies on Alcoholism, 29,* 229–243.

Finney, J. W., Noyes, C. A., Coutts, A. I., & Moos, R. H. (1998). Evaluating substance abuse treatment process models: I. Changes on proximal outcome variables during 12-step and cognitive-behavioral treatment. *Journal of Studies on Alcohol, 59,* 371–380.

Freedberg, E. J., & Johnston, W. E. (1978). *The effects of assertion training within the context of a multi-modal alcoholism treatment program for employed alcoholics.* Toronto: Addiction Research Foundation.

Hedberg, A. G., & Campbell, L. (1974). A comparison of four behavioral treatments of alcoholism. *Journal of Behavior Therapy and Experimental Psychiatry, 5,* 251–256.

Higgins, S. T., & Petry, N. M. (1999). Contingency management: Incentives for sobriety. *Alcohol Research and Health, 23,* 122–127.

Higgins, S. T., & Silverman, K. (1999). *Motivating illicit-drug abusers to change their behavior: Research on contingency management interventions.* Washington, DC: American Psychological Association.

Hodgins, D. C., Leigh, G., Milne, R., & Gerrish, R. (1997). Drinking goal selection in behavioral self-management treatment of chronic alcoholics. *Addictive Behaviors, 22(2),* 247–255.

Holder, H., Longabaugh, R., Miller, W. R., & Rubonis, A. V. (1991). The cost effectiveness of treatment for alcoholism: A first approximation. *Journal of Studies on Alcohol, 52,* 517–540.

Iguchi, M. Y., Belding, M. A., Morral, A. R., Lamb, R. J., & Husband, S. D. (1997). Reinforcing operants other than abstinence in drug abuse treatment: An effective alternative for reducing drug use. *Journal of Consulting and Clinical Psychology, 65,* 421–428.

Irvin, J. E., Bowers, C. A., Dunn, M. E., & Wang, M. C. (1999). Efficacy of relapse prevention: A meta-analytic review. *Journal of Consulting and Clinical Psychology, 67,* 563–570.

Ito, J. R., Donovan, D. M., & Hall, J. J. (1988). Relapse prevention in alcohol aftercare: Effects on drinking outcome, change process, and aftercare attendance. *British Journal of Addictions, 83,* 171–181.

Jones, S. L., Kanfer, R., & Lanyon, R. I. (1982). Skill training with alcoholics: A clinical extension. *Addictive Behaviors, 7,* 285–290.

Jones, S. L., & Lanyon, R. I. (1981). Relationship between adaptive skills and outcome of alcoholism treatment. *Journal of Studies on Alcohol, 42,* 521–525.

Kadden, R. M., Carroll, K., Donovan, D., Cooney, N., Monti, P., Abrams, D., Litt, M., & Hester, R. (Eds.). (1992). *Cognitive-behavioral coping skills therapy manual: A clinical research guide for therapists treating individuals with alcohol abuse and dependence* (Project MATCH Monograph Series Vol. 4; DHHS Publication No. ADM92-1895). Rockville, MD: National Institute on Alcohol Abuse and Alcoholism.

Kadden, R. M., Cooney, N. L., Getter, H., & Litt, M. D. (1989). Matching alcoholics to coping skills or interactional therapies: Posttreatment results. *Journal of Consulting and Clinical Psychology, 57,* 698–704.

Kadden, R. M., Litt, M. D., Cooney, N. L., Kabela, E., & Getter, H. (2001). Prospective matching of alcoholic clients to cognitive-behavioral or interactional group therapy. *Journal of Studies on Alcohol, 62,* 359–369.

Kalman, D., Longabaugh, R., Clifford, P. R., Beattie, M., & Maisto, S. A. (2000). Matching alcoholics to treatment: Failure to replicate finding of an earlier study. *Journal of Substance Abuse Treatment, 19*, 183–187.

Liebson, I., Tommasello, A., & Bigelow, G. (1978). A behavioral treatment of alcoholic methadone patients. *Annals of Internal Medicine, 89*, 342–344.

Litman, G. K., Stapleton, J., Oppenheim, A. N., Peleg, M., & Jackson, P. (1984). The relationship between coping behaviours, their effectiveness and alcoholism relapse and survival. *British Journal of Addiction, 79*, 283–291.

Longabaugh, R., & Morgenstern, J. (1999). Cognitive-behavioral coping skills therapy for alcohol dependence: Current status and future directions. *Alcohol Research and Health, 23*, 78–85.

Longabaugh, R., Rubin, A., Malloy, P., Beattie, M., Clifford, P. R., & Noel, N. (1994). Drinking outcomes of alcohol abusers diagnosed as antisocial personality disorder. *Alcoholism: Clinical and Experimental Research, 18*, 778–785.

Longabaugh, R., Rubin, A., Stout, R. L., Zywiak, W. H., & Lowman, C. (1996). The reliability of Marlatt's taxonomy for classifying relapses. *Addiction, 91*(Suppl.), S73–S88.

Longabaugh, R., Wirtz, P. W., Beattie, M. C., & Noel, N. (1995). Matching treatment focus to patient social investment and support: 18-month follow-up results. *Journal of Consulting and Clinical Psychology, 63*, 296–307.

Maisto, S. A., Connors, G. J., & Zywiak, W. H. (2000). Alcohol treatment, changes in coping skills, self-efficacy, and levels of alcohol use and related problems one year following treatment initiation. *Psychology of Addictive Behaviors, 14*, 257–266.

Marlatt, G. A. (Ed.). (1998). *Harm reduction: Pragmatic strategies for managing high risk behaviors*. New York: Guilford Press.

Marlatt, G. A., & Gordon, J. R. (Eds.). (1985). *Relapse prevention* (1st ed.). New York: Guilford Press.

McCrady, B. S., & Epstein, E. E. (1996). Theoretical bases of family approaches to substance abuse treatment. In F. Rotgers, D. S. Keller, & J. Morgenstern (Eds.), *Treating substance abuse: Theory and technique* (1st ed., pp. 117–142). New York: Guilford Press.

McCrady, B. S., Epstein, E. E., & Hirsch, L. S. (1999). Maintaining change after conjoint behavioral alcohol treatment for men: Outcomes at 6 months. *Addiction, 94*(9), 1381–1396

McKay, J. R., Longabaugh, R., Beattie, M. C., Maisto, S. A., & Noel, N. E. (1993). Does adding conjoint therapy to individually focused alcoholism treatment lead to better family functioning? *Journal of Substance Abuse, 5*, 45–59.

Mee-Lee, D., Shulman, G. D., Fishman, M., Gastfriend, D. R., & Griffith, J. H. (Eds.). (2001). *ASAM patient placement criteria for the treatment of substance-related disorders* (2nd ed., rev.). Chevy Chase, MD: American Society of Addiction Medicine.

Meyer, R. E. (1986). How to understand the relationship between psychopathology and addictive disorders: Another example of the chicken and the egg. In R. E. Meyer (Ed.), *Psychopathology and addictive disorders* (pp. 3–16). New York: Guilford Press.

Meyers, R. J., & Smith, J. E. (1995). *Clinical guide to alcohol treatment: The community reinforcement approach*. New York: Guilford Press.

Miller, P. (1975). A behavioral intervention program for public drunkenness offenders. *Archives of General Psychiatry, 32,* 915–918.

Miller, P. M., Hersen, M., Eisler, R. M., & Watt, J. G. (1974). Contingent reinforcement of lowered blood/alcohol levels in an outpatient chronic alcoholic. *Behavior Research and Therapy, 12,* 261–263.

Miller, P. M., & Mastria, M. A. (1977). *Alternatives to alcohol abuse: A social learning model.* Champaign, IL: Research Press.

Miller, W. R., Brown, J. M., Simpson, T. L., Handmaker, N. S., Bien, T. H., Luckie, L. F., Montgomery, H. A., Hester, R. K., & Tonigan, J. S. (1995). What works? A methodological analysis of the alcohol treatment outcome literature. In R. K. Hester & W. R. Miller (Eds.), *Handbook of alcoholism treatment approaches: Effective alternatives* (2nd ed., pp. 12–44). Boston: Allyn & Bacon.

Miller, W. R., & Muñoz, R. F. (1982). *How to control your drinking.* Albuquerque: University of New Mexico Press.

Miller, W. R., & Pechacek, T. F. (1987). New roads: Assessing and treating psychological dependence. *Journal of Substance Abuse Treatment, 4,* 73–77.

Miller, W. R., & Rollnick, S. (2002). *Motivational interviewing: Preparing people for change* (2nd ed.). New York: Guilford Press.

Miller, W. R., Tonigan, J. S., & Longabaugh, R. (1995). *The Drinker Inventory of Consequences (DrInC): An instrument for assessing adverse consequences of alcohol abuse* (Project MATCH Monograph Series Vol. 4; NIH Publication No. 95-3911). Rockville, MD: National Institute on Alcohol Abuse and Alcoholism.

Miller, W. R., Westerberg, V. S., Harris, R. J., & Tonigan, J. S. (1996). What predicts relapse? Prospective testing of antecedent models. *Addiction, 91,* S155–S171.

Moggi, F., Ouimette, P. C., Moos, R. H., & Finney, J. W. (1999). Dual diagnosis patients in substance abuse treatment: Relationship of general coping and substance-specific coping to one-year outcomes. *Addiction, 94,* 1805–1816.

Monti, P. M., Abrams, D. B., Binkoff, J. A., Zwick, W. R., Liepman, M. R., Nirenberg, T. D., & Rohsenow, D. J. (1990). Communication skills training, communication skills training with family and cognitive behavioral mood management training for alcoholics. *Journal of Studies on Alcohol, 51,* 263–270.

Monti, P. M., Kadden, R. M., Rohsenow, D. J., Cooney, N. L., & Abrams, D. B. (2002). *Treating alcohol dependence: A coping skills training guide.* New York: Guilford Press.

Morgenstern, J., & Longabaugh, R. (2000). Cognitive-behavioral treatment for alcohol dependence: A review of evidence for its hypothesized mechanisms of action. *Addiction, 95,* 1475–1490.

Moser, A. E., & Annis, H. M. (1996). The role of coping in relapse crisis outcome: A prospective study of treated alcoholics. *Addiction, 91,* 1101–1113.

National Institute on Alcohol Abuse and Alcoholism. (1995). *The physicians' guide to helping patients with alcohol problems* (NIH Publication No. 95-3769). Washington, DC: U.S. Government Printing Office.

Oei, T. P. S., & Jackson, P. R. (1980). Long-term effects of group and individual social skills training with alcoholics. *Addictive Behaviors, 5,* 129–136.

Oei, T. P. S., & Jackson, P. (1982). Social skills and cognitive behavioral approaches to the treatment of problem drinking. *Journal of Studies on Alcohol, 43,* 532–547.

O'Farrell, T. J. (1995). Marital and family therapy. In R. K. Hester & W. R. Miller

(Eds.), *Handbook of alcoholism treatment approaches: Effective alternatives* (2nd ed., pp. 195–220). Boston: Allyn & Bacon.

O'Farrell, T. J., Van Hutton, V., & Murphy, C. M. (1999). Domestic violence before and after alcoholism treatment: A two-year longitudinal study. *Journal of Studies on Alcohol, 60,* 317–321.

Pattison, E. M. (1985). The selection of treatment modalities for the alcoholic patient. In J. H. Mendelson & N. K. Mello (Eds.), *The diagnosis and treatment of alcoholism* (2nd ed., pp. 189–294). New York: McGraw-Hill.

Petry, N. M., Martin, B., Cooney, J. L., & Kranzler, H. R. (2000). Give them prizes and they will come: Contingency management for treatment of alcohol dependence. *Journal of Consulting and Clinical Psychology, 68,* 250–257.

Prochaska, J. O., & DiClemente, C. C. (1984). *The transtheoretical approach: Crossing traditional boundaries of therapy.* Homewood, IL: Dow Jones-Irwin.

Project MATCH Research Group. (1997). Matching alcoholism treatments to client heterogeneity: Project MATCH posttreatment drinking outcomes. *Journal of Studies on Alcohol, 58,* 7–29.

Project MATCH Research Group. (1998). Matching alcoholism treatments to client heterogeneity: Treatment main effects and matching effects on drinking during treatment. *Journal of Studies on Alcohol, 59,* 631–639.

Rohsenow, D. J., Monti, P. M., Binkoff, J. A., Liepman, M., Nirenberg, T., & Abrams, D. B. (1991). Patient-treatment matching for alcoholic men in communication skills versus cognitive-behavioral mood management training. *Addictive Behaviors, 16,* 63–69.

Rohsenow, D. J., Monti, P. M., Rubonis, A. V., Gulliver, S. B., Colby, S. M., Binkoff, J. A., & Abrams, D. B. (2001). Cue exposure with coping skills training and communication skills training for alcohol dependence: Six and twelve month outcomes. *Addiction, 96,* 1161–1174.

Rosenthal, R. N., & Westreich, L. (1999). Treatment of persons with dual diagnoses of substance use disorder and other psychological problems. In B. S. McCrady & E. E. Epstein (Eds.), *Addictions: A comprehensive guidebook* (pp. 439–476). New York: Oxford University Press.

Sanchez-Craig, M., & Walker, K. (1982). Teaching coping skills to chronic alcoholics in a coeducational halfway house: I. Assessment of programme effects. *British Journal of Addiction, 77,* 35–50.

Schuckit, M. A., Tipp, J. E., Bergman, M., Reich, W., Hesselbrock, V. M., & Smith, T. L. (1997). Comparison of induced and independent major depressive disorders in 2,945 alcoholics. *American Journal of Psychiatry, 154,* 948–957.

Schutte, K. K., Byrne, F. E., Brennan, P. L., & Moos, R. H. (2001). Successful remission of late-life drinking problems: A 10-year follow-up. *Journal of Studies on Alcohol, 62,* 322–334.

Sjoberg, L., & Samsonowitz, V. (1985). Coping strategies in alcohol abuse. *Drug and Alcohol Dependence, 15,* 283–301.

Smith, J. E., & Meyers, R. J. (2000). CRA: The community reinforcement approach for treating alcohol problems. In M. J. Dougher (Ed.), *Clinical behavior analysis* (pp. 207–230). Reno, NV: Context Press.

Smith, J. E., Meyers, R. J., & Delaney, H. D. (1998). The community reinforcement approach with homeless alcohol-dependent individuals. *Journal of Consulting and Clinical Psychology, 66,* 541–548.

Wells, E. A., Catalano, R. F., Plotnick, R., Hawkins, J. D., & Brattesani, K. A. (1989). General versus drug-specific coping skills and posttreatment drug use among adults. *Psychology of Addictive Behaviors, 3*, 8–21.

Wunschel, S. M., Rohsenow, D. J., Norcross, J. C., & Monti, P. M. (1993). Coping strategies and the maintenance of change after inpatient alcoholism treatment. *Social Work Research and Abstracts, 29*, 18–22.

CHAPTER 4

Relapse Prevention for Smoking

Saul Shiffman
Jon Kassel
Chad Gwaltney
Dennis McChargue

Cigarette smoking remains the most preventable cause of illness and death in our society today. Upwards of 430,000 smokers die in the United States alone each year (Centers for Disease Control and Prevention, 1997), while worldwide over 1,200,000 deaths a year are attributable to smoking-related causes (World Health Organization, 2000). The magnitude of the problem is made even more salient by the realization that relapse is the modal outcome among those attempting to quit smoking (e.g., Garvey, Bliss, Hitchcock, Heinold, & Rosner, 1992; Shiffman, 1982). Whereas the best available treatments yield 1-year abstinence rates of about 30%, even among smokers who successfully quit for a full year, as many as 40% eventually return to regular smoking (U.S. Department of Health and Human Services [USDHHS], 1990). Smokers who attempt to quit on their own fare even less well, with relapse rates ranging from 90 to 97% (Cohen et al., 1989; Hughes et al., 1992).

As such, the importance of preventing relapse among smokers trying to quit (either on their own or through formal interventions) cannot be overstated. In this respect, the relapse prevention (RP) model originally put forth by Marlatt and colleagues (Marlatt & Gordon, 1985) has come to profoundly influence the way we think about smoking cessation. Although formal tests of the model have been relatively few in number within the realm of smoking cessation (Irvin, Bowers, Dunn, & Wang, 1999), the notion that smoking cessation is a *process* that unfolds over time has come to shape the field's attitudes toward smoking interventions. Indeed, the realization that relapse occurs more often than not underscores the sentiments expressed long ago by Mark Twain, who asserted, "Quitting smoking is the easiest thing I ever did. I ought to know. I've done it a thousand times."

The good news is that numerous treatments for cigarette smoking and nicotine dependence appear to work. Several recent reviews (e.g., USDHHS, 2000; World Health Organization [WHO], 2001) have presented findings supporting evidence-based efficacy of both behavioral and pharmacological interventions for smoking cessation. Thus, clinicians now have available to them a variety of therapies from which to choose when treating the smoker who desires to quit (e.g., nicotine replacement, bupropion, behavioral skills training). The treatment literature generally has not made strong or consistent distinctions between relapse prevention—preventing the reoccurrence of smoking after a period of sustained abstinence—and other goals or modalities of treatment. Because so much treatment failure is due to relapse, however, this distinction, though conceptually important, may be practically unimportant. Accordingly, we also do not strictly distinguish between RP and other goals or modalities of treatment. In the sections that follow, we review treatment for smoking cessation, and how the RP model has influenced and informed smoking cessation efforts.

TREATMENT ISSUES IN RELAPSE PREVENTION

Treatment Goals: Abstinence versus Harm Reduction

The central mission of tobacco control is to reduce the morbidity and mortality due to tobacco use (Stratton, Shetty, Wallace, & Bondurant, 2001; Warner, 2002)—abstinence has been the major means, but is not an end in itself. To increase the reach of smoking interventions beyond cessation and prevention, researchers have begun to investigate potential strategies that might reduce tobacco-related harm without necessarily eliminating smoking or tobacco use, or nicotine exposure. Such efforts at tobacco harm reduction (THR) aim to decrease exposure to tobacco toxins. The approaches being investigated include use of potential reduced exposure products (PREPs; Stratton et al., 2001), switching to tobacco products that may lower risk (e.g., smokeless tobacco), and behavioral techniques that reduce the number of cigarettes smoked daily.

Although reduction-focused models of treatment are gaining in popularity, the application of reduction principles in tobacco treatment remains controversial. Two important questions fuel concerns about THR. The first question is What is the effect of adopting a particular PREP on the user's health risk (Shiffman, 1998; Shiffman et al., 2002)? The second question addresses the effect on the population as a whole, and considers the possibility that a "safer" product might increase the numbers of new tobacco users and/or undermine abstinence efforts of current tobacco users, thus resulting in increased harm (Shiffman, 1998; Shiffman et al., 2002). Underlying both questions is the concern of whether the advent of new THR approaches, other than abstinence-focused ones, might unknowingly have an adverse effect on public health or on an individual user's health. Until these questions are adequately answered, THR approaches will remain controversial and risky.

Stepping Down Harmful Consequences (Harm Reduction Goal)

The various potential forms of harm reduction have been discussed elsewhere (Shiffman et al., 2002). In brief, non-abstinence THR approaches fall into four categories: (1) behavioral approaches to reduce number of cigarettes smoked daily, (2) cigarette-like products that are engineered to reduce exposure to harmful toxins, (3) a switch to smokeless tobacco use, and (4) the use of medicinal nicotine (e.g., nicotine replacement therapy) as a partial or complete substitute for smoking. Reviewing the toxicological implications of these approaches is far beyond the scope of this chapter. In this brief section, we aim merely to provide the clinician with some guidance and cautions.

Reducing how much someone smokes has intuitive appeal as a harm reduction strategy, as many (but not all) smoking-related diseases show steep dose–response curves (USDHHS, 1997). However, there are several caveats to be considered in adopting this strategy. First, epidemiological data suggest that reductions in smoking must be maintained over periods of years to have an impact on health (Burns, 2004). Thus, the clinician and smoker should not be too readily comforted by near-term reductions. Second, cigarettes are a very flexible dosing vehicle, with the result that reductions in number of cigarettes smoked may not be accompanied by parallel reductions in actual exposure. Smokers endeavor to keep their nicotine intake constant, so when the number of cigarettes is reduced, they increase their smoking intensity, thereby extracting more toxins from each cigarette, and possibly counteracting the effects of reduced smoking (Stratton et al., 2001; USDHHS, 2001). Thus, reductions in smoking may not be meaningful without some assessment of biological exposures (e.g., through a proxy measure like carbon monoxide). Some data suggest that, with few exceptions (Pickworth, Fant, Nelson, & Henningfield, 1998), behavioral harm reduction strategies do not produce marked reduction in biomarkers used to assess harm exposure (Hurt et al., 2000; Kozlowski, Sweeney, & Pillitteri, 1996). On the other hand, a review by Hughes (2000) suggests that, even though smokers compensate for reduced smoking, some reductions in biochemical exposure can be achieved.

Whether reengineered cigarettes will be able to deliver on the promise of reduced risk remains to be seen. There are already several such products in the marketplace making unproven claims to reduce exposure or risk, but the early evidence is, at best, mixed. For example, the PREP known as "Eclipse" was engineered to reduce pyrolysis or burning as a way of reducing some toxins (Shiffman, Gitchell, Warner, et al., 2002). However, research has shown that the "Eclipse" substantially increases the level of exposure to carbon monoxide and other toxins (Fagerstrom, Hughes, Rasmussen, & Callas, 2000), and introduces a new risk of inhaling glass fibers (Pauly et al., 1998; Pauly, Cummings, & Streck, 2000). In brief, it provides a new chemical cocktail that has not been studied enough to know whether it would be associated with a reduction in disease risk under actual human use conditions.

The history of "light" cigarettes—in which the tobacco industry knowingly promulgated misinformation indicating that the products were safer when they were not (USDHHS, 2001)—suggests the need for healthy skepticism of manufacturer's claims. Absent an independent, science-based, health-focused regulatory authority, it will be hard to know whether any health benefits claimed for reengineered tobacco products can be relied upon.

Some people have advocated the use of oral tobacco as a harm reduction strategy. Evidence does suggest that people who have only used smokeless tobacco have a lower risk of disease compared to cigarette smokers (Foulds, Ramstrom, Burke, & Fagerstrom, 2003). However, relatively few people in the United States switch from cigarettes to smokeless tobacco, and dual use of smokeless tobacco and cigarettes is not known to reduce health risk. Cigarette smokers who delay quitting smoking by using smokeless tobacco when they cannot smoke might actually be increasing their disease risk (Henningfield, Rose, & Giovino, 2002). Moreover, combining smoking and smokeless tobacco use has the potential to increase risk over smoking alone. There is no proven method for switching smokers to exclusive use of smokeless tobacco. Switching to cigars (or even pipes) similarly is not guaranteed to lower risk, as cigarette smokers tend to inhale cigars and pipes (Baker et al., 2000).

Because smokers smoke to get nicotine but are harmed by tobacco-related toxins, another strategy is to provide nicotine, without tobacco toxins, via nicotine replacement therapy (NRT) products. There is good evidence for the safety of nicotine gum over periods as long as 5 years (Murray et al., 1996). Some evidence suggests that use of NRT products can help smokers reduce smoking and reduce toxic exposures (Etter, Laszlo, Zellweger, Perrot, & Perneger, 2002); however, this is not a well-established treatment. It is not clear how NRT might optimally be used for harm reduction, considering that the magnitude of effects is not known and long-term studies are unavailable.

Perhaps more important than any technical considerations of harm reduction strategies are conceptual considerations about the goal of treatment. The benefits of permanent abstinence from smoking and tobacco are well-known and certain (USDHHS, 1990). The possible benefits of THR strategies are speculative. In these circumstances, it is sensible to do everything to encourage complete abstinence, and do nothing to undermine it. This complicates the offer of harm reduction strategies, because it raises the question of whether offering reduction as an option might undermine smokers' interests in cessation (evidence to the contrary is discussed later). On the other hand, when cessation is not an option, and persistent smoking appears to be the only alternative, harm reduction options—especially sustained reductions in smoking—make sense. Fortunately, the clinician working with an individual smoker faces a simpler task than the tobacco control policymaker. The policymaker must be concerned about the broad implication of policy across populations, and must consider the effect of communication across diverse groups of smokers. In contrast, the clinician is primarily concerned with the well-being of the particular smoker in front of him or her, about whom the clinician has a good deal of information. Clinicians can target their advice to a particular smoker without concern about spillover effects and can follow a patient to monitor for unintended consequences.

Accordingly, the clinician confronted with a relapsing smoker who seems to be headed inexorably toward resuming high rates of smoking might reasonably guide the smoker toward harm reduction, promoting reduced tobacco consumption through both behavioral and pharmacological strategies (importantly, this use of pharmacological aids has not been thoroughly tested and is not approved by the Food and Drug Administration). Conversely, though, it would not be appropriate to offer a harm reduction alternative to smokers who are interested in quitting completely, lest they be diverted from what all agree is the best alternative. Finally, a clinician confronted with a smoker who indicates little interest in quitting, but who is willing to attempt smoking reduction may be well advised to engage the smoker in a smoking-reduction program. Several studies suggest that smokers who undertake reduction have an enhanced likelihood of quitting (Carpenter, Hughes, & Keeley, 2003; Hughes, 2000). In a striking study, Carpenter et al. (2003) selected smokers who declined cessation treatment, even when they were offered free NRT, and offered them smoking reduction with NRT. These smokers engaged in at least as much cessation activity as a group that was diligently prompted to quit smoking. Thus, responding to smokers who are not ready to quit by accepting them as they are and engaging them in reduction efforts may ironically be an effective means to encourage cessation. The tobacco control community is now assessing the viability of harm reduction strategies, so the options and outcomes should become clearer in the coming years. For now, attempts at harm reduction are fraught with complexity and risk.

Assessment and Treatment Planning

Over 15 years ago, we observed that clinical assessment instruments related to smoking cessation have prognostic value, yet such information has been of little clinical utility because it has had no obvious implications for treatment decisions (Shiffman, 1988). The state of the science has not changed much, and similar sentiments were expressed more recently by the authors of the U.S. Public Health Service Clinical Practice Guideline (Fiore et al., 2000).

The bottom line is that the available database does not generally support a linkage between treatment approaches and specialized assessment. At the same time, it must be noted that smokers are very heterogeneous and that some effective interventions (e.g., problem solving) implicitly assume treatment tailoring based on systematic assessment of individual patient characteristics (Fiore et al., 2000). Accordingly, although systematic algorithms for treatment matching are not available, the clinician may find it useful to undertake formal assessments to get to know his or her patient better.

In individual treatment, prognostic information may be useful, if only to determine the intensity of treatment that might be appropriate (e.g., giving more attention to high-risk cases). Many variables predict outcome, and a review is beyond the scope of this chapter. A more thorough treatment of assessment is available in Shadel and Shiffman (2005; see also Kassel & Yates, 2002).

The severity of nicotine dependence is an important prognostic indicator. The Fagerstrom Tolerance Questionnaire (FTQ) and Fagerstrom Test for Nicotine Dependence (FTND) (Fagerstrom, 1978; Heatherton, Kozlowski, Frecker, & Fagerstrom, 1991) are the most widely used assessments. A newer scale, the Nicotine Dependence Syndrome Scale (NDSS; Shiffman, Waters, & Hickcox, 2004), provides a more differentiated, multidimensional assessment of dependence. Motivation to quit can be assessed straightforwardly using a single face-valid item.

Other assessments can help identify particular vulnerabilities or deficits that may guide treatment. Deficits in social support can be assessed using measures of either global support (Cohen & Hoberman, 1983), or specific support for smoking cessation (Mermelstein, Lichtenstein, & McIntyre, 1983). Assessing comorbid psychopathology may also be useful. Smoking is particularly linked to depression (Breslau, 1995), and some authors have suggested that smokers with a history of depression are vulnerable to emergent depression (Glassman, Covey, Stetner, & Rivelli, 2001) and to relapse (Covey, Glassman, Stetner, & Becker, 1993). Generally, smokers with comorbid depression should receive treatment (cognitive-behavioral and/or pharmacological) for depression along with treatment for smoking cessation.

Self-efficacy for smoking cessation is a robust predictor of outcome, and smokers with low efficacy warrant efficacy-boosting interventions. Situationally based efficacy ratings can also help identify situations in which the smoker may be at high risk for lapsing, and thus help guide treatment. Smokers should be vigilant for and try to avoid such situations, and should work on developing coping strategies to cope with temptations in those situations. The Relapse Situation Self-Efficacy Questionnaire (Gwaltney et al., 2001) is designed to capture such situational variance, and has been shown to predict the situations in which smokers first lapse (Gwaltney et al., 2002). The smoker's coping repertoire may be assessed with coping checklists or interviews. It is essential to cover all three kinds of coping (Shiffman, 1988): (1) *anticipatory coping* (in which the patient anticipates and plans for an encounter with a high-risk situation, for example, a party at which others are smoking); (2) *immediate coping*, which is synonymous with temptation coping, and refers to coping with an urge or craving to smoke; and (3) *restorative coping*, which reflects the ability of the patient to cope with a smoking lapse. The Coping with Temptation Inventory (Shiffman, 1988) can be used for this purpose. In sum, assessment of situational risk and coping can have direct implications for tailored interventions and RP planning.

COMORBID PERSONALITY AND PSYCHOPATHOLOGY

Although there is evidence that personality factors are associated with smoking, such associations are relatively weak, and have no evident implications for treatment. However, smoking and nicotine dependence demonstrate comorbidity with a variety of psychopathological conditions (Hughes, Hatsukami, Mitchell, & Dahlgren, 1986). Comorbid psychopathology represents an important issue to address in nicotine dependence research because these individuals report excessive dependence levels and extreme difficulty quitting (Hughes et al., 1986; McChargue, Gulliver, & Hitsman, 2002a, 2002b). The treatment implications are unclear, but clinicians should consider concomitant treatment of psychiatric conditions.

Many smokers report that they smoke in order to manage negative affect. However, the evidence that smoking is in fact associated with negative affect is mixed (e.g., see Kassel, Stroud, & Paronis, 2003; Shiffman, Gwaltney, et al., 2002), and the evidence that smoking or nicotine actually ameliorates negative affect is even weaker (Kassel et al., 2003). Accordingly, smokers should be advised to challenge their beliefs in the relaxing powers of smoking. Those who demonstrate deficits in appropriate coping with affective distress may need some focus on affect management (see "Pre-Quit Interventions" section for discussion of challenging smoking expectancies).

TREATMENT COMPONENTS AND INTERVENTION STRATEGIES

Proximal Interventions

The RP model emphasizes the importance of specific high-risk situations in the relapse process. The theoretical model (Marlatt & Gordon, 1985), partially validated by empirical research (Shiffman, 1982; Shiffman, Paty, et al., 1996), suggests that lapses to smoking are likely to occur in particular situational contexts, such as under stress and negative affect, when alcohol is consumed, when other smokers are present, and so on. However, even when these situational cues are encountered, smoking is not inevitable; smokers can sometimes forestall a lapse by performing appropriate coping. This account implies that avoiding exposure to such high-risk situations, minimizing their impact, and successfully coping with them are keys to RP. This conceptualization has profoundly influenced the development of nicotine dependence interventions: Nearly every nonpharmacological cessation treatment includes a component where smokers identify high risk for relapse situations and develop or improve coping skills needed to negotiate these situations without smoking. (These components of treatment will be called "skills training" here.) Indeed, based on meta-analyses of the treatment outcome literature (Irvin et al., 1999; Stead, Lancaster, & Perera, 2003), federal and expert treatment guidelines recommend the inclusion of skills training in nicotine dependence interventions (e.g., Abrams et al., 2003; Fiore et al., 2000).

In this section, we review the steps involved in skills training. A recent treatment handbook carefully describes the skills training component of RP (Abrams et al., 2003); the reader is referred to that manual for greater detail. In addition to reviewing the "how to" of skills training, relevant empirical research addressing skills training appearing since the 1985 publication of *Relapse Prevention* is discussed. Cue exposure therapy, another influential proximal intervention, is also be reviewed.

Identification of High-Risk Situations

The initial step in skills training involves identifying situations that may pose challenges to maintaining abstinence—high-risk situations or relapse crises. These situations may involve combinations of affect states (including cigarette craving), activities (e.g., alcohol consumption), and environmental contexts (e.g., others smoking). Several methods are available to identify high-risk situations: (1) smokers may simply be asked to identify high-risk situations in an open-ended format; (2) smokers may identify situations or motives associated with *ad lib.* smoking prior to the quit attempt using questionnaires or self-monitoring strategies[1]; or (3) smokers, using a self-efficacy questionnaire or related instrument, may identify contexts in which they have low confidence in their ability to abstain. In addition, treatment facilitators should emphasize certain situations that have documented relationships with lapsing, including negative affect, intense craving, alcohol consumption, and being around other smokers or other smoking cues (Shiffman, 1982; Shiffman, Gnys et al., 1996; Shiffman, Paty, Gnys, Kassel, & Richards, 1996).

Lapses tend to occur soon after initial cessation (Brandon, Herzog, & Webb, 1990; Garvey et al., 1992; Shiffman, Paty, et al., 1996). Therefore, identification of high-risk situations (and related coping strategies, discussed later) should begin before the target quit date and continue beyond it (Brown, 2003). Further, smokers should identify as many high-risk situations as possible.

Coping Skills Training

The balance between the excitatory "pull" of the high-risk situation (e.g., cigarette craving) and the inhibitory effects of coping will determine the outcome of a relapse crisis. Therefore, development of effective coping responses is at the core of RP. Communicating the importance of coping to smokers in treatment not only will serve as the beginning of coping skills training, but also can foster a sense of control in the client: He or she is not at the mercy of withdrawal and craving—there are tools that can be used to successfully maintain abstinence.

As noted earlier, the first step in coping skills training requires an assessment of the smoker's existing coping repertoire. This assessment can be accomplished via open-ended questions, comprehensive measures, such as the Coping with Temptation Inventory (Niaura & Shadel, 2003), or even simulated high-risk situations (Abrams et al., 1987; Drobes, Meier, & Tiffany, 1994; Shiffman, Read, Maltese, Rapkin, & Jarvik, 1985). These assessments can therefore identify strengths and weaknesses in the smoker's coping repertoire.

Coping strategies can be either cognitive or behavioral in nature. Rather than reprint a comprehensive inventory of coping responses that can be found elsewhere (e.g., Niaura & Shadel, 2003; Shiffman, 1988), Table 4.1 provides a listing of self-quitters' nine most frequently used coping strategies in the first 10 days after quitting (O'Connell et al., 1998). In general, self-quitters report using behavioral skills more frequently than cognitive skills. Coping responses used to prevent a lapse can be anticipatory (anticipating and preventing or avoiding high-risk situations) or immediate (coping performed during a high-risk situation). For example, anticipating that one may be tempted by offers of cigarettes at a bar and then avoiding the bar is an example of anticipatory coping, while assertively declining offers to smoke in a bar is an example of immediate coping.

Once coping skill deficits or needs have been identified, skills training is necessary. This training can take many forms, from "brainstorming" and

TABLE 4.1. Coping Skill Categories and Representative Examples

	Examples	Frequency rank
	Behavioral strategies	
Behavioral distraction	• Kept busy with work. • Doodled on the phone instead of smoking.	1
Breathing exercises	• Took three deep breaths. • Pretended to inhale on a cigarette.	2
Food and drink	• Drank a glass of water. • Ate a piece of candy.	3
Oral ingestion	• Chewed gum. • Kept cinnamon toothpicks in mouth.	6
Stimulus control	• Sat in nonsmoking section of restaurant. • Didn't drink coffee in the morning because I always smoke when I drink coffee.	8
Informal exercise	Got up and took a walk down the hall.	9
	Cognitive strategies	
Self-encouragement	• Thought: I can do it. • Visualizing self as nonsmoker.	4
Cognitive distraction	• Thought about what I needed to do for work.	5
Thinking of smoking's negative effects	• Thought: It would be nice for kids to have fresh air. • Thought of cancer.	7

Note. Data from O'Connell et al. (1998).

identifying skills that can be used in high-risk situations to rehearsing these strategies in the treatment clinic, prior to using them in the real world. Early studies (Bliss, Garvey, Heinold, & Hitchcock, 1989; Curry & Marlatt, 1985) suggested that cognitive and behavioral coping strategies may be equally effective and their combination may be ideal (Curry & Marlatt, 1985; Shiffman, 1984). More recent work (Shiffman, Paty, et al., 1996), using improved real-time data collection (Stone & Shiffman, 1994) rather than retrospective self-report, suggests that cognitive coping responses may actually be more efficacious. In this analysis, combining cognitive and behavioral coping did not seem to yield incremental efficacy. This is important, given the previously mentioned finding that self-quitters tend to rely on behavioral coping strategies that may be less effective.

However, the coping data clearly show that the real impact of coping on the outcome of high-risk situations comes from the superiority of coping versus not coping at all. This suggests that the emphasis in treatment should be on learning a few coping responses well, so that they are easily triggered and executed, rather than on developing a large coping repertoire or sophisticated systems for matching a coping response to particular challenges.

There are several other reasons why learning a few coping responses well may be superior to superficially learning many coping responses. Using coping skills requires cognitive effort: Resources are needed to identify the high-risk situation and coping response, and to plan and execute the response. Unfortunately, such cognitive resources may be drained by repeated use (Muraven & Baumeister, 2000). Frequent coping with cigarette craving may exhaust self-regulatory "strength," leaving the individual more vulnerable to relapse (Piasecki, Fiore, McCarthy, & Baker, 2002). Beyond this, cognitive resources can be consumed by drug urges and cravings (Sayette, 1999; Sayette & Hufford, 1994). Therefore, it may be most difficult to use coping skills precisely at the times when they are most needed. By overlearning a few coping responses and making them more "automatic" (e.g., Bargh & Ferguson, 2000), their use may require less self-regulatory effort. Thus, they may be less vulnerable to the influence of craving and self-regulatory fatigue.

Incorporating coping response rehearsal (via role-playing analogues; Shiffman et al., 1985) into RP treatment may also make coping less effortful and more automatic. For example, a smoker could repeatedly practice assertively asking a friend to sit in the no-smoking section of a restaurant (an example of anticipatory coping), with the therapist or a group member playing the part of the smoker's friend. In addition to making the coping response more automatic and less effortful, coping rehearsal may strengthen self-regulatory resources, allowing them to be used more frequently and vigorously (Muraven & Baumeister, 2000).

The Surgeon General's Report (USDHHS, 2000) concludes that coping skill acquisition during treatment predicts cessation outcome (e.g., Zelman, Brandon, Jorenby, & Baker, 1992). Though important, these findings do not directly assess whether coping responses used in high-risk situations prevent lapsing. Other studies comparing coping in lapses and temptations may be more informative. As previously mentioned, Shiffman et al. (1996), using real-time data collection, found that coping was more common in temptations than in lapses. This finding is consistent with other studies comparing lapses and temptations, using retrospective summaries (Baer, Kamarck, Lichtenstein, & Ransom, 1989; Bliss, Garvey, & Ward, 1999). Although coping may be less frequent in lapses, the Shiffman, Paty, et al. (1996) study still suggests that it is relatively common, with coping responses used in 81% of all first lapses (vs. 99% of all temptations). Thus, while coping may frequently defuse high-risk situations, it may also frequently fail.

Basic research on coping and the relationship between coping and urge to smoke or negative affect has not progressed much in the last 15 years. Much is still unknown about coping. Renewed empirical study of coping may lead to improved interventions. In the interim, treatment should ensure that smokers master and automatize a few basic coping strategies that can be reliably enacted when abstinence is threatened.

USE OF "RESCUE" MEDICATION

A new development in proximal interventions to prevent lapses is the potential use of acute pharmacological treatment. Specifically, it appears that use of relatively fast-acting nicotine medications such as nicotine gum or nicotine nasal spray (discussed later) can be helpful in preventing lapses. For example, Shiffman et al. (2003) modeled the intense craving of high-risk situations in the laboratory (by exposing abstinent smokers to a lit cigarette) and showed that chewing nicotine gum could blunt the craving in the course of minutes. Niaura et al. (2003) showed that a faster-acting gum could provide even faster craving relief, and Hurt et al. (1998) showed that nicotine nasal spray also acutely reduced craving. Thus, these medications (and possibly other acute forms of medicine) can be used as a pharmacological coping strategy when smokers are confronted with intense temptations to smoke.

Cue Exposure Therapy

Cue exposure therapy (CET) is based on the premise that cues associated with drug use—especially the sight and smell of the drug—can produce conditioned reactions, and these reactions can predispose the individual to relapse (Niaura et al., 1988). The conditioned reactions include drug craving and physiological activation (e.g., salivation). Social-cognitive variables important in the RP model—outcome expectancies, self-efficacy, coping, and attributions—are also believed to be affected when cues are encountered during a quit attempt. One goal of CET is to extinguish the link between the cues and the conditioned responses, by repeatedly exposing the smoker to smoking cues without following them with actual smoking. Another goal is to have the smoker practice coping skills in the presence of smoking cues. This qualifies as a proximal intervention, because its goal is to reduce craving and positive-outcome expectancies and increase self-efficacy expectancies and coping skills in high-risk situations.

As CET involves exposure to situations likely to promote lapsing, practical considerations arise regarding how to achieve exposure to a range of relevant situations. This has been accomplished *in vivo*, via laboratory analogues (e.g., having a confederate smoke in the presence of the participant) and via imagery (e.g., imagining a fight with a friend where you feel urges to smoke and negative affect; Drobes et al., 1994); more recently, virtual reality has been explored as a vehicle for cue exposure (Kuntze et al., 2001; Lee et al., 2003).

CET, in combination with skills training, reduces relapse to other drugs, most notably alcohol (Rohsenow, Monti, & Abrams, 1995). However, CET has largely failed to live up to its promise with regards to smoking cessation. Niaura et al. (1999) found no incremental benefit of adding CET to other empirically supported treatments (CBT and nicotine gum). This finding is significant because this was a rigorously controlled, carefully implemented trial. Additionally, it comes on the heels of smaller studies with similar disappointing results (reviewed in Niaura et al., 1988). Thus, whereas CET should not be added to RP treatments at this time (see also USDHHS, 2000) it likely warrants further development and exploration.

Distal Interventions

In addition to emphasizing the importance of episodic high-risk situations, the RP model also highlights influences that may set the stage for high-risk situations. Specifically, the RP model suggests that an addict's lifestyle may be dominated by aversive, externally imposed tasks and hassles ("shoulds"), while pleasurable, hedonistic behaviors ("wants") are relatively absent. This lifestyle imbalance, while not proximally causing a challenge to abstinence, is posited to increase the smoker's "relapse proneness" (Shiffman, 1988). The RP model recommends balancing the addict's lifestyle by increasing the ratio of "wants" to "shoulds." This balancing can involve the substitution of positive "addictions," such as exercise, prayer, or meditation. The RP model also suggests that accessing and utilizing support from one's social network can buffer the stress-inducing effects of daily hassles, further decreasing the probability of relapse. In this section, studies addressing lifestyle modification interventions for smoking cessation are reviewed. Because most empirical research has addressed social support and exercise interventions, we focus on these techniques.

Other important aspects of RP treatment may need to take place before initial cessation occurs, in order to increase the likelihood of initial cessation and decrease the probability of experiencing high-risk situations. These components, loosely grouped together here as "pre-quit interventions," include motivational enhancement, stimulus control, expectancy challenge, and cigarette/nicotine fading procedures.

Social Support Interventions

Two levels of social support have been conceptualized in the empirical and clinical literature. Global social support refers to the availability of others for social contact, activities, and help and the availability of others to supportively listen to one's troubles (Cohen & Hoberman, 1983). These functions have no specific relationship to smoking. Specific support for smoking cessation refers to the involvement of others in emotionally or concretely supporting one's efforts to quit smoking. In our review, we emphasize smoking cessation support, both because the evidence for beneficial effects of such support is fairly strong and also because clinicians are more likely to be able to intervene in this specific form of support.

Social support is hypothesized to increase motivation to quit smoking, provide positive reinforcement for achieving and maintaining abstinence (Abrams et al., 2003), and buffer the effects of stressors (Brown, 2003; Cohen, 1988). Enlisting social support in RP treatment can be accomplished in several ways. One method involves actually bringing a partner or "buddy" (someone who will quit smoking at the same time and provide support and encouragement; e.g., Janis & Hoffman, 1971) into treatment with the smoker (e.g., Gruder et al., 1993; McIntyre-Kingsolver, Lichtenstein, & Mermelstein, 1986). In treatment, identification of situations where support is needed and methods for requesting and accessing this support can be reviewed and practiced. Helpful partner behaviors can also be identified and practiced. Alternatively, the smoker in treatment can perform similar activities (recognition of situations requiring support and methods for accessing support) in the absence of the partner (Brown, 2003). Finally, as treatments move toward being more portable and easily disseminated, self-help guidelines can include instructions and exercises for eliciting support from partners as well as strategies to be read and implemented by the social support network (Orleans et al., 1991).

Empirical studies have identified behaviors of significant others, particularly behaviors by spouses or other romantic partners, that may facilitate abstinence. "Positive" support behaviors, such as complimenting and reinforcing abstinence, are associated with better outcomes (Coppotelli & Orleans, 1985; Mermelstein et al., 1983), whereas "negative" support behaviors, such as nagging or shunning, are associated with increased relapse rates (Glasgow, Klesges, & O'Neill, 1986). Further, the frequency of positive and negative support behaviors may not be as predictive as their ratio (Cohen & Lichtenstein, 1990), suggesting that one's general sense of a positive supportive environment may be more important than how often these behaviors are enacted by the spouse or partner. This suggests that smokers should be coached in how to assertively ask for the helpful behaviors, and "buddies" should be trained in delivering them. There is often a risk that support will diminish over time, even though it is still needed. Smokers and buddies must be prompted to maintain positive behaviors for several months.

Despite the endorsement by the U.S. Public Health Service and other expert treatment manuals (Abrams et al., 2003), there is still doubt about the efficacy of social support interventions for smoking cessation. A meta-analysis by the Cochrane Review group suggests that social support interventions failed to increase abstinence rates over control interventions

(Park, Schultz, Tudiver, Campbell, & Becker, 2003). Prior to this, other qualitative reviews reached similar conclusions (Lichtenstein, Glasgow, & Abrams, 1986). This may reflect the difficulty in changing established patterns of interaction between the smoker and their (potential) support persons. Thus, although social support interventions have been officially recommended in U.S. smoking cessation treatment guidelines, their efficacy is still unclear.

Most social support research has addressed social support occurring outside of treatment. However, support occurring within treatment sessions may also be important (Fiore et al., 2000). Recommendations for increasing intratreatment support are presented in Table 4.2 (see also Abrams et al., 2003). Some support may come merely from going through the process with others who are experiencing similar challenges. However, it often requires planning, effort, and modeling from a group leader to ensure a supportive group environment, as well as deliberate interventions at key points during the group to elicit mutual support from the members.

Exercise and Weight Control Interventions

Prescribing exercise as a component of a RP cessation treatment has much intuitive appeal. Exercise can be used as a "positive addiction" that can substitute for smoking. Second, exercise can improve one's mood, protecting the smoker against withdrawal symptoms and episodic mood disturbances (Bock, Marcus, King, Borrelli, & Roberts, 1999; Ussher, Nunziata, Cropley, & West, 2001). Finally, it has been suggested that weight gain, a common occurrence following smoking cessation, or concerns about weight gain may be a risk factor for relapse, particularly among women (Swan, Ward, Carmelli, & Jack, 1993). Exercise may prevent weight gain and, therefore, prevent relapse. Thus, another reason for the appeal of exercise interventions is that they may provide particular benefits to women smokers, who are generally less successful at quitting smoking (Perkins, Donny, & Caggiula, 1999).

Despite the appeal of exercise interventions, there is surprisingly little evidence that exercise prevents relapse. Both quantitative and qualitative reviews of weight control interventions found little evidence supporting the efficacy of exercise interventions (Fiore et al., 2000; Ussher, West, McEwen, Taylor, & Steptoe, 2003). However, two recent studies of interventions designed to enhance exercise (Marcus et al., 1999) and reduce weight concerns (Perkins et al., 2001) in women both yielded positive findings. Thus, interventions designed to address women's concerns about weight gain following smoking cessation, as well as those that incorporate exercise into standard cognitive-behavioral treatments for smoking cessation, show promise in reducing relapse rates.

TABLE 4.2. Common Elements of Intra- and Extratreatment Support Interventions

Supportive treatment component	Examples
	Intratreatment support
Encourage the patient in the quit attempt.	1. Note the effective tobacco dependence treatments that are now available. 2. Note that one-half of all people who have ever smoked have now quit. 3. Communicate belief in the patient's ability to quit.
Communicate caring and concern.	1. Ask how the patient feels about quitting. 2. Directly express concern and willingness to help. 3. Be open to the patient's expression of fears of quitting, difficulties experienced, and ambivalent feelings.
Encourage the patient to talk about the quitting process.	Ask about: 1. Reasons the patient wants to quit. 2. Concerns or worries about quitting. 3. Success the patient has achieved. 4. Difficulties encountered while quitting.
	Extratreatment support
Train the patient in support-solicitation skills.	1. Show videotapes that model support skills. 2. Practice requesting social support from family, friends, and coworkers. 3. Aid the patient in establishing a smoke-free home.
Prompt support seeking.	1. Help the patient identify supportive others. 2. Call the patient to remind him or her to seek support. 3. Inform patients of community resources such as hotlines and helplines.
Clinician arranges outside support.	1. Mail letters to supportive others. 2. Call supportive others. 3. Invite others to cessation sessions. 4. Assign patients to be "buddies" for one another.

Note. From Fiore et al. (2000).

Pharmacological Interventions

Although behavioral treatments have long predominated the smoking cessation field, recent advances in the pharmacotherapy of smoking and nicotine dependence are providing new and effective means of helping the smoker achieve abstinence and prevent relapse (Hughes, Goldstein, Hurt, & Shiffman, 1999). There is no contradiction between behavioral and pharmacological approaches. Indeed, the two work well together, and there is every reason to include pharmacological interventions in behavioral treatment programs. Research (Hughes, 1995) shows that the effects of the two approaches are additive. That is, the combination of the two approaches yields the highest success rates, but each modality is also effective on its own. We provide a brief review of medications, but refer readers to sources such as the USPHS guidelines (Fiore et al., 2000) for a more thorough review of medications.

NICOTINE REPLACEMENT THERAPIES

Perhaps the most dramatic shift in the landscape of smoking cessation treatment over the last 20 years has been the advent and dissemination of nicotine replacement therapies (NRTs). The basic premise governing NRT is that nicotine is the psychoactive constituent of cigarette smoke most responsible for motivating tobacco use (Benowitz, 1999). As such, providing nicotine in pure form should ease the transition to abstinence by lessening the severity of withdrawal symptoms and, hence, enhancing the likelihood of successful cessation. Five NRTs are proven effective (Fiore et al., 2000).

NICOTINE PATCH

The nicotine patch delivers nicotine throughout the day using a passive delivery system. The absorption of nicotine is slow (Jarvis & Sutherland, 1998), resulting in peak levels of nicotine being achieved between 4 to 9 hours after administration (Fant, Henningfield, Shiffman, Strahs, & Reitberg, 2000). The patch is available in either 24-hour or 16-hour doses. One direct comparative study showed that the 24-hour patch can yield better control of morning craving (Shiffman, Elash, et al., 2000), which has been associated with relapse risk (Shiffman, Engberg, et al., 1997). Nicotine patches are available over the counter, without a prescription.

NICOTINE GUM

Nicotine gum is an over-the-counter oral form of NRT that must be self-administered repeatedly throughout the day. Use on a regular schedule is recommended (Ockene, Kristeller, & Donnelly, 1999). Compared to patch, gum is relatively fast-acting, reaching peak blood-nicotine levels within 20–30 minutes (Hatsukami & Lando, 1999). As such, it also lends itself to reactive use to control cravings during high-risk situations (Shiffman et al., 2003). Importantly (and as a rare example of a patient X treatment interaction), evidence shows that 4-mg nicotine gum is more efficacious than 2-mg gum among heavy or highly dependent smokers (e.g., Herrera et al., 1995).

NICOTINE LOZENGE

A nicotine lozenge has recently been introduced and demonstrated to be effective (Shiffman, Dresler, et al., 2002). It is also available in 2- and 4-mg doses, and smokers are allocated to dose based on how soon they smoke their first cigarette of the day (an indicator of dependence). The kinetics of the lozenge resemble those of nicotine gum, but the lozenge delivers somewhat more nicotine at the same nominal dose.

NICOTINE INHALATOR

The nicotine inhalator is a device (prescription-only in the United States, nonprescription in the United Kingdom) that resembles a cigarette holder with a nicotine-containing sponge inside, and delivers volatilized nicotine when the user puffs on it. The nicotine is deposited in the mouth, so the device is not a true inhaler, and its pharmacokinetics resemble those of nicotine gum. Frequent and vigorous puffing is required to achieve substantial nicotine delivery, so robust compliance is called for.

NICOTINE NASAL SPRAY

Nicotine *nasal spray* is another acute NRT form, but is available by prescription only (Fiore et al., 2000). The nasal spray results in the fastest nicotine absorption of current NRT forms, and has been demonstrated to reduce acute craving (Hurt et al., 1998).

NRT COMBINATIONS

Finally, several studies have found that combining patch, which delivers slow steady-state nicotine levels, with an acute delivery form (e.g., gum, spray) can increase success rates (see Sweeney, Fant, Fagerstrom, McGovern, & Henningfield, 2001). This is likely due to the ability to combine effortless steady nicotine dosing to dampen craving and withdrawal, with acute use of "rescue" doses when the user is confronted with intense craving in a high-risk situation. Combinations of NRT are not approved by the Food and Drug Administration, although the literature suggests they are safe and effective (Sweeney et al., 2001).

NON-NICOTINE THERAPIES

Three other prescription medications have been deemed efficacious (Fiore et al., 2000). These include bupropion, nortriptyline, and clonidine. Among these, bupropion, an antidepressant, should be viewed as the first choice (Fiore et al., 2000; Hays et al., 2001), and is the only non-nicotine medication approved by the Food and Drug Administration for use in the treatment of smoking. Nortriptyline (also an antidepressant; Hall et al., 1998) and clonidine both appear somewhat effective, but are considered second-line treatments (due to potential side effects and lack of Food and Drug Administration sanction as smoking cessation aids).

Some evidence suggests that antidepressant medications may be particularly suitable for smokers with a history of depression, who appear more likely to benefit from either bupropion (Hayford et al., 2000) or nortriptyline (Hall et al., 1998). Smokers with weight-gain concerns may find that either bupropion (Chengappa et al., 2001) or nicotine gum (Doherty, Militello, Kinnunen, & Garvey, 1996) delays the onset of weight gain. Otherwise, selection of a particular modality of pharmacological treatment is largely a matter of patient preference.

BEHAVIORAL INTERVENTIONS FOR COMPLIANCE

For medications to be effective for smoking cessation, they have to be used, and used in the proper dose and for the proper interval. Noncompliance and underdosing is often considered to be the biggest factor in the failure of drug therapy. Patient instruction and behavioral treatment have an important role in promoting compliance. This is particularly important for the acute dosing forms of NRT (gum, lozenge, nasal spray, and inhalator), which require repeated dosing for effectiveness. As with any medication, the behavioral burden of repeated self-dosing discourages adequate use. In this case, smokers' beliefs and attitudes present additional barriers to compliance. Most smokers harbor misconceptions about the potential risks of taking nicotine, and are thus reluctant to use the recommended amount. Smokers also prefer to "do it on their own" and thus are ready to discontinue their medications as soon as they believe they have achieved some stability. It is important, therefore, that smokers be given accurate information about the safety of nicotine medications and that there be systematic intervention to promote compliance. This should include self-monitoring of compliance, along with goal setting and incentives for appropriate compliance.

Pre-Quit Interventions

MOTIVATIONAL INTERVIEWING

The decision to quit using any drug is often marked by ambivalence. For this reason, there has been a surge of interest in interventions designed to increase individuals' motivation to change. Perhaps the most influential treatment designed to reduce ambivalence and move people toward change is motivational interviewing (Emmons, 2003; Miller & Rollnick, 2002). Motivational interviewing involves innovations in both style and content. Treatment sessions are nonconfrontational and client-centered, reflecting the intervention's philosophy that the locus of behavior change resides in the patient, not the counselor. The content of motivational interviewing involves developing a discrepancy between where the drug user currently sees him- or herself and where the user would like to be, through providing objective feedback (e.g., carbon monoxide levels) or exploring pros and cons of continuing or quitting smoking. As Emmons (2003) notes, many smokers find that there are more things they dislike about smoking than things they like. Abrams et al. (2003) provide a decisional worksheet that can be used to explore pros and cons. Few studies have addressed the efficacy of motivational interviewing for smoking cessation, but initial results are promising (e.g., Colby et al., 1998).

EXPECTANCY CHALLENGE

Although not necessarily conceptualized as motivation enhancement treatments, expectancy challenge interventions may also increase the likelihood of successful behavior change by debunking beliefs about drug use. Smokers often hold favorable views about the effects of smoking (e.g., negative affect reduction; Copeland, Brandon, & Quinn, 1995) and negative views about the difficulty involved in quitting (Shiffman et al., 1985). Challenging these beliefs may increase both motivation and self-efficacy to maintain abstinence. For example, smokers who viewed a videotape of ill smokers discussing smoking-related illnesses increased their expectancies for negative health effects from smoking and reduced their smoking over a 3-month follow-up period (Copeland & Brandon, 2000). Assessment of smoking expectancies (Copeland et al., 1995) can provide a basis for expectancy challenges. Additionally, Shiffman et al. (1985) presented a list of common "myths" regarding smoking cessation that can be challenged during treatment. For example, if smokers believe that "craving for cigarettes lasts forever," they can be instructed that individual cravings are relatively brief in duration and should decrease in frequency over time, although their intensity may change more slowly.

STIMULUS CONTROL

Stimulus control techniques are a centerpiece of behavioral smoking-cessation interventions. Stimulus control refers to altering or avoiding environmental cues that are conducive to smoking. Thus, as with coping skills training, the initial step in stimulus control involves identifying situations that are associated with smoking. Next, prior to quitting smoking, the individual is instructed to alter these environmental cues. This can involve a number of activities, including (1) changing routines, such that smoking occurs in situations not previously associated with smoking; (2) storing cigarettes in relatively inaccessible places, so that the automatic behavior chain of reaching for and lighting a cigarette is broken; and (3) doing activities, such as eating dinner, in nonsmoking areas. These changes serve to both break conditioned associations between smoking and the environment and provide some experience with using coping skills. Recent studies (e.g., Cinciripini et al., 1995) suggest that stimulus control procedures (specifically uncoupling smoking from usual cues) may enhance cognitive-behavioral smoking-cessation treatments.

CIGARETTE FADING

Cigarette fading involves gradually reducing the frequency of smoking prior to a quit attempt. However, a meta-analysis of studies addressing the efficacy of cigarette fading suggests that it works no better than no treatment at all (Fiore et al., 2000). This failure may be due to the use of unstructured instructions for reduction. Cinciripini and colleagues (1995) have demonstrated that structured reduction, in which the intercigarette interval is very systematically lengthened, yields good clinical results.

Other Distal Interventions

Perhaps the most basic distal intervention is to decrease smoking among individuals in the smoker's social network. For example, Mermelstein, Cohen, Lichtenstein, Baer, and Kamarck (1986) report that having other smokers in one's household or in the social network (e.g., friends, coworkers) increased the probability of relapse 1 year following cessation treatment. Indeed, in a randomized intervention study, Janis and Hoffman (1971) found that pairs of smokers trying to quit who had daily contact smoked significantly fewer cigarettes in the subsequent year than subjects who either had fewer or no contacts with other smokers who were quitting. Reducing the number of smokers in the social environment may be an important, fundamental aspect of RP interventions.

The original RP guidelines suggest that relaxation techniques (e.g., meditation, progressive muscle relaxation) may decrease relapse. Relaxation is proposed to reduce relapse through decreasing stress. However, a recent analysis of stress in the days leading up to a lapse suggested that daily stress levels were in fact unrelated to lapse risk (Shiffman & Waters, 2004). It has also been suggested that deep relaxation might generate a "high" that can substitute for positive drug effects. However, a recent meta-analysis (Fiore et al., 2000) suggests that relaxation and deep breathing interventions do not prevent relapse and may even result in lower abstinence rates than no treatment at all.

Coping with Lapses

The distinction between a lapse (a distinct episode of smoking) and relapse (return to regular smoking) is a central tenet of the RP model. Indeed, this distinction sharply differentiates the RP model from other conceptualizations of addictive disorders, such as 12-step models ("1 drink = drunk"). Studies of the natural history of cessation and relapse have shown that about 85% of lapses lead to relapse (Kenford et al., 1994). According to the RP model, cognitive-emotional reactions to lapses, rather than stable characteristics of the individual (e.g., physiological disease, personality), largely determine whether or not abstinence will be restored. If the lapse is attributed to internal, stable, global, and uncontrollable factors (e.g., willpower) and if smoking violates a strong commitment to abstinence, affect disturbance (e.g., guilt) and decreases in self-efficacy may result. This constellation of responses has been termed the abstinence violation effect (AVE). The AVE is hypothesized to increase the likelihood of subsequent smoking and, ultimately, relapse. In this section, intervention techniques designed to prevent or reduce the AVE are reviewed. Empirical research addressing the AVE is also discussed.

Research has shown that smokers do indeed react to lapses with negative affect, self-blame, and reduced efficacy (Shiffman, Hickox, Paty, Gnys, et al., 1997). Some retrospective research had suggested that more severe AVE reactions were associated with relapse (e.g., Curry, Marlatt, & Gordon, 1987). However, these studies were based on retrospective reports of attributions and emotional responses following a lapse. These reports are particularly prone to autobiographical memory bias (Shiffman, Hufford, et al., 1997), in part based on the subsequent course of events: Relapsers have strong evidence that the causes of their initial lapse were internal, stable, global, and uncontrollable—their subsequent smoking and ultimate relapse confirm this. However, a prospective follow-up of smokers who reported their responses to a first lapse soon after the event found that intensity of AVE reactions (negative affect, loss of efficacy, or attributions) did not predict progression to relapse (Shiffman, Hickcox, et al., 1996). There was some relationship between feeling like giving up and progression (Shiffman, Hickcox, et al., 1996), and decreasing self-efficacy did accompany the downward slide into relapse (Shiffman et al., 2000), providing support for the RP account of the relapse process. Although interventions aspiring to weaken the AVE process may still be worthwhile, these results suggest caution in placing too much confidence in such interventions to restore abstinence following a lapse. Avoidance of lapses is still the mainstay of RP.

Recent treatment manuals (Abrams et al., 2003; see also Brandon, 2000) provide a detailed description of how smokers can be inoculated against experiencing the AVE (called "AVE training" here). Because lapses tend to occur quickly (e.g., Brandon, Tiffany, Obremski, & Baker, 1990; Garvey et al., 1992; Shiffman, Paty, et al., 1996), AVE training should begin either before or soon after initial cessation (Abrams et al., 2003). The first step in AVE training is educational: Smokers are told that (1) although abstinence is the goal, slips may occur; (2) slips are not equal to relapses; (3) if slips occur, one may experience guilt and/or depression; and (4) these feelings may arise from thinking that one is a failure or "has blown it" by smoking (Brown, 2003). In group treatment settings, group members may discuss their own previous reactions to lapses. The second step involves identifying strategies for preventing or minimizing the AVE following a slip. These techniques are listed in Table 4.3. Each of these strategies is an example of "restorative coping" (Shiffman & Wills, 1985). In intensive behavioral treatments (i.e., cessation clinics), it is recommended that AVE principles and coping strategies be reviewed multiple times both before and after the quit attempt (Brown, 2003).

Discussing the AVE in treatment raises a thorny clinical issue: Framing slips as "mistakes" that can be overcome may make slips seem permissible. Thus, the "Don't do it! . . . But if you do . . . " message could be confusing to patients. Brandon (2000) presents an excellent analogy that could prove useful in describing the AVE to patients. In this analogy, the AVE is compared to discussing fire safety with children. Although fire prevention is important, it is clearly beneficial for children to know exit routes from home or school or how to use a fire extinguisher should a fire occur. Having this knowledge about what to do in case of fire in no way indicates that it is permissible for children to play with matches; they still need to prevent fire at all costs. Having a cigarette after quitting is like playing with fire— one must know what to do once the fire starts.

AVE training is commonly a component of RP treatments evaluated in empirical studies. Although this attests to its appeal, it complicates assessment of its efficacy, because its effect is often confounded with the effects of other treatment strategies incorporated in multicomponent treatments. Only one study, to our knowledge, has addressed the unique contribution of AVE training (Supnick & Colletti, 1984). In this study, participants were randomly assigned to receive AVE training or an absolute abstinence message (where participants were taught that one slip invariably does lead to relapse). Surprisingly, individuals who received AVE training actually smoked significantly *more* cigarettes in the 6-month follow-up period than did individuals given an absolute abstinence message. Although this counterintuitive finding could be due to methodological limitations (e.g., many participants never achieved initial abstinence, making AVE training irrelevant), it also may reflect the difficulty of discussing how to deal with a lapse without apparently giving permission to lapse.

Even if AVE counseling does not have an effect in slowing the progression from a lapse to a relapse, helping smokers deal with their slips and relapses can help prompt cessation in the long term. Many smokers have to quit several times before succeeding. This makes it important to inoculate them against demoralization following a "failure," so that they are better able to bounce back and make another quit attempt. One study looked at the influence of attributions and cognitive-emotional reactions to quit failures (failing to achieve even a day of abstinence) on subsequent quit attempts (recycling; Spanier, Shiffman, Maurer, Reynolds, & Quick, 1996).

TABLE 4.3. Suggestions for Preventing and Coping with the Abstinence Violation Effect (AVE)

Brown (2003)

- "Think of the slip as a mistake rather than as evidence that you are weak or are a failure."
- "Respond to the slip as you would to other mistakes (i.e., use it as a learning experience, figure out what you did wrong and how to correct it or avoid doing it next time)."
- "Realize that one cigarette does not mean that you are a smoker unless you allow it to."
- "Redouble your coping efforts, reminding yourself of all the successful, hard work you have put in so far."
- "Do not smoke the next cigarette and realize that the depressed, guilty, angry feelings will decrease with each passing hour and day of abstinence."

Brandon (2000)

- "Put it out and get rid of any cigarettes."
- "Think of that cigarette as a 'slip,' and not a 'relapse.' It does not have to mean that all is lost."
- "Even though you may be upset with yourself, do not 'beat yourself up.' "
- "Use behavioral and mental coping strategies right away. Renew your commitment to quitting, leave the situation, call a friend?. . . . "
- "Make that cigarette your last. Do not put off quitting again until tomorrow, next week, or next year. The sooner you commit yourself to quitting again, the easier it will be, because your body will not yet have readjusted itself to nicotine."
- "Learn from your slip. What led up to your smoking? You now know this is a high-risk situation that will need better preparation the next time."

Attributing the failure to quit to stable causes and reporting lower self-efficacy after the failed attempt were associated with a decreased likelihood of making a subsequent quit attempt.

If AVE training is included in RP treatments, it seems prudent to strongly encourage complete abstinence from smoking. Brandon's (2000) self-help materials may serve as a useful guide for implementing such a strategy. In addition to guidelines for coping with cognitive and emotional AVE responses, these recommendations also emphasize immediate behavioral strategies (throwing away all cigarettes) for regaining abstinence, and they encourage immediate commitment to become a nonsmoker again. The message should be loud and clear: "DON'T SMOKE AGAIN."

Pharmacotherapy and Lapses

There is some evidence that pharmacotherapies for smoking cessation may dampen the progression from lapse to relapse. For example, long-term bupropion use (vs. placebo) improves point-prevalence abstinence rates more robustly and consistently than continuous abstinence rates (Hays et al., 2001). This suggests that some bupropion users lapsed and then returned to abstinence. Further, one study showed that nicotine patches slowed progression from lapse to relapse (Shiffman et al., 2003). Therefore, an additional aspect of AVE training may involve encouraging patients to continue using their medications even after lapsing. Smokers in RP treatment should be told that they should continue using medications even after lapses, but if they return to regular smoking and no longer wish to quit, obviously these medications should be discontinued.

The apparently inexorable progression from limited lapses to relapse is one of the greatest challenges in clinical treatment of smoking and other addictions. No interventions have yet proven very potent in avoiding this progression, which reinforces the importance of preventing lapses in the first place.

TREATMENT MODALITY AND FORMAT ISSUES

We have thus far addressed the *content* of treatment, and framed delivery of treatment in the context of a traditional face-to-face encounter between a clinician and a client or group of clients. However, face-to-face treatment poses significant barriers to widespread use of treatment. Face-to-face treatment is expensive and is largely rejected by smokers, with the result that very, very few smokers receive treatment this way. As a result, behavioral treatment has had minimal *impact*. Impact has been defined as the number of ex-smokers produced, which is a function of *efficacy* (the percentage who succeed) times *reach* (the number of smokers who undertake treatment; Shiffman, Mason, & Henningfield, 1998). The need to increase treatment impact has driven the development of novel *channels* for delivering treatment content to a greater number and greater variety of people. These have generally entailed using technology to deliver treatment without face-to-face contact.

Telephone Counseling

Telephone counseling for smokers has received wide acceptance over the past 20 years. Such counseling has the potential to supplement face to face support, or to substitute for in-person contact. Telephone counseling can take one of two forms (Lichtenstein, Glasgow, Lando, Ossip-Klein, & Boles, 1996). Reactive counseling is provided via telephone "hotlines" (e.g., Shiffman et al., 1985; Zhu, Anderson, Johnson, Tedeschi, & Roeseler, 2000) that offer counseling to those who want it on demand. In proactive counseling, the counselor initiates contact in order to provide support in making a quit attempt or avoiding relapse.

Based on an analysis of 27 trials, the Cochrane Review Group (Stead et al., 2003) recently reported that proactive counseling can be effective compared to an intervention without personal contact. Successful interventions typically involved multiple contacts timed around a quit attempt. The content of treatment in proactive telephone counseling often closely resembles that of traditional face-to-face treatment. Telephone hotlines aim to "be there" for the smoker when he or she is facing an immediate crisis or high-risk situation, and have been in use for more than 20 years (Shiffman, 1982). Evidence suggests they are effective (Ossip-Klein & McIntosh, 2003). However, smokers fail to make much use of hotlines when they are made available, which suggests the advantage of a proactive approach to telephone counseling.

Self-Help Materials

Self-help programs for smoking cessation are often embodied in reading materials that can be widely disseminated. Such written materials, therefore, have several clear advantages: They can embody the content of empirically validated behavioral programs; they can be disseminated to areas in which therapist-led interventions are unavailable; they are relatively inexpensive; and they allow the smoker to seek help in the privacy of his or her own home. In addition to written materials, self-help interventions may also include use of videotapes and, more recently, the Internet (see next section). Unfortunately, systematic reviews of the literature (Lancaster & Stead, 2003) show that typical self-help materials had only modest efficacy.

One exception to this gloomy conclusion has been the data on tailored materials. Whereas typical print materials are "one-size-fits-all," computer technology increasingly allows for materials to be customized based on the intended user's characteristics and needs. Two studies have demonstrated the efficacy of tailored print materials as adjuncts to pharmacological therapy (Shiffman et al., 2000; Shiffman, Paty, Rohay, Di Marino, & Gitchel, 2001). Other studies suggest that tailored cessation materials are superior to untailored materials (Strecher, Wang, Derry, Wildenhaus, & Johnson, 2002). Well-designed tailored materials may mimic a therapist's skill in selecting interventions that are most relevant or appropriate for a particular client.

Another exception has been the success of a set of RP materials developed and tested by Brandon and colleagues (Brandon, Collins, Juliano, & Lazev, 2000; Brandon et al., 2003). A novel aspect of Brandon et al.'s work is that they focused specifically on RP, rather than initial quitting. They offered self-help materials on RP to smokers who had already quit, some for a year or more. Mailing of eight RP booklets was demonstrated to be effective, particularly for those abstinent for 3 months or less. A subsequent study showed that it was the treatment content, and not the repeated mail contact, that influenced outcome. This suggests that well-designed (and tested) treatment materials can have a clinical impact and specifically shows that a focus on RP can help smokers who have already achieved abstinence.

Internet Approaches

The Internet provides new opportunities for making material readily available (e.g., via a website), for reaching out proactively to smokers (e.g., via e-mail), and for implementing tailoring (because the content is naturally computer-driven). As Internet use and access has increased, the Internet is becoming a viable medium for treatment delivery. Several authors (Etter, le Houezec, & Landfeldt, 2003; Feil, Noell, Lichtenstein, Boles, & McKay, 2003; Lenert et al., 2003) have described creative use of Internet resources to offer smoking cessation treatment. While initial findings are encouraging, thorough and robust assessments of specific programs are still lacking. However, a randomized trial of a web-based tailored behavioral program, offered as a supplement to nicotine patch use, has demonstrated efficacy, when compared to a control condition using nicotine patch plus untailored web material (Strecher et al., 2003). This suggests that we may be on the cusp of a new era in sophisticated treatment tailoring and delivery via the Internet.

Stepped-Care Models

Although we have discussed different treatment modalities in isolation, there is a compelling argument for integrating different modalities and intensities of treatment into a systematic treatment system. The stepped-care model draws upon specialized assessment and then matches patients to interventions that vary in their intensity (see Abrams et al., 1996; Monti, Niaura, & Abrams, 2003). Thus, the underlying philosophy governing this approach is to target the largest number of smokers possible and offer the most easily disseminated treatment. If a less intensive treatment proves ineffective, the smoker would be "stepped-up" to the next level of intervention intensity. Of course, critical to the stepped-care approach is the algorithm used to guide treatment matching. As a hypothetical example, Abrams et al. (1996) proposed the following algorithm: Smokers with low nicotine dependence, no comorbidity, and no past treatment failures would be assigned to a minimal care, self-help intervention. Those with high dependence and no comorbidity would receive moderate care, including brief professional treatment, nicotine replacement, skills training and support, and follow-up visits. Finally, the most intensive intervention would be for those smokers with high dependence and comorbid disorders. Such individuals would receive maximal specialized care in either an outpatient or inpatient clinic. Although the stepped-care approach is intuitively appealing, to date it has received little empirical substantiation (Smith et al., 2001).

CONCLUSIONS

In sum, the smoking cessation landscape has changed dramatically over the last 20 years, shaped, in no small part, by the influential RP model. As discussed throughout this chapter, many components integral to state-of-the-art cognitive-behavioral interventions for smoking cessation derive from the RP approach to the treatment of addictive disorders. Concurrently, effective pharmacological treatments have been developed, and these can be used in ways that are consistent with the RP approach. At the same time, treatment success rates continue to be modest, and appear to be declining (Irvin et al., 1999). There has been relatively little innovation in behavioral treatment (Shiffman, 1993), and many challenges remain. Continued innovation, development, and research is essential to address RP for smokers. Their lives depend on it.

AUTHOR NOTES

Saul Shiffman consults to GlaxoSmithKline exclusively on matters related to smoking cessation. He also has an interest in a new smoking cessation product, and is a cofounder of invivodata, inc., which markets electronic diaries for clinical trials.

NOTE

1. The validity of retrospective measures designed to capture smoking motives and cues has been challenged (Shiffman, 1993). See the second edition of *Assessment of Addictive Behaviors* (Donovan & Marlatt, 2005) for a more thorough discussion of this issue.

REFERENCES

Abrams, D. B., Monti, P. M., Pinto, R., Elder, J. P., Brown, R. A., & Jacobus, S. I. (1987). Psychosocial stress and coping in smokers who relapse or quit. *Health Psychology, 6,* 289–304.

Abrams, D. B., Niaura, R., Brown, R. A., Emmons, K. M., Goldstein, M. G., & Monti, P. M. (2003). *The tobacco dependence treatment handbook: A guide to best practices.* New York: Guilford Press.

Abrams, D. B., Orleans, C. T., Niaura, R., Goldstein, M., Prochaska, J., & Velicer, W. (1996). Integrating individual and public health perspectives for treatment of tobacco dependence under managed health care: A combined stepped-care and matching model. *Annals of Behavioral Medicine, 18,* 290–304.

Baer, J. S., Kamarck, T., Lichtenstein, E., & Ransom, C. C. (1989). Prediction of smoking relapse: Analyses of temptations and transgressions after initial cessation. *Journal of Consulting and Clinical Psychology, 57,* 623–627.

Baker, F., Ainsworth, S. R., Dye, J. T., Crammer, C., Thun, M. J., Hoffman, D., et al.

(2000). Health risks associated with cigar smoking. *Journal of the American Medical Association, 284,* 735–740.

Bargh, J. A., & Ferguson, M. J. (2000). Beyond behaviorism: On the automaticity of higher mental processes. *Psychological Bulletin, 126,* 925–945.

Benowitz, N. L. (1999). Nicotine addiction. *Primary Care, 26,* 611–631.

Bliss, R. E., Garvey, A. J., Heinold, J. W., & Hitchcock, J. L. (1989). The influence of situation and coping on relapse crisis outcomes after smoking cessation. *Journal of Consulting and Clinical Psychology, 57*(3), 443–449.

Bliss, R. E., Garvey, A. J., & Ward, K. D. (1999). Resisting temptations to smoke: Results from within-subjects analyses. *Psychology of Addictive Behaviors, 13,* 143–151.

Bock, B. C., Marcus, B. H., King, T. K., Borrelli, B., & Roberts, M. R. (1999). Exercise effects on withdrawal and mood among women attempting smoking cessation. *Addictive Behaviors, 24*(3), 399–410.

Brandon, T. H. (2000). *Forever free.* Tampa, FL: H. Lee Moffitt Cancer Center and Research Institute, University of South Florida.

Brandon, T. H., Collins, B. N., Juliano, L. M., & Lazev, A. B. (2000). Preventing relapse among former smokers: A comparison of minimal interventions through telephone and mail. *Journal of Consulting and Clinical Psychology, 68,* 103–113.

Brandon, T. H., Herzog, T. A., & Webb, M. S. (2003). It ain't over till it's over: The case for offering relapse-prevention interventions to former smokers. *American Journal of Medical Sciences, 326,* 197–200.

Brandon, T. H., Tiffany, S. T., Obremski, K. M., & Baker, T. B. (1990). Postcessation cigarette use: The process of relapse. *Addictive Behaviors, 15,* 105–114.

Breslau, N. (1995). Psychiatric comorbidity of smoking and nicotine dependence. *Behavior Genetics, 25,* 95–101.

Brown, R. A. (2003). Intensive behavioral treatment. In *The tobacco dependence treatment handbook: A guide to best practices* (pp. 118–177). New York: Guilford Press.

Burns, D. M. (2004, February). Estimating the benefits of reducing exposure to smoke as a harm reduction strategy. In S. Shiffman (Chair), *Can nicotine replacement products be used for harm reduction?* Symposium presented at the annual meeting of the Society for Research on Nicotine and Tobacco, Scottsdale, AZ.

Carpenter, M. J., Hughes, J. R., & Keely, J. P. (2003). Effect of smoking reduction on later cessation: A pilot experimental study. *Nicotine and Tobacco Research, 5,* 155–162.

Centers for Disease Control and Prevention. (1997). Cigarette smoking among adults—United States, 1995. *Morbidity and Mortality Weekly Report, 46,* 1217–1230.

Chengappa, K. N., Kambhampati, R. K., Perkins, K., Nigam, R., Anderson, T., Brar, J. S., et al. (2001). Bupropion sustained release as a smoking cessation treatment in remitted depressed patients maintained on treatment with selective serotonin reuptake inhibitor antidepressants. *Journal of Clinical Psychiatry, 62,* 503–508.

Cinciripini, P. M., Lapitsky, L., Seay, S., Wallfisch, A., Kitchens, K., & Van Vunakis, H. (1995). The effects of smoking schedules on cessation outcome: Can we improve on common methods of gradual and abrupt nicotine withdrawal? *Journal of Consulting and Clinical Psychology, 63*(3), 388–399.

Cohen, S. (1988). Psychosocial models of the role of social support in the etiology of physical disease. *Health Psychology, 7*(3), 269–297.

Cohen, S., & Hoberman, H. (1983). Positive events and social supports as buffers of life change stress. *Journal of Applied Social Psychology, 13*, 99–125.

Cohen, S., & Lichtenstein, E. (1990). Partner behaviors that support quitting smoking. *Journal of Consulting and Clinical Psychology, 58*(3), 304–309.

Cohen, S., Lichtenstein, E., Prochaska, J. O., Rossi, J. S., Gritz, E. R., Carr, C. R., et al. (1989). Debunking myths about self-quitting: Evidence from 10 prospective studies of persons who attempt to quit smoking by themselves. *American Psychologist, 44*, 1355–1365.

Colby, S. M., Monti, P. M., Barnett, N. P., Rohsenow, D. J., Weissman, K., Spirito, A., et al. (1998). Brief motivational interviewing in a hospital setting for adolescent smoking: A preliminary study. *Journal of Consulting and Clinical Psychology, 66*(3), 574–578.

Copeland, A. L., & Brandon, T. H. (2000). Testing the causal role of expectancies in smoking motivation and behavior. *Addictive Behaviors, 25*(3), 445–449.

Copeland, A. L., Brandon, T. H., & Quinn, E. P. (1995). The Smoking Consequences Questionnaire—Adult: Measurement of smoking outcome expectancies of experienced smokers. *Psychological Assessment, 7*, 484–494.

Coppotelli, H. C., & Orleans, C. T. (1985). Partner support and other determinants of smoking cessation maintenance among women. *Journal of Consulting and Clinical Psychology, 53*(4), 455–460.

Covey, L. S., Glassman, A. H., Stetner, F., & Becker, J. (1993). Effect of history of alcoholism or major depression on smoking cessation. *American Journal of Psychiatry, 150*, 1546–1547.

Curry, S. G., & Marlatt, G. A. (1985). Unaided quitters' strategies for coping with temptations to smoke. In S. Shiffman & T. A. Wills (Eds.), *Coping and substance abuse* (pp. 243–266). Orlando, FL: Academic Press.

Curry, S., Marlatt, G. A., & Gordon, J. R. (1987). Abstinence violation effect: Validation of an attributional construct with smoking cessation. *Journal of Consulting and Clinical Psychology, 55*(2), 145–149.

Doherty, K., Militello, F. S., Kinnunen, T., & Garvey, A. J. (1996). Nicotine gum dose and weight gain after smoking cessation. *Journal of Consulting and Clinical Psychology, 64*, 799–807.

Donovan, D. M., & Marlatt, G. A. (Eds.). (2005). *Assessment of addictive behaviors* (2nd ed.). New York: Guilford Press.

Drobes, D. J., Meier, E. A., & Tiffany, S. T. (1994). Assessment of the effects of urges and negative affect on smokers' coping skills. *Behavior Research Therapy, 32*(1), 165–174.

Emmons, K. M. (2003). Increasing motivation to stop smoking. In *The tobacco dependence treatment handbook: A guide to best practices* (pp. 73–100). New York: Guilford Press.

Etter, J. F., Laszlo, E., Zellweger, J. P., Perrot, C., & Perneger, T. V. (2002). Nicotine replacement to reduce cigarette consumption in smokers who are unwilling to quit: A randomized trial. *Journal of Clinical Psychopharmacology, 22*, 487–495.

Etter, J. F., le Houezec, J., & Landfeldt, B. (2003). Impact of messages on concomitant use of nicotine replacement therapy and cigarettes: A randomized trial on the Internet. *Addiction, 98*, 941–950.

Fagerstrom, K. O. (1978). Measuring degree of physical dependence to tobacco smoking with reference to individualization of treatment. *Addictive Behaviors, 3*, 235–241.

Fagerstrom, K. O., Hughes, J. R., Rasmussen, T., & Callas, P. W. (2000). Randomized trial investigating effect of a novel nicotine delivery service (Eclipse) and a nicotine oral inhaler on smoking behaviour, nicotine and carbon monoxide exposure, and motivation to quit. *Tobacco Control, 9*, 327–333.

Fant, R. V., Henningfield, J. E., Shiffman, S., Strahs, K. R., & Reitberg, D. P. (2000). A pharmacokinetic crossover study to compare the absorption characteristics of three transdermal nicotine patches. *Pharmacology, Biochemistry and Behavior, 67*, 479–482.

Feil, E. G., Noell, J., Lichtenstein, E., Boles, S. M., & McKay, H. G. (2003). Evaluation of an Internet-based smoking cessation program: Lessons learned from a pilot study. *Nicotine and Tobacco Research, 5*, 189–194.

Fiore, M. C., Bailey, W. C., Cohen, S. J., Dorfman, S. F., Gritz, E. R., Heyman, R. B., et al. (2000). *Treating tobacco use and dependence: Clinical practice guideline.* Rockville, MD: U.S. Department of Health and Human Services, Public Health Service.

Foulds, J., Ramstrom, L., Burke, M., & Fagerstrom, K. (2003). Effect of smokeless tobacco (snus) on smoking and public health in Sweden. *Tobaco Control, 12*, 349–359.

Garvey, A. J., Bliss, R. E., Hitchcock, J. L., Heinold, J. W., & Rosner, B. (1992). Predictors of smoking relapse among self-quitters: A report from the normative aging study. *Addictive Behaviors, 17*, 367–377.

Glasgow, R. E., Klesges, R. C., & O'Neill, H. K. (1986). Programming social support for smoking modification: An extension and replication. *Addictive Behaviors, 11*(4), 453–457.

Glassman, A. H., Covey, L. S., Stetner, F., & Rivelli, S. (2001). Smoking cessation and course of major depression: A follow-up study. *Lancet, 357*, 1929–1932.

Gruder, C. L., Mermelstein, R. J., Kirkendol, S., Hedeker, D., Wong, S. C., Schreckengost, J., et al. (1993). Effects of social support and relapse prevention training as adjuncts to a televised smoking-cessation intervention. *Journal of Consulting and Clinical Psychology, 61*(1), 113–120.

Gwaltney, C. J., Shiffman, S., Norman, G. J., Paty, J. A., Kassel, J. D., Gnys, M., et al. (2001). Does smoking abstinence self-efficacy vary across situations? Identifying context-specificity within the Relapse Situation Efficacy questionnaire. *Journal of Consulting and Clinical Psychology, 69*, 516–527.

Gwaltney, C. J., Shiffman, S., Paty, J. A., Liu, K. S., Kassel, J. D., Gnys, M., et al. (2002). Using self-efficacy judgments to predict characteristics of lapses to smoking. *Journal of Consulting and Clinical Psychology, 70*, 1140–1149.

Hall, S. M., Reus, V. I., Munoz, R. F., Sees, I. L., Humfleet, G., Hartz, D. T., et al. (1998). Nortriptyline and cognitive-behavioral therapy in the treatment of cigarette smoking. *Archives of General Psychiatry, 55*, 692–693.

Hatsukami, D. K., & Lando, H. (1999). Smoking cessation. In P. J. Ott, R. E. Tarter & R. T. Ammerman (Eds.), *Sourcebook on substance abuse: Etiology, epidemiology, assessment, and treatment* (pp. 399–415). Boston: Allyn & Bacon.

Hayford, K. E., Patten, C. A., Rummans, T. A., Schroeder, D. R., Offord, K. P., Croghan, I. T., et al. (2000). Efficacy of bupropion for smoking cessation in smokers with a former history of major depression or alcoholism. *British Journal of Psychiatry, 177*, 87–88.

Hays, J. T., Hurt, R. D., Rigotti, N. A., Niaura, R., Gonzales, D., Durcan, M. J., et al. (2001). Sustained-release bupropion for pharmacologic relapse prevention after smoking cessation. A randomized, controlled trial. *Annals of Internal Medicine, 135*, 423–433.

Heatherton, T. F., Kozlowski, L. T., Frecker, R. C., & Fagerstrom, K. O. (1991). The Fagerstrom Test for Nicotine Dependence: A revision of the Fagerstrom Tolerance Questionnaire. *British Journal of Addiction, 86*, 1119–1127.

Henningfield, J. E., Rose, C. A., & Giovino, G. A. (2002). Brave new world of tobacco disease prevention: Promoting dual product use? *American Journal of Preventive Medicine, 23*, 226–228.

Herrera, N., Franco, R., Herrera, L., Partidas, A., Rolando, R., & Fagerstrom, K. O. (1995). Nicotine gum, 2 and 4 mg, for nicotine dependence. A double-blind placebo-controlled trial within a behavior modification support program. *Chest, 108*, 447–451.

Hughes, J. R. (1995). Combining behavioral therapy and pharmacotherapy for smoking cessation: An update. *NIDA Research Monograph, 150*, 92–109.

Hughes, J. R. (2000). Reduced smoking: An introduction and review of the evidence. *Addiction, 95*(Suppl. 1), S3–S7.

Hughes, J. R., Goldstein, M. G., Hurt, R. D., & Shiffman, S. (1999). Recent advances in the pharmacotherapy of smoking. *Journal of the American Medical Association, 282*, 72–76.

Hughes, J. R., Gulliver, S. B., Fenwick, J. W., Valliere, W. A., Cruser, K., Pepper, S., et al. (1992). Smoking cessation among self-quitters. *Health Psychology, 11*, 331–334.

Hughes, J. R., Hatsukami, D. K., Mitchell, J. E., & Dahlgren, L. A. (1986). Prevalence of smoking among psychiatric outpatients. *America Journal of Psychiatry, 143*, 993–997.

Hurt, R. D., Croghan, G. A., Wolter, T. D., Croghan, I. T., Offord, K. P., Williams, G. M., et al. (2000). Does smoking reduction result in reduction of biomarkers associated with harm? A pilot study using a nicotine inhaler. *Nicotine and Tobacco Research, 2*, 327–336.

Hurt, R. D., Offord, K. P., Croghan, I. T., Croghan, G. A., Gomez-Dahl, L. C., Wolter, T. D., et al. (1998). Temporal effects of nicotine nasal spray and gum on nicotine withdrawal symptoms. *Psychopharmacology, 140*, 98–104.

Irvin, J. E., Bowers, C. A., Dunn, M. E., & Wang, M. C. (1999). Efficacy of relapse prevention: A meta-analytic review. *Journal of Consulting and Clinical Psychology, 67*, 563–570.

Janis, I. L., & Hoffman, D. (1971). Facilitating effects of daily contact between partners who make a decision to cut down on smoking. *Journal of Personality and Social Psychology, 17*(1), 25–35.

Jarvis, M., & Sutherland, G. (1998). Tobacco smoking. In D. W. Johnston & M. Johnston (Eds.), *Comprehensive clinical psychology* (pp. 645–674). New York: Elsevier Science.

Kassel, J. D., Stroud, L. R., & Paronis, C. A. (2003). Smoking, stress, and negative affect: Correlation, causation, and context across stages of smoking. *Psychological Bulletin, 129,* 270–304.

Kassel, J. D., & Yates, M. (2002). Is there a role for assessment in smoking cessation treatment? *Behaviour Research and Therapy, 40,* 1457–1470.

Kenford, S. L., Fiore, M. C., Jorenby, D. E., Smith, S. S., Wetter, D., & Baker, T. B. (1994). Predicting smoking cessation: Who will quit with and without the nicotine patch. *Journal of the American Medical Association, 271*(8), 589–594.

Kozlowski, L. T., Sweeney, C. T., & Pillitteri, J. L. (1996). Blocking cigarette filter vents with lips more than doubles carbon monoxide intake from ultra-low tar cigarettes. *Experimental and Clinical Psychopharmacology, 4,* 404–408.

Kuntze, M. F., Stoermer, R., Mager, R., Roessler, A., Mueller-Spahn, F., & Bullinger, A. H. (2001). Immersive virtual environments in cue exposure. *CyberPsychology and Behavior, 4,* 497–501.

Lancaster, T., & Stead, L. F. (2003). Self-help interventions for smoking cessation (Cochrane Review). In *The Cochrane library* (Issue 3). Oxford, UK: Update Software.

Lee, J. H., Lim, Y., Graham, S. J., Kim, G., Wiederhold, B. K., Wiederhold, M. D., et al. (2003). Experimental application of virtual reality for nicotine craving through cue exposure. *CyberPsychology and Behavior, 6,* 275–280.

Lenert, L., Munoz, R. F., Stoddard, J., Delucchi, K., Bansod, A., Skoczen, S., et al. (2003). Design and pilot evaluation of an Internet smoking cessation program. *Journal of the American Medical Informatics Association, 10,* 16–20.

Lichtenstein, E., Glasgow, R. E., & Abrams, D. B. (1986). Social support in smoking cessation: In search of effective interventions. *Behavior Therapy, 17,* 607–619.

Lichtenstein, E., Glasgow, R. E., Lando, H. A., Ossip-Klein, D. J., & Boles, S. M. (1996). Telephone counseling for smoking cessation—Rationales and metaanalytic review of evidence. *Health Education Research, 11,* 243–257.

Marcus, B. H., Albrecht, A. E., King, T. K., Parisi, A. F., Pinto, B. M., Roberts, M., et al. (1999). The efficacy of exercise as an aid for smoking cessation in women: A randomized controlled trial. *Archives of Internal Medicine, 159*(11), 1229–1234.

Marlatt, G. A., & Gordon, J. R. (Eds.). (1985). *Relapse prevention* (1st ed.). New York: Guilford Press.

McChargue, D. E., Gulliver, S. B., & Hitsman, B. (2002a). A reply to the commentaries on schizophrenia and smoking treatment: More research is needed. *Addiction, 97,* 785–793.

McChargue, D. E., Gulliver, S. B., & Hitsman, B. (2002b). Would smokers with schizophrenia benefit from a more flexible approach to smoking treatment? *Addiction, 97*(799–800).

McIntyre-Kingsolver, K., Lichtenstein, E., & Mermelstein, R. J. (1986). Spouse training in a multicomponent smoking-cessation program. *Behavior Therapy, 17,* 67–74.

Mermelstein, R., Cohen, S., Lichtenstein, E., Baer, J. S., & Kamarck, T. (1986). Social support and smoking cessation and maintenance. *Journal of Consulting and Clinical Psychology, 54,* 447–453.

Mermelstein, R., Lichtenstein, E., & McIntyre, K. (1983). Partner support and relapse in smoking-cessation programs. *Journal of Consulting and Clinical Psychology, 51,* 465–466.

Miller, W. R., & Rollnick, S. (2002). *Motivational interviewing: Preparing people for change* (2nd ed.). New York: Guilford Press.

Monti, P. M., Niaura, R., & Abrams, D. B. (2003). Ongoing research and future directions. In *The tobacco dependence treatment handbook: A guide to best practices* (pp. 277–295). New York: Guilford Press.

Muraven, M., & Baumeister, R. F. (2000). Self-regulation and depletion of limited resources: Does self-control resemble a muscle? *Psychological Bulletin, 126*(2), 247–259.

Murray, R. P., Bailey, W. C., Daniels, K., Bjornson, W. M., Kurnow, K., Connett, J. E., et al. (1996). Safety of nicotine polacrilex gum used by 3,094 participants in the Lung Health Study. *Chest, 109*, 438–445.

Niaura, R., Abrams, D. B., Shadel, W. G., Rohsenow, D. J., Monti, P. M., & Sirota, A. D. (1999). Cue exposure treatment for smoking relapse prevention: A controlled clinical trial. *Addiction, 94*(5), 685–695.

Niaura, R. S., Rohsenow, D. J., Binkoff, J. A., Monti, P. M., Pedraza, M., & Abrams, D. B. (1988). Relevance of cue reactivity to understanding alcohol and smoking relapse. *Journal of Abnormal Psychology, 97*(2), 133–152.

Niaura, R., Sayette, M., Shiffman, S., Nides, M., Shelanski, M., Shadel, W., Robbins, B., & Sorentino, J. (2003, February). *Comparative efficacy of rapid-release nicotine gum vs. Nicorette(r) in relieving smoking cue-provoked craving.* Paper presented at the annual meeting of the Society for Research on Nicotine and Tobacco, New Orleans, LA.

Niaura, R., & Shadel, W. G. (2003). Assessment to Inform Smoking Cessation Treatment. In *The tobacco dependence treatment handbook: A guide to best practices* (pp. 27–72). New York: Guilford Press.

Ockene, J. K., Kristeller, J. L., & Donnelly, G. (Eds.). (1999). *The American Psychiatric Press textbook of substance abuse treatment* (2nd ed). Washington, DC: American Psychiatric Association.

O'Connell, K. A., Gerkovich, M. M., Cook, M. R., Shiffman, S., Hickcox, M., & Kakolewski, K. E. (1998). Coping in real time: Using Ecological Momentary Assessment techniques to assess coping with the urge to smoke. *Research in Nursing and Health, 21*(6), 487–497.

Orleans, C. T., Schoenbach, V. J., Wagner, E. H., Quade, D., Salmon, M. A., Pearson, D. C., et al. (1991). Self-help quit smoking interventions: effects of self-help materials, social support instructions, and telephone counseling. *Journal of Consulting and Clinical Psychology, 59*(3), 439–448.

Ossip-Klein, D. J., & McIntosh, S. (2003). Quitlines in North America: Evidence base and applications. *American Journal of Medical Sciences, 326*, 201–205.

Park, E. W., Schultz, J. K., Tudiver, F., Campbell, T., & Becker, L. (2003). Enhancing partner support to improve smoking cessation (Cochrane Review). In *The Cochrane library* (Issue 3). Oxford, UK: Update Software.

Pauly, J. L., Cummings, K. M., & Streck, R. J. (2000). More about safe cigarette alternatives? Industry critics say "not yet." *Journal of the National Cancer Institute, 92*, 660.

Pauly, J. L., Lee, J. H., Hurley, E. L., Cummings, K. M., Lesses, J. D., & Streck, R. J. (1998). Glass fiber contamination of cigarette filters: An additional health risk to the smoker? *Cancer Epidemiology, Biomarkers and Prevention, 7*, 967–979.

Perkins, K. A., Donny, E., & Caggiula, A. R. (1999). Sex differences in nicotine effects and self-administration: Review of human and animal evidence. *Nicotine and Tobacco Research, 1,* 301–315.

Perkins, K. A., Marcus, M. D., Levine, M. D., D'Amico, D., Miller, A., Broge, M., et al. (2001). Cognitive-behavioral therapy to reduce weight concerns improves smoking cessation outcome in weight-concerned women. *Journal of Consulting and Clinical Psychology, 69*(4), 604–613.

Piasecki, T. M., Fiore, M. C., McCarthy, D. E., & Baker, T. B. (2002). Have we lost our way? The need for dynamic formulations of smoking relapse proneness. *Addiction, 97*(9), 1093–1108.

Pickworth, W. B., Fant, R. V., Nelson, R. A., & Henningfield, J. E. (1998). Effects of cigarette smoking through a partially occluded filter. *Pharmacology, Biochemistry and Behavior, 60,* 817–821.

Rohsenow, D. J., Monti, P. M., & Abrams, D. B. (1995). Cue exposure treatment in alcohol dependence. In D. C. Drummond, S. T. Tiffany, S. Glautier, & B. Remington (Eds.), *Addictive behaviour: Cue exposure theory and practice* (pp. 169–196). Oxford, UK: Wiley.

Sayette, M. A. (1999). Cognitive theory and research. In K. E. Leonard & H. T. Blane (Eds.), *Psychological theories of drinking and alcoholism* (2nd ed., pp. 247–291). New York: Guilford Press.

Sayette, M. A., & Hufford, M. R. (1994). Effects of cue exposure and deprivation on cognitive resources in smokers. *Journal of Abnormal Psychology, 103*(4), 812–818.

Shadel, W. G., & Shiffman, S. (2005). Assessment and smoking behavior. In D. M. Donovan & G. A. Marlatt (Eds.), *Assessment of addictive behaviors* (pp. 113–154). New York: Guilford Press.

Shiffman, S. (1982). Relapse following smoking cessation: A situational analysis. *Journal of Consulting and Clinical Psychology, 50,* 71–86.

Shiffman, S. (1984). Coping with temptations to smoke. *Journal of Consulting and Clinical Psychology, 52,* 261–267.

Shiffman, S. (1988). Smoking behavior: Behavioral assessment. In D. M. Donovan & G. A. Marlatt (Eds.), *Assessment of addictive behaviors* (1st ed., pp. 139–188). New York: Guilford Press.

Shiffman, S. (1993). Smoking cessation treatment: Any progress? *Journal of Consulting and Clinical Psychology, 61,* 718–722.

Shiffman S. (1998). Population risks of less deadly cigarettes: Beyond toxicology. In *Report of Canada's Expert Committee on Cigarette Toxicity Reduction* (pp. 1–13). Toronto, Canada: Health Canada.

Shiffman, S., Dresler, C. M., Hajek, P., Gilburt, S. J., Targett, D. A., & Strahs, K. R. (2002). Efficacy of a cotinine lozenge for smoking cessation. *Archives of Internal Medicine, 162,* 1267–1276.

Shiffman, S., Elash, C. A., Paton, S., Gwaltney, C. J., Paty, J. A., Clark, D. B., Liu, K. S., & Di Marino, M. E. (2000). Comparative efficacy of 24-hour and 16-hour transdermal nicotine replacement for relief of morning craving. *Addiction, 95*(8), 1185–1195.

Shiffman, S., Engberg, J. B., Paty, J. A., Perz, W. G., et al. (1997). A day at a time: Predicting smoking lapse from daily urge. *Journal of Abnormal Psychology, 106*(1), 104–116.

Shiffman, S., Gitchell, J. G., Warner, K. E., Slade, J., Henningfield, J. E., & Pinney, J.

M. (2002). Tobacco harm reduction: Conceptual structure and nomenclature for analysis research. *Nicotine and Tobacco Research*, 4(Suppl. 2), S113–S129.

Shiffman, S., Gnys, M., Richards, T. J., Paty, J. A., Hickcox, M., & Kassel, J. D. (1996). Temptations to smoke after quitting: A comparison of lapsers and maintainers. *Health Psychology*, 15(6), 455–461.

Shiffman, S., Gwaltney, C. J., Balabanis, M. H., Liu, K. S., Paty, J. A., Kassel, J. D., Hickcox, M., & Gnys, M. (2002). Immediate antecedents of cigarette smoking: An analysis from ecological momentary assessment. *Journal of Abnormal Psychology*, 111(4), 531–545.

Shiffman, S., Hickcox, M., Paty, J. A., Gnys, M., Kassel, J. D., & Richards, T. J. (1996). Progression from a smoking lapse to relapse: Prediction from abstinence violation effects, nicotine dependence, and lapse characteristics. *Journal of Consulting and Clinical Psychology*, 64(5), 993–1002.

Shiffman, S., Hickcox, M., Paty, J. A., Gnys, M., Kassel, J. D., & Richards, T. J. (1997). The abstinence violation effect following smoking lapses and temptations. *Cognitive Therapy and Research*, 21, 497–523.

Shiffman, S., Hickcox, M., Paty, J. A., Gnys, M., Richards, T., & Kassel, J. D. (1997). Individual differences in the context of smoking lapse episodes. *Addictive Behaviors*, 22, 797–811.

Shiffman, S., Hufford, M., Hickcox, M., Paty, J. A., Gnys, M., & Kassel, J. D. (1997). Remember that? A comparison of real-time versus retrospective recall of smoking lapses. *Journal of Consulting and Clinical Psychology*, 65, 292–300.

Shiffman, S., Mason, K. M., & Henningfield, J. E. (1998). Tobacco dependence treatments: Review and prospects. *Annual Reviews of Public Health*, 19, 335–358.

Shiffman, S., Paty, J. A., Gnys, M., Kassel, J. A., & Hickcox, M. (1996). First lapses to smoking: Within-subjects analysis of real-time reports. *Journal of Consulting and Clinical Psychology*, 64(2), 366–379.

Shiffman, S., Paty, J. A., Rohay, J. M., Di Marino, M. E., & Gitchell, J. (2000). The efficacy of computer-tailored smoking cessation material as a supplement to nicotine polacrilex gum therapy. *Archives of Internal Medicine*, 160, 1675–1681.

Shiffman, S., Paty, J. A., Rohay, J. M., Di Marino, M. E., & Gitchell, J. G. (2001). The efficacy of computer-tailored cessation material as a supplement to nicotine patch therapy. *Drug and Alcohol Dependence*, 64, 35–46.

Shiffman, S., Read, L., Maltese, J., Rapkin, D., & Jarvik, M. E. (1985). Preventing relapse in ex-smokers: A self-management approach. In G. A. Marlatt & J. R. Gordon (Eds.), *Relapse prevention* (1st ed., pp. 472–520). New York: Guilford Press.

Shiffman, S., Shadel, W. G., Niaura, R., Khayrallah, M. A., Jorenby, D. E., Ryan, C. F., et al. (2003). Efficacy of acute administration of nicotine gum in relief of cue-provoked cigarette craving. *Psychopharmacology (Berlin)*, 166(4), 343–350.

Shiffman, S., & Waters, A. J. (2004). Negative affect and smoking lapses: A prospective analysis. *Journal of Consulting and Clinical Psychology*, 72(2), 192–201.

Shiffman, S., Waters, A.J., & Hickcox, M. (2004). The Nicotine Dependence Syndrome Scale: A multi-dimensional measure of nicotine dependence. *Nicotine and Tobacco Research*, 6, 327–348.

Shiffman, S., & Wills, T. A. (Eds.). (1985). *Coping and substance use*. Orlando, FL: Academic Press.

Smith, S. S., Jorenby, D. E., Fiore, M. C., Anderson, J. E., Mielke, M. M., Beach, K. E., et al. (2001). Strike while the iron is hot: Can stepped-care treatments resurrect relapsing smokers? *Journal of Consulting and Clinical Psychology, 69*, 429–439.

Spanier, C. A., Shiffman, S., Maurer, A., Reynolds, W., & Quick, D. (1996). Rebound following failure to quit smoking: The effects of attributions and self-efficacy. *Experimental and Clinical Psychopharmacology, 4*, 191–197.

Stead, L. F., Lancaster, T., & Perera, R. (2003). *Telephone counselling for smoking cessation (Cochrane Review).* In *The Cochrane library* (Vol. 3). Oxford, UK:, Update Software.

Stone, A. A., & Shiffman, S. (1994). Ecological momentary assessment in behavioral medicine. *Annals of Behavioral Medicine, 16*, 199–202.

Stratton, K., Shetty, P., Wallace, R., & Bondurant, S. (Eds.). (2001). *Clearing the smoke: Assessing the science base for tobacco harm reduction.* Washington, DC: National Academy Press.

Strecher, V., Wang, C., Derry, H., Wildenhaus, K., & Johnson, C. (2002). Tailored interventions for multiple risk behaviors. *Health Education Research, 17*, 619–626.

Supnick, J. A., & Colletti, G. (1984). Relapse coping and problem solving training following treatment for smoking. *Addictive Behaviors, 9*(4), 401–404.

Swan, G. E., Ward, M. N., Carmelli, D., & Jack, L. M. (1993). Differential rates of relapse in subgroups of male and female smokers. *Journal of Clinical Epidemiology, 46*, 1041–1053.

Sweeney, C. T., Fant, R. V., Fagerstrom, K. O., McGovern, J. F., & Henningfield, J. E. (2001). Combination nicotine replacement therapy for smoking cessation: Rationale, efficacy and tolerability. *CNS Drugs, 15*, 453–467.

U.S. Department of Health and Human Services. (1990). *The health benefits of smoking cessation: A report of the Surgeon General* (DHHS Publication No. CDC 90-8416). Atlanta: Public Health Service, Centers for Disease Control, National Center for Chronic Disease Prevention and Health Promotion, Office on Smoking and Health.

U.S. Department of Health and Human Services. (1997). *Changes in cigarette related disease risks and their implication for prevention and control* (Smoking and Tobacco Control Monograph No. 8; NIH Publication No. 97-4213). Bethesda, MD: U.S. Public Health Service.

U.S. Department of Health and Human Services. (2000). *Reducing tobacco use: A report of the Surgeon General—Executive Summary.* Atlanta: U.S. Department of Health and Human Services, Centers for Disease Control and Prevention, National Center for Chronic Disease Prevention and Health Promotion, Office on Smoking and Health.

U.S. Department of Health and Human Services. (2001). *Risks associated with smoking cigarettes with low machine-measured yields of tar and nicotine* (Smoking and Tobacco Control Monograph No. 13; NIH Publication No. 02-5047). Bethesda, MD: U.S. Public Health Service.

Ussher, M., Nunziata, P., Cropley, M., & West, R. (2001). Effect of a short bout of exercise on tobacco withdrawal symptoms and desire to smoke. *Psychopharmacology (Berlin), 158*(1), 66–72.

Ussher, M., West, R., McEwen, A., Taylor, A., & Steptoe, A. (2003). Efficacy of exercise counselling as an aid for smoking cessation: A randomized controlled trial. *Addiction, 98*(4), 523–532.

Warner, K. E. (2002). Tobacco harm reduction: Promise and perils. *Nicotine and Tobacco Research*, 4, 61–72.

World Health Organization. (2000). *Partnership to reduce tobacco dependence.* Copenhagen: Author.

World Health Organization. (2001). *WHO evidence based recommendations on the treatment of tobacco dependence.* Copenhagen: Author.

Zelman, D. C., Brandon, T. H., Jorenby, D. E., & Baker, T. B. (1992). Measures of affect and nicotine dependence predict differential response to smoking cessation treatments. *Journal of Consulting and Clinical Psychology*, 60, 943–952.

Zhu, S. H., Anderson, C. M., Johnson, C. E., Tedeschi, G., & Roeseler, A. A. (2000). A centralized telephone service for tobacco cessation: The California experience. *Tobacco Control*, 9(Suppl. 2), 48.

CHAPTER 5

Relapse Prevention
for Stimulant Dependence

Kathleen M. Carroll
Richard A. Rawson

The application of relapse prevention (RP) skill training approaches to stimulant dependence disorders represents a particularly, and perhaps uniquely, fortuitous match of a complex disorder with a theoretical model and treatment approach. RP approaches as a whole are one of very few behavioral therapies that have been consistently demonstrated to be effective in the treatment of stimulant use disorders (including, for the purposes of this chapter, cocaine, amphetamine, and methamphetamine). This achievement is all the more remarkable if one considers the comparative recency of the increase in individuals seeking treatment for stimulant use problems in the United States, compared with those seeking treatment for alcohol, smoking, and opioid use problems. This chapter provides a brief summary of the range of RP approaches that have been applied to stimulant-using populations, reviews the empirical evidence supporting the efficacy of these approaches with stimulant-using populations, and ends by touching on areas that are deserving of more attention by researchers and clinicians interested in this area.

COCAINE, AMPHETAMINE, AND METHAMPHETAMINE: A BRIEF REVIEW

Cocaine and methamphetamine (for simplicity, methamphetamine will be the primary amphetamine discussed, since it currently is the most widely abused drug in this category) are both powerful psychostimulants. They share many similarities in their pharmacology, routes of administration, acute and chronic effects, the pathologies that result from their use, abuse and dependence and the manner in which users should be assessed and treated (Jaffe, Ling, & Rawson, 2004; Jaffe, Rawson, & Ling, 2004).

Cocaine (and "crack," its smokable form) is a derivative of the coca plant and is imported into the United States from Central and South America. Methamphetamine ("crystal," "crank," "speed," or "ice," its smokable form) is primarily a domestically produced compound, manufactured from readily available household ingredients in large volume, West Coast superlabs or in small quantities in personal, amateur, home "labs" located throughout rural and suburban areas of the Western and Midwestern United States. During the 1980s and 1990s, the view of cocaine transformed from being a high-status drug associated with wealthy upper-income users, to an inner-city drug associated with poverty and crime. In contrast, methamphetamine has been the predominant illicit drug used in Hawaii and the Western states of the United States and more recently has migrated into the Midwestern and Southeastern United States, especially in rural areas.

Both drugs can be injected, smoked, snorted, or ingested orally. The intensity and duration of the "rush" that accompanies the use of these stimulants is a result of the release of high levels of dopamine into the brain, and depends, in part, on the method of administration. Specifically, the effect is almost instantaneous when smoked or injected, while it takes approximately 5 minutes after snorting or 20 minutes after oral ingestion. The half-life of cocaine is about 1 hour, giving a short-lived high of 20–30 minutes, while the half-life of methamphetamine is 12 hours, giving a duration of effect ranging from 8 to 24 hours.

The immediate effects produced by the use of cocaine and methamphetamine include euphoria; increased energy; increased blood pressure, body temperature, heart rate, sex drive, and breathing rate; and decreased fatigue and appetite. Negative side effects include tremor, high body temperature, stroke, and cardiac arrhythmia, along with anxiety, insomnia, paranoia, and hallucinations. Prolonged use of cocaine and methamphetamine may result in a tolerance for the drug and increased use at higher dosage levels, which may produce dependence. Chronic use of these stimulants also can produce severe weight loss, fatigue, headaches, powerful craving, and an intense preoccupation with the acquisition and use of the drug, In addition, chronic use produces a sensitization in some areas of the brain, and for some individuals this results in an almost immediate, severe paranoia. Discontinuing use of cocaine and methamphetamine often results in a state of depression, as well as irritability, fatigue, anergia, anhedonia, and some types of cognitive impairment that last anywhere from 2 days to several months.

HETEROGENEITY OF RELAPSE PREVENTION
APPROACHES FOR STIMULANT DEPENDENCE

As has been highlighted elsewhere in this volume, RP approaches in no way represent a unitary approach to treatment. Within the general category of "cognitive-behavioral approaches," RP approaches encompass an extremely broad range of interventions, from those where behavioral principles are used in extinction paradigms for conditioned cravings for drugs (Monti et al., 1993; Rohsenow, Niaura, Childress, Abrams, & Monti, 1990/1991), to short-term focused cognitive-behavioral skills training approaches (Carroll, 1998; Monti, Rohsenow, Michalec, Martin, & Abrams, 1997), to more comprehensive and intensive multimodal broad-spectrum approaches (Azrin et al., 1996; Budney & Higgins, 1998; Rawson et al., 1995). The fundamental assumptions of these approaches include the following (Rotgers, 1996):

- Much of human behavior is largely learned (although etiology does not necessarily dictate treatment).
- The same learning processes that create problem behaviors can be used to change them.
- Behavior is largely determined by contextual and environmental factors.
- Covert behaviors such as thoughts and feelings are subject to change through the application of learning principles.
- Actually engaging in new behaviors in the contexts in which they are to be performed is a critical part of behavior change.
- Each client is unique and must be assessed as an individual in a particular context.
- The cornerstone of adequate treatment is a thorough behavioral assessment.

Major Components of Relapse Prevention Approaches with Stimulant Users

Several RP approaches have been developed and evaluated with stimulant users (Annis & Davis, 1989; Azrin et al., 1996; Carroll, 1998; Marques & Formigoni, 2001; Monti et al., 1997; Rawson et al., 1995). While these vary with respect to breadth, intensity, format, and specific focus, there are a number of essential components they have in common.

Assessment

A thorough behavioral assessment is at the heart of RP with stimulant users, and specific assessment tools and procedures used in the clinical assessment of cocaine and methamphetamine users, are described in the second edition of *Assessment of Addictive Behaviors* (Donovan & Marlatt, 2005). Assessment is typically organized around a functional analysis of the individual's substance use, which is simply an exploration of substance use with respect to its antecedents and consequences. Early in treatment, the functional analysis plays a critical role in helping the client and therapist assess the determinants of the individual's substance use, set goals for treatment, prioritize problems, select the type and sequence of interventions to be used, and monitor progress in meeting treatment goals.

Thus, effective application of RP requires that the patient and therapist have a thorough understanding of the following areas (see Table 5.1):

1. What are the particular determinants of this person's substance use? What is the severity of this person's stimulant use (intensity, quantity/ frequency, and route of administration)? What are his or her individual patterns of use (weekends only, every day, binge use)? What are his or her conditioned cues, or "triggers" for stimulant use? Does this person use by him- or herself or with other people? Where does this person buy and use stimulants? Where does he or she acquire the money to buy drugs? What were the specific events and cognitions leading to this person's most recent episode of use? What circumstances were at play when the stimulant use began or became problematic? How does this person describe the substance and its effects on him or her? What roles, both positive and negative, does cocaine, amphetamines, or methamphetamine use play in this individual's life?

2. In evaluating the environmental context of the individual's substance use, therapists typically cover at least the following general domains:

   a. *Social*: With whom does the individual spend most of his or her time? With whom does he or she use stimulants? Does he or she have relationships with those individuals outside of substance use? Does the individual live with someone who is a substance abuser? How has the patient's social network changed since drug use began or escalated?

   b. *Environmental*: What are the particular environmental "cues" for this patient's stimulant use (e.g., money, alcohol use, particular times of day, particular neighborhoods)? What is the level of this person's day-to-day exposure to these cues? Can some of these cues be easily avoided? Which cues are "fixed" in the individual's environment and hence difficult to change (e.g, living with another substance user)?

   c. *Emotional*: Affect states commonly precede substance use or craving. These include both negative (depression, anxiety, boredom, anger) and positive (excitement, joy) affect states. Because many

TABLE 5.1. Areas for Assessment for Relapse Prevention

The particular determinants of substance use

- Severity of abuse or dependence
- Patterns
- Triggers and cues
- Sources of access to drugs
- Access to money
- Roles stimulant use may play in the person's life

The context of substance use

Social
- With whom does the individual spend most of his or her time?
- With whom does he or she use stimulants?
- Does he or she have relationships with those individuals outside of substance use?
- Does the individual live with someone who is a substance abuser?
- How has the patient's social network changed since drug use began or escalated?

Environmental
- What are the particular environmental "cues" for this patient's stimulant use?
- What is the level of this person's day-to-day exposure to these cues?
- Can some of these cues be easily avoided?
- Which cues are "fixed" in the individual's environment and hence difficult to change (e.g, living with another substance user)?

Emotional
- What are the affect states that precede substance use or craving?

Cognitive
- What are the particular sets of thoughts or cognitions that also frequently precede stimulant use (e.g., "I need to escape," "I can't deal with this unless I'm high," "The hell with it," "I deserve to get high")?

Skills and resources

- What skills or resources does the individual lack and what concurrent problems may be obstacles to becoming abstinent?
- Has this person been able to recognize the need to reduce availability of stimulants?
- Has the patient been able to recognize important conditioned cues?
- Has he or she been able to achieve even brief periods of abstinence?
- Has he or she been able to tolerate periods of craving or emotional distress without resorting to drug use?
- Does he or she recognize the relationship of his or her other substance use (especially alcohol) in maintaining this pattern of stimulant dependence?
- Are there people in the patient's social network who do not use or supply drugs?
- What skills or strengths has the patient demonstrated during any previous periods of abstinence?
- What is his or her coping style? Has he or she been able to maintain a job or positive relationships during substance use?
- What family/social supports and resources may be available to bolster the patient's efforts to become abstinent?
- How does he or she spend time when not using drugs or recovering from their effects?
- What was this person's highest level of functioning before using drugs?
- What brought this person to treatment now?
- How ready is this individual to change problem behavior?

patients initially have difficulty linking particular states to their substance use (or do so, but only at a surface level), affective antecedents of substance use typically are more difficult to identify in the initial stages of treatment.

    d. *Cognitive*: Particular sets of thought or cognitions also frequently precede stimulant use ("I need to escape," "I can't deal with this unless I'm high," "The hell with it," "I deserve to get high"). These cognitions often have a sense of urgency and hence, if unrecognized by the individual, can lead to a chain of behaviors that can result in relapse.

    3. What skills or resources does the individual lack and what concurrent problems may be obstacles to becoming abstinent? Has this person been able to recognize the need to reduce availability of substances? Has the patient been able to recognize important conditioned cues? Has he or she been able to achieve even brief periods of abstinence? Has he or she recognized events that have led to relapse? Has he or she been able to tolerate periods of craving or emotional distress without resorting to drug use? Does he or she recognize the relationship of his or her other substance use (especially alcohol) in maintaining this pattern of stimulant dependence? Are there people in the patient's social network who do not use or supply drugs? Does he or she have a concurrent psychiatric disorder or other problems (e.g., medical, legal, familial, employment) that might confound his or her efforts to change behavior?

    4. What skills and strengths does the individual have? What skills or strengths has the patient demonstrated during any previous periods of abstinence? What is his or her coping style? Has he or she been able to maintain a job or positive relationships during substance use? What family/social supports and resources may be available to bolster the patient's efforts to become abstinent? How does he or she spend time when not using drugs or recovering from their effects? What was this person's highest level of functioning before using drugs? What brought this person to treatment now? How ready is this individual to change problem behavior?

Setting Treatment Goals

As for other substance users, treatment goals in RP with stimulant users are highly individualized, and typically reflect a collaborative process between the client and clinician. Goals of moderation or risk reduction have been more typical of RP approaches for alcohol use disorders than among treatments for stimulant use disorders, in part because of the illicit nature of drug use, as well as the comparative risks and serious morbidities associated with HIV, tuberculosis, hepatitis, and other medical complications of stimulant use.

    Treatment goals should be highly focused and typically depend on the nature of the specific treatment approach. For example, cue exposure and extinction approaches are intended primarily to reduce reactivity to specific cues (e.g., cocaine paraphernalia), and may not generalize to other cues (e.g., affect states), nor affect other substance-related problems (Childress et al., 1993; Modesto-Lowe & Kranzler, 1999; Weiss et al., 2001). The goal of "RP" as applied to many treatment-seeking cocaine abusers has in fact been "abstinence initiation" rather than "RP" (Carroll, 1996), where the primary initial focus is in initiating a stable period of abstinence. Conversely, in broad-spectrum cognitive-behavioral treatments (Azrin et al., 1996; Rawson et al., 1995), the patient and therapist may select a wide range of target behaviors in addition to a treatment goal of abstinence or harm reduction, including improved social skills or social functioning, reduced psychiatric symptoms, and reduced social isolation or entry into the work force.

One example of a broad-spectrum approach is the manualized, 16-week Matrix Model, used as an intensive outpatient approach for the treatment of stimulant users for over 15 years (Rawson et al., 1989, 1995, 2002; Shoptaw et al., 1994). The foundation of the model is based primarily on the cognitive-behavioral principles described in Marlatt and Gordon (1985; Chapter 1, this volume). This treatment approach attempts to (1) teach immediate skills needed to stop drug (and alcohol) use; (2) provide an understanding of factors critical to sustaining abstinence/avoiding relapse; (3) educate family members affected by addiction and recovery; (4) explicitly reinforce and support positive behavior change; (5) familiarize patients with self-help programs; and (6) monitor drug/alcohol use by urine toxicology and breath alcohol testing. The Matrix Model is designed to integrate several interventions into a comprehensive approach. Elements of the program include individual cognitive-behavioral therapy (CBT) sessions, CBT materials presented in a group setting, family education groups, urine testing, and encouragement to participate in self help activities. Content of the treatment program is tailored to individual needs (particularly in the individual session), although basic program elements are structured and manualized.

One aspect of the Matrix Model is that much of the CBT content is delivered within a group setting. The RP groups are led by a nonjudgmental leader who serves as a teacher/coach and who maintains the focus of the group on the CBT content material and how it applies to the current behavior of individual clients (Rawson & Obert, 2002). There is an extensive use of verbal praise from the group leader and peers for positive behavioral change. The focus of the RP prevention group is the dissemination of RP information to group members and their utilization of it, in contrast to focusing on the feelings and emotional expressions of the group members, as is characteristic in traditional substance abuse groups.

The purpose of the RP group is to provide a forum in which people in substance abuse treatment can receive assistance with the issue of relapse. This is accomplished through the use of didactic materials and by applying the CBT principles to group members' immediate challenges in achieving and sustaining abstinence. The specific goals of the RP group are different from the goals of the group therapies used in many traditional inpatient settings. Specific RP group goals are (1) to allow clients to interact with other people with common problems; (2) to provide a forum for the presentation of specific CBT concepts and skills; (3) to promote some group cohesion and allow peer to peer reinforcement among group members; and (4) to alleviate the isolation that many newly abstinent individuals experience as a result of loss of drug-using friends Although there are some issues that require individual attention and are not effectively addressed in these groups (e.g., some relationship conflicts, some aspects of sexual behavior), combining these group sessions with individual sessions appears to be a useful clinical technique.

Structure of Treatment

RP approaches tend to be more highly structured in comparison to other approaches for substance use disorders. That is, these treatment approaches are typically comparatively brief (12–24 weeks) and organized closely around well-specified treatment goals. There is typically an articulated agenda for each session and discussion remains focused around issues directly related to substance use. Progress toward treatment goals is monitored closely and frequently, and the therapist takes an active stance throughout treatment. In broad spectrum cognitive-behavioral approaches, sessions are often organized roughly in thirds (the "20/20/20" rule; Carroll, 1998), with the first third of the session devoted to assessment of substance use and general functioning in the past week, as well as opportunity for the patient to report current concerns and problems; the second third is more didactic and devoted to skills training and practice; and the final third allows time for therapist and patient to plan for the week ahead and discuss how new skills will be implemented. Practice of new skills outside of sessions is generally seen as an integral part of treatment in relapse prevention approaches.

Major Techniques and Intervention

Techniques and interventions used in RP vary with the setting, population, and specific "version" used. There are a variety of manuals and protocols available which describe the techniques associated with each approach (Carroll, 1998; Monti, 1989; Rawson, 1989). For example, cue exposure RP approaches typically begin with a thorough assessment of cues, or stimuli, associated with conditioned craving, and development of a hierarchy of cues. This is followed by repeated exposure to those cues (through actual exposure to or handling of a conditioned cue, videotapes, or imagery) in a laboratory or other controlled setting, which prevents the patient from having access to the substance. The patient's physiological and subjective responses to the stimuli are typically assessed both before and after each exposure session. Extinction of craving associated with a specific stimulus typically takes place in 20 sessions or fewer (Childress et al., 1993).

Broad-spectrum approaches include a range of skills to foster or maintain abstinence. These typically include strategies for (1) reducing availability and exposure to cocaine and related cues (these vary widely across users, including, for example, alcohol, cocaine paraphernalia, and cash), (2) fostering resolution to stop cocaine use through exploring positive and negative consequences of continued use, (3) self-monitoring to identify high-risk situations and to conduct functional analyses of substance use, (4) recognition of conditioned craving and development of strategies for coping with craving, (5) identification of seemingly irrelevant decisions that can culminate in high-risk situations, (6) preparation for emergencies and coping with a relapse to substance use, (7) cocaine refusal skills, and (8) identifying and confronting thoughts about cocaine. Material discussed during sessions is typically supplemented with extrasession tasks (i.e., homework) intended to foster practice and mastery of coping skills. These approaches may also expand to include interventions directed to other problems in the individual's life that are seen as functionally related to substance use. These may include general problem-solving skills, assertiveness training, strategies for coping with negative affect, awareness of anger and anger management, coping with criticism, increasing pleasant activities, enhancing social support networks, job-seeking skills, and so on.

EMPIRICAL SUPPORT FOR RELAPSE PREVENTION WITH STIMULANT USERS

Over the past 10 years, there has been steadily growing and consistent support for RP approaches with stimulant users. Since the body of literature is still comparatively small, we describe many of the recent well-controlled randomized trials and their implications in some detail in the following sections.

Relapse Prevention/Cognitive-Behavioral Therapy and Outpatient Cocaine Abusers

Our group at Yale has been involved in a programmatic series of studies on the effectiveness of CBT, alone and in combination with pharmacotherapy, for the past 15 years. As our understanding of this population and this treatment has deepened over time, this series of studies has been marked by progressively larger effect sizes for CBT over the comparison or control conditions, which suggests that as our experience grows with this approach, we are developing a more potent form of CBT. For example, in our first randomized trial, we conducted a direct comparison of CBT with another active therapy, interpersonal psychotherapy (IPT; Rounsaville, Gawin, & Kleber, 1985), adapted for cocaine users. In that trial, CBT was not found to have a main effect over IPT, but was significantly more effective among the more severely dependent cocaine abusers (Carroll, Rounsaville, & Gawin, 1991).

Severity of cocaine dependence as a moderator of CBT effects was replicated in our next study (Carroll, Rounsaville, Gordon, et al., 1994), which used a 2 × 2 factorial design, and which was also the first to report on increasing effectiveness for CBT at a 1-year follow-up (the "sleeper effect") (Carroll, Rounsaville, Nich, et al., 1994). This in turn led to increasing interest in mechanisms that might underlie this effect, with skills training and behavioral practice through homework assignments as prime candidates.

Thus, in our next study, which was the first to report a significant main effect for CBT over supportive clinical management (Carroll, Nich, Ball, McCance-Katz, & Rounsaville, 1998) and which replicated the "sleeper effect" for CBT over a 1-year follow-up (Carroll, Nich, Ball, et al., 2000), we also evaluated the acquisition of coping skills in CBT and their relationship to outcome in this population. We developed and validated a role-play task for assessing the acquisition of coping skills in CBT (Carroll, Nich, Frankforter, & Bisighini, 1999), and then used it to demonstrate (1) significantly increased coping skills after CBT, (2) differential acquisition of specific behavioral and cognitive coping strategies in CBT with respect to alternate behavioral therapies (12-step facilitation and clinical management), and (3) that greater acquisition of CBT-specific behavioral and cognitive coping skills was associated with significantly less cocaine use over the 1-year follow-up (Carroll, Nich, Ball, et al., 2000).

In our most recently completed trial (Carroll, Fenton, et al., 2004), 121 cocaine-dependent individuals were randomized to one of four conditions in a 2 × 2 factorial design: disulfiram (250 mg/day) plus CBT, disulfiram plus IPT, placebo plus CBT, and placebo plus IPT. Across outcome measures and for the full intention-to-treat sample (as well as across all subsamples, including treatment initiators and treatment completers), patients assigned to CBT reduced their cocaine use significantly more than those assigned to IPT, and patients assigned to disulfiram reduced their cocaine use significantly more than those assigned to placebo. Effects of CBT plus placebo were comparable to those of the CBT–disulfiram combination. This was our first trial to identify a significant main effect for CBT over another active behavioral therapy (IPT). Furthermore, although retention was a significant predictor of better drug use outcomes, the CBT × time effect remained statistically significant after controlling for retention.

Matching Studies

Maude-Griffin and colleagues (1998) randomized 128 cocaine users to either CBT or 12-step facilitation (TSF), a manualized disease model (Nowinski, Baker, & Carroll, 1992) counseling approach, in order to test several a priori matching hypotheses. Treatment was delivered in both group and individual sessions. Results suggested that CBT was more effective than TSF overall. In addition, several matching hypotheses were supported. For example, CBT was differentially effective for individuals with a history of depression, while TSF was more effective for participants with low levels of abstract reasoning skills.

Coping Skills Training/Relapse Prevention as an Adjunct to Inpatient Treatment

Monti and colleagues (1997) evaluated the effectiveness of adding individual sessions of coping skills training to 128 cocaine users who were enrolled in an inpatient program or an intensive partial hospitalization program. Compared with an attention placebo-control condition (manualized meditation relaxation training), CBT was more effective in reducing the frequency of cocaine use and length of relapse episodes (when they occurred) through a 3-month follow-up. A 9-month follow-up study indicated treatment effects on cocaine use were sustained through 6 months; however, differential effects of treatment on alcohol use outcomes and matching effects for gender, severity, sociopathy, or depression were not found.

Relapse Prevention as Continuing Care

McKay and colleagues (1997) evaluated the effectiveness of individualized RP as continuing care following completion of an intensive outpatient program for cocaine dependence. Ninety-eight cocaine-dependent patients were randomly assigned to either standard group counseling or RP. At the end of the 6-month trial, rates of complete abstinence were higher in the standard counseling condition than in RP, but for those who relapsed, the RP condition was associated with less severe relapses, particularly during the earlier months of the intervention. McKay also evaluated a series of matching hypotheses with this group, and found that relapse prevention was associated with better outcomes for those individuals who did not maintain stable abstinence during the initial intensive outpatient program as well as those individuals whose initial treatment goal was total abstinence. The latter effect was sustained through a 2-year follow-up.

Relapse Prevention with Methamphetamine versus Cocaine Users

The literature evaluating the efficacy and effectiveness of RP with stimulant users has been nearly all conducted with cocaine users as the study participants. This is primarily because cocaine use escalated across in the United States during the 1980s, while methamphetamine emerged about a decade later in a much more limited geographic area. The preponderance of data with cocaine users raises the question concerning the generalizability of RP research findings to the treatment of methamphetamine users.

One set of data provides support for the view that the response to RP treatments is quite comparable between cocaine dependent individuals and those dependent upon methamphetamine (Rawson et al., 2000). In a large open trial, 500 methamphetamine users were treated in the same outpatient clinic over the same time period, by the same staff using the identical Matrix treatment protocol, as a group of 224 cocaine users. Although there were very substantial differences in baseline participant characteristics, the treatment response of the two groups was comparable. The mean number of days in treatment, the number and type of treatment sessions attended, the in-treatment urinalysis results and the proportion of participants completing the treatment protocol were virtually identical for both groups. The comparison of the treatment response between these two groups of outpatients suggests that cocaine and methamphetamine users respond in a very similar manner to the Matrix treatment approach.

Matrix Treatment Approach for Methamphetamine Users: A Multisite Trial

One evaluation of a broad-spectrum treatment approach with a methamphetamine-dependent population was conducted within an eight-site, Center for Substance Abuse Treatment (CSAT)-sponsored study assessing the effectiveness of the Matrix treatment protocol versus "treatment as usual" in the eight community treatment organizations (Rawson et al., 2004). In this study, conducted in sites in Montana, Hawaii, and six California locations, 978 methamphetamine-dependent individuals were randomly assigned to outpatient treatment with either the Matrix 16-week protocol, or to the treatment approach that was routinely used by the eight treatment organizations.

The study results provided support for the superior treatment response of methamphetamine users treated with the Matrix approach. These participants were retained significantly longer in treatment, attended more scheduled sessions, and attended a higher percentage of scheduled treatment sessions. Higher proportion of individuals in the Matrix condition completed the scheduled treatment episode. In addition, individuals in the Matrix condition gave more urine samples negative for methamphetamine, and a higher percentage were able to achieve 3 consecutive weeks of abstinence from methamphetamine. Although the differential superiority of the Matrix approach was not reflected by data collected at posttreatment follow-up points, the in-treatment gains made by participants treated with the Matrix approach suggest the treatment approach has positive empirical evidence for treating methamphetamine-dependent individuals when compared to a heterogeneous group of community treatment protocols.

Cognitive-Behavioral Therapy/Relapse Prevention Contrasted and Combined with Contingency Management

A particularly exciting development in the field of treatment of cocaine dependence has been the very strong empirical support for contingency management (CM) approaches, where participants receive incentives (i.e., vouchers redeemable for goods and services, chances to draw prizes from a bowl) contingent on demonstrating acquisition of treatment goals (e.g., submitting drug-free urine specimens, attending treatment sessions) (Higgins et al., 1991, 1994, 2003; Petry & Martin, 2002; Silverman et al., 1996). CM has strong immediate effects on targeted behavior that tend to weaken somewhat when the contingencies are terminated, whereas RP tends to have more modest effects on initial treatment retention and reduction of cocaine use, with its effects strengthening after treatment ends. Therefore, the relative strengths and weaknesses of these approaches, in contrast and combination, are of great interest.

Rawson and colleagues (2002) recently compared group CBT, voucher CM, and a CBT/CM combination in conjunction with standard methadone maintenance treatment for cocaine-using methadone maintenance patients. During the acute phase of treatment, the group assigned to CM had significantly better cocaine use outcomes. However, during the follow-up period, a CBT "sleeper" effect emerged again, where the group assigned to CBT had better outcomes at the 26-week and 52-week follow-up than the CM group (Rawson et al., 2002).

Epstein and colleagues (Epstein, Hawkins, Covi, Umbricht, & Preston, 2003), conducted a similar study, again in the context of intensive methadone maintenance, where participants were offered CM, group CBT, or a combination, in addition to standard individual counseling. Results were largely parallel to the Rawson study in that the investigators reported large initial effects for CM, with drop-off after the termination of the contingencies, and best 1-year outcomes for the CM + CBT combination.

Individual versus Group Cognitive-Behavioral Therapy

Two trials have directly compared the delivery of RP in individual versus group format. Schmitz and colleagues (1997) compared outcomes following 12 sessions of either group or individually delivered RP among 32 cocaine-dependent individuals as aftercare after hospitalization. No significant differences were found in outcome through a 6-month follow-up. Given the small sample size, it should be noted that the groups were also small (three to seven members) and thus may have offered substantial individual attention. In a larger study involving 155 both alcohol- and drug-using individuals (Marques & Formigoni, 2001), Marques and colleagues also found no differences in outcome for group- versus individually-delivered CBT. While preliminary, these studies suggest that CBT/RP can be effectively implemented in either format.

RELAPSE PREVENTION FOR STIMULANT USE: WHERE ARE WE AND WHERE SHOULD WE BE GOING?

Although the burgeoning literature supporting CBT/RP's efficacy as treatment for stimulant dependence is impressive, the field is still comparatively new, and several important issues have not yet received much attention in the literature. For example, there has been comparatively little focus on the optimal dose and intensity of CBT for different types of stimulant users; how CBT can best be combined with medications to enhance outcomes; components of CBT that may be differentially effective (e.g., how best to select from the menu of skills and techniques that comprises CBT), and many others. Next, we consider two issues that we believe are particularly deserving of greater consideration by clinicians and researchers: first, understanding the role of practice of skills and the importance of homework assignments as a means of fostering skill development and implementation, and, second, the need to understand the effect of cognitive functioning and its effect on response to CBT.

Homework and Skills Acquisition as a Possible Mediator of Cognitive-Behavioral Therapy

Understanding the mechanisms of action of CBT and other empirically validated therapies has heretofore received very little attention in the literature (Kraemer, Wilson, Fairburn, & Agras, 2002; Morgenstern & Longabaugh, 2000; Weisz, Hawley, Pilkonis, Woody, & Follette, 2000), but it is an area of great importance. Understanding treatment mechanisms not only can advance the development of more effective treatment strategies, but also result in more powerful, efficient, and ultimately less expensive treatments (Kraemer et al., 2002; Wilson, Fairburn, Agras, Walsh, & Kraemer, 2002).

The converging evidence suggesting that CBT is a particularly durable approach has led to increased focus on its unique or distinctive aspects that might account for its durability; encouraging clients to implement and practice skills outside of sessions via homework assignments is one possible mechanism for this effect. Homework encourages practice of skills outside sessions and possibly generalization of skills to other problems (Beck, Rush, Shaw, & Emery, 1979; Edelman & Chambliss, 1995; Primakoff, Epstein, & Covi, 1986) and emphasis on extrasession practice assignments is a unique feature of CBT (Blagys & Hilsenroth, 2002). Moreover, investigators evaluating CBT in nonsubstance psychiatric disorders have noted the importance of homework in CBT's effectiveness, with some recent work suggesting that homework compliance may have a causal effect on symptom reduction in CBT for depression (Addis & Jacobson, 2000; Burns & Spangler, 2000) and that ratings of the quality of the patient's homework predicts outcome in CBT for panic disorder (Schmidt & Woolaway-Bickel, 2000).

The relationship of homework compliance, skills acquisition, and outcome in CBT has received very little attention in the substance abuse literature. Thus, in a recent trial (Carroll et al., in press), we evaluated homework completion in detail, collecting data on the specific type of homework assigned and how well it was done (e.g., fully, partially, no attempt made) at every session. We found strong relationships between homework compliance and outcome. Compared with the participants assigned to CBT who did not do homework or who did it only rarely, the participants who did homework consistently *stayed in treatment significantly longer, had more consecutive days of cocaine abstinence* (a strong predictor of long-term outcome) (Carroll, Rounsaville, Nich, et al., 1994; Higgins, Wong, Badger, Haug-Ogden, & Dantona, 2000), *and had significantly more days of abstinence and fewer cocaine-positive urines during treatment*. Similar effects were found for the subset of participants who completed treatment in this study, suggesting that the effects of homework compliance on better substance use outcomes were not completely accounted for by differential retention. In addition, we found strong relationships between homework compliance and acquisition of coping skills, as well as between homework completion and participants' ratings of their confidence in avoiding use in a variety of high-risk situations. Participants who completed homework had significant increases over time in their self-reported confidence in handling a variety of high-risk situations, while scores for the subgroup that did not do homework did not change over time.

Farabee, Rawson, and McCann (2002) evaluated the extent to which cocaine users reported engaging in a series of specific drug-avoidance activities (e.g., avoiding drug-using friends and places where cocaine would be available, exercising, using thought-stopping) after CBT versus alternate treatments (e.g., CM and a control condition). They found that, by the end of treatment, participants assigned to CBT reported more frequent engagement in drug-avoidance activities than participants in the comparison treatments. *Furthermore, the frequency of drug-avoidance activities was strongly related to better cocaine use outcomes over the 1-year follow-up.* Taken together, these studies suggest that CBT interventions that foster the patients' engagement in active behavior change may play a key role in CBT's comparative durability and should be pursued in future research.

Neuropsychological Functioning and Cognitive-Behavioral Therapy

Another significant gap in the CBT/RP literature is failure to attend to cognitive functioning in understanding treatment effects and outcomes with drug users (Carroll & Ball, 2005). Given clear evidence of cognitive impairment among chronic cocaine users (Bolla, Funderburk, & Cadet, 2000; DiSclafani, Tolou-Shams, Price, & Fein, 2002; Fals-Stewart & Bates, 2003; Gottschalk, Beauvais, Hart, & Kosten, 2001), this omission is particularly significant, as CBT's emphasis on learning and applying complex, abstract, and often novel concepts and strategies assumes comparatively intact attention, memory, as well as problem-solving, decision-making, and reasoning skills.

To our knowledge, there is only one study linking substance abusers' neuropsychological functioning and outcomes in CBT for stimulant users. Aharmovich and colleagues (Aharonovich, Nunes, & Hasin, 2003) reported that cocaine users with higher levels of neuropsychological impairment were less likely to complete CBT. It is an important but under-investigated question whether specific neuropsychological strengths and deficits may predict response to CBT. There is as yet no data regarding, for example, whether individuals with problems in attention, memory, verbal processing, and executive cognitive control may have difficulty learning and implementing skills taught in CBT.

Conversely, specific skills taught in CBT may also improve some aspects of executive functioning (e.g., attentional bias, decision-making and problem-solving skills, impulse control, response to specific aspects of craving) by either improving cognitive dysfunction itself or by enhancing the individual's ability to skillfully compensate for executive dysfunction. Again, however, there is virtually no data regarding how CBT may improve cognitive functioning in clients who have specific deficits. It is also possible that focused neuropsychological assessments may help detect treatment effects and thus broaden our understanding of how CBT exerts its effects. One implication of this line of research, if fruitful, is that the efficacy of CBT could be enhanced through clinical assessment of patients' cognitive functioning, which would enable the clinician to be aware of the individuals pattern of cognitive strengths and weaknesses, and, where indicated, to modify treatment appropriately (e.g., through repeating material, presenting it in different formats, or by providing cognitive rehabilitative interventions prior to CBT).

CONCLUSIONS

There has been tremendous progress and growth in the application of RP cognitive-behavioral approaches to stimulant-using populations in the past 10 years. Even with a great deal of variability across the various approaches and the specific populations to which they have been applied, empirical support is generally consistent. It is imperative that we, as clinicians and researchers, now build on these approaches to foster the strength, applicability, and generalizability of this very promising group of approaches.

ACKNOWLEDGMENTS

Support was provided by National Institute on Drug Abuse Grant Nos. K05-DA 00457 (to Kathleen M. Carroll) and P50-DA09241, and by the U.S. Department of Veterans Affairs VISN 1 Mental Illness Research, Education, and Clinical Center. Support for the preparation of this chapter was provided by the National Institute on Drug Abuse through the Methamphetamine Clinical Trials Group (N01DA08804) and by the CSAT ATTC Program (UD1TI13594), Pacific Southwest Addiction Technology Transfer Center, and CSAT Methamphetamine Abuse Treatment— Special Studies (270-01-7089).

REFERENCES

Addis, M. E., & Jacobson, N. S. (2000). A closer look at the treatment rationale and homework compliance in cognitive-behavioral therapy for depression. *Cognitive Therapy and Research, 24,* 313–326.

Aharonovich, E., Nunes, E. V., & Hasin, D. (2003). Cognitive impairment, retention and abstinence among cocaine abusers in cognitive-behavioral treatment. *Drug and Alcohol Dependence, 71,* 207–211.

Annis, H. M., & Davis, C. S. (1989). Relapse prevention. In R. K. Hester & W. R. Miller (Eds.), *Handbook of alcoholism treatment approaches* (pp. 170–182). New York: Pergamon Press.

Azrin, N. H., Acierno, R., Kogan, E. S., Donohue, B., Besalel, V. A., & McMahon, P. T. (1996). Follow-up results of supportive versus behavioral therapy for illicit drug use. *Behaviour Research and Therapy, 34,* 41–46.

Beck, A. T., Rush, A. J., Shaw, B. F., & Emery, G. (1979). *Cognitive therapy of depression.* New York: Guilford Press.

Blagys, M. D., & Hilsenroth, M. J. (2002). Distinctive activities of cognitive behavioral therapy: A review of the comparative psychotherapy process literature. *Clinical Psychology Review, 22,* 671–706.

Bolla, K. I., Funderburk, F. R., & Cadet, J. L. (2000). Differential effects of cocaine and cocaine + alcohol on neurocognitive performance. *Neurology, 54,* 2285–2292.

Budney, A. J., & Higgins, S. T. (1998). *A community reinforcement plus vouchers approach: Treating cocaine addiction.* Rockville, MD: National Institute on Drug Abuse.

Burns, D. D., & Spangler, D. L. (2000). Does psychotherapy homework lead to improvements in depression in cognitive-behavioral therapy or does improvement lead to increased homework compliance? *Journal of Consulting and Clinical Psychology, 68,* 46–56.

Carroll, K. M. (1996). Relapse prevention as a psychosocial treatment approach: A review of controlled clinical trials. *Experimental and Clinical Psychopharmacology, 4,* 46–54.

Carroll, K. M. (1998). *A cognitive-behavioral approach: Treating cocaine addiction.* Rockville, MD: National Institute on Drug Abuse.

Carroll, K. M., & Ball, S. A. (2005). Assessment of cocaine abuse and dependence. In D. M. Donovan & G. A. Marlatt (Eds.), *Assessment of addictive behaviors* (2nd ed.). New York: Guilford Press.

Carroll, K. M., Fenton, L. R., Ball, S. A., Nich, C., Frankforter, T. L., Shi, J., et al. (2004). Efficacy of disulfiram and cognitive-behavioral therapy in cocaine-dependent outpatients. *Archives of General Psychiatry, 64,* 264–272.

Carroll, K. M., Nich, C., & Ball, S. A. (in press). Practice makes progress: Homework assignments and outcome in treatment of cocaine dependence. *Journal of Consulting and Clinical Psychology.*

Carroll, K. M., Nich, C., Ball, S. A., McCance-Katz, E. F., Frankforter, T. F., & Rounsaville, B. J. (2000). One year follow-up of disulfiram and psychotherapy for cocaine–alcohol abusers: Sustained effects of treatment. *Addiction, 95,* 1335–1349.

Carroll, K. M., Nich, C., Ball, S. A., McCance-Katz, E., & Rounsaville, B. J. (1998). Treatment of cocaine and alcohol dependence with psychotherapy and disulfiram. *Addiction, 93,* 713–728.

Carroll, K. M., Nich, C., Frankforter, T. L., & Bisighini, R. M. (1999). Do patients change in the way we intend? Treatment-specific skill acquisition in cocaine-dependent patients using the Cocaine Risk Response Test. *Psychological Assessment, 11,* 77–85.

Carroll, K. M., Rounsaville, B. J., & Gawin, F. H. (1991). A comparative trial of psychotherapies for ambulatory cocaine abusers: Relapse prevention and interpersonal psychotherapy. *American Journal of Drug and Alcohol Abuse, 17,* 229–247.

Carroll, K. M., Rounsaville, B. J., Gordon, L. T., Nich, C., Jatlow, P. M., Bisighini, R. M., et al. (1994). Psychotherapy and pharmacotherapy for ambulatory cocaine abusers. *Archives of General Psychiatry, 51,* 177–197.

Carroll, K. M., Rounsaville, B. J., Nich, C., Gordon, L. T., Wirtz, P. W., & Gawin, F. H. (1994). One year follow-up of psychotherapy and pharmacotherapy for cocaine dependence: Delayed emergence of psychotherapy effects. *Archives of General Psychiatry, 51,* 989–997.

Childress, A. R., Hole, A. V., Ehrman, R. N., Robbins, S. J., McLellan, A. T., & O'Brien, C. P. (1993). Cue reactivity and cue reactivity interventions in drug dependence. *National Institute on Drug Abuse Research Monograph Series, 137*, 73–95.

DiSclafani, V., Tolou-Shams, M., Price, L. J., & Fein, G. (2002). Neuropsychological performance of individuals dependent on crack cocaine or crack cocaine and alcohol, at 6 weeks and 6 months of abstinence. *Drug and Alcohol Dependence, 66*, 161–171.

Donovan, D. M., & Marlatt, G. A. (Eds.). (2005). *Assessment of addictive behaviors* (2nd ed.). New York: Guilford Press.

Edelman, R. E., & Chambliss, D. L. (1995). Adherence during sessions and homework in cognitive-behavioral group treatment of social phobia. *Behaviour Research and Therapy, 33*, 573–577.

Epstein, D. E., Hawkins, W. E., Covi, L., Umbricht, A., & Preston, K. L. (2003). Cognitive behavioral therapy plus contingency management for cocaine use: Findings during treatment and across 12-month follow-up. *Psychology of Addictive Behaviors, 17*, 73–82.

Fals-Stewart, W., & Bates, M. E. (2003). The neuropsychological test performance of drug-abusing patients: An examination of latent cognitive abilities and risk factors. *Experimental and Clinical Psychopharmacology, 11*, 34–45.

Farabee, D., Rawson, R. A., & McCann, M. (2002). Adoption of drug avoidance activities among patients in contingency management and cognitive-behavioral treatments. *Journal of Substance Abuse Treatment, 23*, 343–350.

Gottschalk, C. H., Beauvais, J., Hart, R., & Kosten, T. R. (2001). Cognitive function and cerebral perfusion during cocaine abstinence. *American Journal of Psychiatry, 158*, 540–545.

Higgins, S. T., Budney, A. J., Bickel, W. K., Foerg, F. E., Donham, R., & Badger, G. J. (1994). Incentives improve outcome in outpatient behavioral treatment of cocaine dependence. *Archives of General Psychiatry, 51*, 568–576.

Higgins, S. T., Delany, D. D., Budney, A. J., Bickel, W. K., Hughes, J. R., Foerg, F., et al. (1991). A behavioral approach to achieving initial cocaine abstinence. *American Journal of Psychiatry, 148*, 1218–1224.

Higgins, S. T., Sigmon, S. C., Wong, C. J., Heil, S. H., Badger, G. J., Donham, R., et al. (2003). Community reinforcement therapy for cocaine-dependent outpatients. *Archives of General Psychiatry, 60*, 1043–1052.

Higgins, S. T., Wong, C. J., Badger, G. J., Haug-Ogden, D. E., & Dantona, R. L. (2000). Contingent reinforcement increases cocaine abstinence during outpatient treatment and one year follow-up. *Journal of Consulting and Clinical Psychology, 68*, 64–72.

Jaffe, J. A., Ling, W., & Rawson, R. A. (2004). Amphetamine-related disorders. In B. J. Sadock & V. A. Sadock (Eds.), *Kaplan and Sadock's comprehensive textbook of psychiatry* (pp. 1188–1200). Baltimore: Lippincott.

Jaffe, J. A., Rawson, R. A., & Ling, W. L. (2004). Cocaine-related disorders. In B. J. Sadock & V. A. Sadock (Eds.), *Kaplan and Sadock's comprehensive textbook of psychiatry* (pp. 1220–1237). Baltimore: Lippincott.

Kraemer, H. C., Wilson, G. T., Fairburn, C. G., & Agras, W. S. (2002). Mediators and moderators of treatment effects in randomized clinical trials. *Archives of General Psychiatry, 59*, 877–883.

Marlatt, G. A., & Gordon, J. R. (Eds.). (1985). *Relapse prevention: Maintenance strategies in the treatment of addictive behaviors* (1st ed.). New York: Guilford Press.

Marques, A. C., & Formigoni, M. L. (2001). Comparison of individual and group cognitive behavioral therapy for alcohol and/or drug dependent patients. *Addiction, 96,* 835–846.

Maude-Griffin, P. M., Hohenstein, J. M., Humfleet, G. L., Reilly, P. M., Tusel, D. J., & Hall, S. M. (1998). Superior efficacy of cognitive-behavioral therapy for crack cocaine abusers: Main and matching effects. *Journal of Consulting and Clinical Psychology, 66,* 832–837.

McKay, J. R., Alterman, A. I., Cacciola, J. S., Rutherford, M. J., O'Brien, C. P., & Koppenhauer, J. (1997). Group counseling versus individualized relapse prevention aftercare following intensive outpatient treatment for cocaine dependence. *Journal of Consulting and Clinical Psychology, 65,* 778–788.

Modesto-Lowe, V., & Kranzler, H. R. (1999). Using cue reactivity to evaluate medications for treatment of cocaine-dependence: A critical review. *Addiction, 94,* 1639–1651.

Monti, P. M., Abrams, D. B., Kadden, R. M., & Cooney, N. L. (1989). *Treating alcohol dependence: A coping skills training guide.* New York: Guilford Press.

Monti, P. M., Rohsenow, D. J., Michalec, E., Martin, R. A., & Abrams, D. B. (1997). Brief coping skills treatment for cocaine abuse: Substance abuse outcomes at three months. *Addiction, 92,* 1717–1728.

Monti, P. M., Rohsenow, D. J., Rubnis, A. V., Niaura, R. S., Sirota, A. D., Colby, S. M., et al. (1993). Cue exposure with coping skills treatment for male alcoholics: A preliminary investigation. *Journal of Consulting and Clinical Psychology, 61,* 1011–1019.

Morgenstern, J., & Longabaugh, R. (2000). Cognitive-behavioral treatment for alcohol dependence: A review of the evidence for its hypothesized mechanisms of action. *Addiction, 95,* 1475–1490.

Nowinski, J., Baker, S., & Carroll, K. M. (1992). *Twelve-step facilitation therapy manual: A clinical research guide for therapists treating individuals with alcohol abuse and dependence.* Rockville, MD: National Institute on Alcohol Abuse and Alcoholism.

Petry, N. M., & Martin, B. (2002). Low-cost contingency management for treating cocaine- and opioid abusing methadone patients. *Journal of Consulting and Clinical Psychology, 70,* 398–405.

Primakoff, L., Epstein, N., & Covi, L. (1986). Homework compliance: An uncontrolled variable in cognitive therapy outcome research. *Behavior Therapy, 17,* 433–446.

Rawson, R. A., Huber, A., Brethen, P. B., Obert, J. L., Gulati, V., Shoptaw, S., & Ling, W. (2000). Methamphetamine and cocaine users: Differences in characteristics and treatment retention. *Journal of Psychoactive Drugs, 32,* 233–238.

Rawson, R. A., Huber, A., McCann, M. J., Shoptaw, S., Farabee, D., Reiber, C., et al. (2002). A comparison of contingency management and cognitive-behavioral approaches during methadone maintenance for cocaine dependence. *Archives of General Psychiatry, 59,* 817–824.

Rawson, R. A., & the Methamphetamine Treatment Project Corporate Authors.

(2004). A multi-site comparison of psychosocial approaches for the treatment of methamphetamine dependence. *Addiction, 99,* 708–717.

Rawson, R. A., & Obert, J. L. (2002). Relapse prevention groups. In D. W. Brook & H. I. Spitz (Eds.), *Group psychotherapy of substance abuse* (pp. 322–348). Washington, DC: American Psychological Association.

Rawson, R. A., Obert, J. L., McCann, M. J., Smith, D. P., & Scheffey, E. H. (1989). *The neurobehavioral treatment manual.* Beverly Hills, CA: Matrix.

Rawson, R. A., Shoptaw, S. J., Obert, J. L., McCann, M. J., Hasson, A. L., Marinelli Casey, P. J., et al. (1995). An intensive outpatient approach for cocaine abuse treatment: The Matrix Model. *Journal of Substance Abuse Treatment, 12,* 117–127.

Rohsenow, D. J., Niaura, R. S., Childress, A. R., Abrams, D. B., & Monti, P. M. (1990/1991). Cue reactivity in addictive behaviors: Theoretical and treatment implications. *International Journal of the Addictions, 25,* 957–993.

Rotgers, F. (1996). Behavioral theory of substance abuse treatment: Bringing science to bear on practice. In F. Rotgers, D. S. Keller, & J. Morgenstern (Eds.), *Treating substance abusers: Theory and technique* (pp. 174–201). New York: Guilford Press.

Rounsaville, B. J., Gawin, F. H., & Kleber, H. D. (1985). Interpersonal psychotherapy adapted for ambulatory cocaine abusers. *American Journal of Drug and Alcohol Abuse, 11,* 171–191.

Schmidt, N. B., & Woolaway-Bickel, K. (2000). The effects of treatment compliance on outcome in cognitive-behavioral therapy for panic disorder: Quality versus quantity. *Journal of Consulting and Clinical Psychology, 68,* 13–18.

Schmitz, J. M., Oswald, L. M., Jacks, S., Rustin, T., Rhoades, H. M., & Grabowski, J. (1997). Relapse prevention treatment for cocaine dependence: Group versus individual format. *Addictive Behaviors, 22,* 405–418.

Shoptaw, S., Rawnson, R. A., McCann, M. J., & Obert, J. L. (1994). The Matrix Model of Outpatient Stimulant Abuse Treatment: Evidence of efficacy. *Journal of Addictive Diseases, 13*(4), 129–141.

Silverman, K., Higgins, S. T., Brooner, R. K., Montoya, I. D., Cone, E. J., Schuster, C. R., et al. (1996). Sustained cocaine abstinence in methadone maintenance patients through voucher-based reinforcement therapy. *Archives of General Psychiatry, 53,* 409–415.

Weiss, F., Martin-Fardon, R., Ciccocioppo, R., Kerr, T. M., Smith, D. L., & Ben-Sharar, O. (2001). Enduring resistance to extinction of cocaine-seeking behavior induced by drug-related cues. *Neuropsychopharmacology, 25,* 361–372.

Weisz, J. R., Hawley, K. M., Pilkonis, P. A., Woody, S. R., & Follette, W. C. (2000). Stressing the (other) three Rs in the search for empirically supported treatments: Review procedures, research quality, relevance to practice and the public interest. *Clinical Psychology: Science and Practice, 7,* 243–258.

Wilson, G. T., Fairburn, C. G., Agras, W. S., Walsh, B. T., & Kraemer, H. C. (2002). Cognitive-behavioral therapy for bulimia nervosa: Time course and mechanisms of change. *Journal of Consulting and Clinical Psychology, 70,* 267–274.

CHAPTER 6

Relapse Prevention
for Opioid Dependence

Nancy A. Haug
James L. Sorensen
Valerie A. Gruber
Yong S. Song

Heroin is the most widely abused opioid in the United States, with rising prevalence among young adults and affluent communities (National Institute on Drug Abuse, 2000). In 1997, 87% of new heroin users were under age 26 (National Institute on Drug Abuse, 1997). Snorting and smoking heroin are growing in popularity as alternatives to injection; this is likely related to increased purity, misconceptions about its addictive qualities, and fear of AIDS (Substance Abuse and Mental Health Services Administration, 2001). Abuse of narcotic analgesics—natural or synthetic opioids derived for relieving pain (e.g., Darvon, Demerol, Dilaudid, OxyContin, Percodan, and Vicodin)—has also increased dramatically from 1994 to 2002, as indicated by the incidence of emergency department visits (Substance Abuse and Mental Health Services Administration, 2004). In 2002, 20% percent of teens (4.7 million) reported they had used prescription painkillers without a doctor's prescription, and 40% of 12th graders did not see great risk in using heroin once or twice (Johnston, O'Malley, & Bachman, 2002). A recent 33-year longitudinal study of 600 heroin abusers demonstrates high mortality rates and severe negative consequences, such as high levels of health problems, criminal behavior, incarceration, and public assistance associated with long-term heroin use (Hser, Hoffman, Grella, & Anglin, 2001). Other known consequences related to opioid abuse include HIV/AIDS, hepatitis, tuberculosis, and even death from overdose or medical complications. Treatment admission rates for primary heroin abuse have increased in publicly funded substance abuse treatment programs across the country between 1993 and 1999 (Substance Abuse and Mental Health Services Administration, 2002b). The reality is that a majority of opioid abusers relapse after completing or leaving treatment, and many cycle through the drug treatment system for years.

This chapter describes relapse prevention (RP) strategies for opioid dependence, with a focus on both abstinence-based and harm reduction orientations. It will also discuss psychiatric and medical comorbidity, strategies for preventing or dealing with lapse and relapse, the role of coping, and substance-related cues. Motivational interventions are flexibly employed for RP as well as reduction of harmful behaviors. Cognitive-behavioral techniques are utilized to modify thinking and increase coping skills, enabling clients to manage difficult situations. Contingency management uses a voucher-based system where patients earn incentives based on drug abstinence and treatment participation. Other effective treatment approaches for opioid addiction include long-term treatment in residential facilities, therapeutic communities, self-help groups, and outpatient treatment programs. Methadone is the medication used most frequently to treat heroin addiction. Other pharmacological approaches include levo-alpha-acetylmethadol (LAAM), naltrexone, and buprenorphine, a recently approved office-based medical management drug. Alternative therapies such as acupuncture and spiritual interventions are presented as complements for existing treatments. The information provided in this chapter is both clinically and empirically informed to provide practical and comprehensive RP strategies for opioid dependence in a variety of settings.

TREATMENT ISSUES IN OPIOID DEPENDENCE

Goals: Abstinence versus Harm Reduction

Because drug dependence by definition involves drug use that has escalated out of control (American Psychiatric Association, 1994), total separation from the addictive substances is the goal in most drug treatment programs. Abstinence from illicit opioids is associated with improved medical, social, and legal outcomes; relapse to illicit opioid use reverses these benefits. One study reported that opioid-dependent patients who endorsed "never use again" as their heroin abstinence goal demonstrated lower risk of relapse compared to patients with less stringent goals (Wasserman, Weinstein, Havassy, & Hall, 1998). Abstinence from other drugs commonly abused by opioid-dependent individuals has positive outcomes. Moreover, medication adherence is clearly better on abstinent days than days when illicit drugs are used (Rosen, Rigsby, Dieckhaus, & Cramer, 2003). It is very difficult for people to use intoxicating drugs and at the same time take other prescribed medications regularly.

Although drug-free goals are associated with positive outcomes, abstinence as a treatment goal has major limitations. Many individuals seeking drug treatment are ambivalent about stopping their drug use. They cannot imagine giving up drugs, or do not see sufficient benefit of doing so for their particular situation. While providers may have seen many people achieve abstinence and experience the benefits thereof, many opioid users do not believe giving up drugs will really lead to a better life for them. This attitude is reinforced by long histories of trauma and by a peer group who share numerous negative treatment experiences (e.g., real or perceived prejudice) and who often glorify opioids and "the hustle" required to get them (Zweben, 1991).

Despite the benefits of being drug-free, all clients may not be able to commit to a treatment goal of total abstinence. If clients with drug use goals other than abstinence are not alienated or discharged from treatment, services can be made available to a larger proportion of those with treatment needs. In addition, by developing shared treatment goals between client and provider, early dropout can be reduced (Heinssen, Levendusky, & Hunter, 1995). For these reasons, Marlatt, Blume, and Parks (2001) advocated using a harm reduction approach in substance abuse treatment. The harm reduction approach parallels recent innovations in care of chronic medical illness. State-of-the-art medical care for chronic illness acknowledges that patients and their families are the principal caregivers, and therefore need to be collaboratively involved in managing their illness in ways that work for them (Bodenheimer, Wagner, & Grumbach, 2002). Adherence to treatment regimens is better if patients choose their treatment goals based on evaluation of treatment options available to them (Meichenbaum & Turk, 1987).

The harm reduction approach is compatible with the transtheoretical model (DiClemente & Prochaska, 1998) and motivational interventions, which have demonstrated effectiveness with various addictive behaviors including opioid dependence (Saunders, Wilkinson, & Phillips, 1995). This approach fully respects the client, even if he or she chooses to reduce harmful patterns of use and not commit to total abstinence. Harm reduction methods were developed to reduce health and other damages incurred by drug users and their communities. When using a harm reduction orientation, treatment goals can range from administering drugs more safely (harm reduction), changing amount of use (quantity reduction), or cessation of one or more drugs used (prevalence reduction) (MacCoun, 1998). Using drugs in less harmful ways (administration method, setting, associated risk behaviors) has been shown to yield health benefits to individuals and society. For example, needle and syringe exchange programs, and safer use educational campaigns have reduced the spread of HIV and other infectious diseases (Des Jarlais et al., 1996). Thus, harm reduction is inclusive of abstinence as a goal; this factor is sometimes overlooked when harm reduction is contrasted with more traditional abstinence-based approaches. On the other hand, abstinence-based treatment approaches usually do not include harm reduction as a viable treatment goal. In fact, repeated relapse to drugs may be justification for terminating the counseling or treatment process. The Minnesota Model and 12-step facilitation are examples of abstinence-based treatments. In these self-help models, heroin addiction is viewed as a chronic and progressive disease, not caused by other factors, and requiring abstinence. Nonetheless, both abstinence and harm reduction approaches recognize that a slip or lapse can serve as a catalyst to help the client identify the problem.

Comorbidity Considerations

Clinicians will find that a significant proportion of patients who present to treatment for opioid dependence have coexisting psychiatric and medical disorders. Up to 47% of patients in treatment for opioid dependence will meet DSM-IV the diagnostic criteria for coexisting psychiatric conditions of the *Diagnostic and Statistical Manual of Mental Disorders*, fourth edition (DSM-IV; American Psychiatric Association, 1994) (Brooner, King, Kidorf, Schmidt, & Bigelow, 1997) and many patients have significant medical problems (Cherubin & Sapira, 1993). These coexisting conditions, when untreated, may pose substantial barriers to effective treatment outcomes among patients with opioid dependence. Thus, assessment and treatment for these co-occurring conditions should be considered in a comprehensive RP plan for these clients.

Psychiatric Disorders

Studies of patients in methadone maintenance treatment show significant rates of psychiatric disorders. Research has revealed that upwards of 74% of patients had at one point in their life met diagnostic criteria for any psychiatric disorder, with 39% of patients in methadone treatment exhibiting a current psychiatric disorder (Brooner et al., 1997; Rounsaville, Weissnam, Kleber, & Wilber, 1982). The etiological and enduring relationship between illicit drug use and psychiatric symptomatology is complex, multifaceted, and variable over time. Proper assessment and treatment for these psychiatric disorders will aid the substance abuse treatment and subsequent RP for such patients. Since the vast majority of opioid-abusing patients are polysubstance dependent, clinicians should tease apart symptoms of intoxication and withdrawal associated with both opioids and non-opioids (e.g., stimulants, benzodiazepines) by evaluating potential psychiatric symptoms from both substance-induced/related and psychiatric etiologies. (See "Relapse Prevention for Opioid Dependence" in Donovan & Marlatt, 2005).

In addition to the DSM-IV Axis I psychiatric syndromes, patients who present to treatment for opioid dependence may also exhibit other psychosocial problems that may affect their ability to fully engage in treatment, thereby contributing to potential relapse. Research has shown a strong association between substance use disorders and personality disorders. Studies of patients in methadone treatment for opioid dependence have reported prevalence rates for antisocial personality disorder of 25 to 27% and borderline personality disorder of 5 to 18% (Brooner et al., 1997; Rounsaville et al., 1998). Treatment studies show that clients with personality disorders can have positive treatment outcomes; however, these individuals may require special treatment considerations to optimize effective treatment engagement (Cecero, Ball, Tennen, Kranzler, & Rounsaville, 1999).

Medical Conditions

Unlike cocaine and alcohol, opioid use has not been significantly associated with chronic medical comorbidities; however, when heroin is administered by injection, there are significant medical complications (O'Connor & Selwyn, 1997). Among opioid users, the efficient transmission of bloodborne infections through injection drug use has been associated with increased incidence of HIV infection, hepatitis C virus (HCV), and bacterial infections (Cherubin & Sapira, 1993). Injecting heroin has been associated with the development of soft-tissue infections, including abscesses, cellulitis, and necrotizing fasciitis (Biderman & Hiatt, 1987), as well as more significant cardiovascular complications such as infectious endocarditis (Abrams, Sklaver, Hoffman, & Greenman). These conditions may require treatments that range from antibiotic treatment to open-heart surgery for replacing damaged cardiac valves.

HIV infection among injection drug users has received considerable attention in the literature. Although the incidence rate of human immunodeficiency virus (HIV) has decreased since the 1980s, depending on the geographic region of the country, approximately 10 to 50% of injection drug users are HIV-positive. Despite medical advances in treating HIV and the development of effective antiretroviral agents to combat it, many infected injection drug users are unable to appropriately adhere to their medical treatments (Samet et al., 1992; Wall et al., 1995). Given the importance of treatment for this high-risk population, clinicians should examine the use of adherence enhancing strategies, such as provision of on-site HIV primary care within methadone treatment programs or providing directly observed therapy to patients who may have difficulty with adherence issues. Approximately 53% of substance abuse treatment facilities in the United States offer HIV/AIDS education, counseling, or support services (Substance Abuse and Mental Health Services Administration, 2000).

In addition to HIV, chronic hepatitis C (HCV) virus is proving to be another emerging epidemic among injection drug users. Among the 2.7 million Americans with chronic HCV, 60% of new infections are among injection drug users (Williams, 1999). Among patients enrolled in methadone maintenance treatment programs, up to 95% are HCV-positive, with approximately 40% showing evidence of ongoing liver damage (McCarthy & Flynn, 2001). Treatment for HCV is available to few patients with histories of opioid dependence due to a variety of factors, including the aversive nature of the current treatment, unwillingness of physicians to treat injection drug users, and the prohibitive cost of pegylated interferon treatment (Edlin et al., 2001). It is important for clinicians to consider the role of health status and chronic illness in RP treatment. Clients with histories of opioid dependence may pose complicated psychiatric and medical comorbidities, which put them at higher risk for lapse and relapse.

FACTORS RELATED TO OPIOID LAPSE AND RELAPSE

Relapse generally involves use of a substance such as heroin following a week or more of abstinence, or one day of heavy use during a period in which the individual has been drug-free and is attempting to maintain abstinence. Slips or lapses, as limited episodes of use, have been distinguished from full-blown relapses. Catastrophic interpretation of a lapse, via cognitive distortions such as all-or-nothing thinking, magnification, or self-blame, can interfere with use of RP skills, such as seeking support from others. The end result of these maladaptive thinking patterns is an increased risk of relapse. Relapse among opioid abusers has been investigated as both lapse from abstinence as well as lapses to other illicit drugs (e.g., cocaine, benzodiazepines) during methadone maintenance treatment (Unnithan, Gossop, & Strang, 1992). With opioid drugs, lapses may lead to prolonged episodes of use, so intervening early in the process is critical (Wasserman et al., 1998). In fact, high rates of relapse to heroin (50% and greater) have been reported among heroin abusers exiting treatment, and the rapidity of initial lapse has been well documented (Gossop, Stewart, Brown, & Marsden, 2002). One study showed most initial lapses occurred within 3 days to 1-week posttreatment, demonstrating the existence of this "critical period" after treatment (Gossop, Green, Phillips, & Bradley, 1989). Because of the high risk for relapse at this time, enhancing coping skills during treatment and aftercare services is crucial.

Proximal, Intermediate, and Distal Factors

The occurrence of relapse has been associated with a range of different variables and categories. Vulnerability to relapse is increased by long-standing, distal, personal factors such as frequency and severity of substance use, situational patterns of use, and psychiatric comorbidity. Intermediate background factors include lack of social support, poor coping skills, low self-efficacy, and negative expectancies, all of which may be stable or slow-changing. Proximal variables include negative affect, craving, cues, and high-risk situations. Marlatt (1985) places emphasis on proximal variables, specifically maladaptive coping responses to high-risk situations: negative emotional states, social pressure, and interpersonal conflict. Among heroin users specifically, the social context related to using drugs was found to increase probability of relapse (Westermeyer, 1989). Cognitions, negative mood states, and external events had the greatest association with relapse among treated heroin users (Bradley, Phillips, Green, & Gossop, 1989). In a study of 100 hospital-treated heroin addicts, Vaillant (1988) reports four factors related to being without relapse for a year or more: compulsory supervision (e.g., parole, employment); substitute dependence (i.e., methadone); new, stable relationships; and inspirational group membership (i.e., self-help groups, Narcotics Anonymous).

Coping Skills

Most literature on treatment and RP for opioid abusers indicates consensus that use of coping skills leads to better outcome. Gossop et al. (2002) compared three groups of heroin-dependent individuals: (1) relapse group who used heroin after treatment and continued to use regularly; (2) lapse group who used heroin post-treatment but did not go back to regular use; and (3) abstinent group who did not use heroin during the follow-up period of 1 year. Findings indicated significant differences in the amount of change between the three groups in cognitive, avoidance, and distraction coping responses from intake to follow-up, with the abstinent group employing the greatest use of coping responses, followed by the lapse group. Coping skills are defined as "any class of cognitive or overt behavior patterns that would deal effectively with problematic situations" (Goldfried, 1980). In this study, coping was measured using the Process of Change questionnaire (Prochaska, Velicer, DiClemente, & Fava, 1988) items on avoidance (e.g., people, places, things), cognitive (e.g., self-talk), and distraction (e.g., activities). The use of coping responses when faced with temptation to use heroin is a choice and, in some situations, clients may choose not to employ their learned coping responses (Gossop et al., 1989) or they may employ them and still fail. RP targeting client motivation, decision making, and consequences of relapse may impact decisions regarding use of coping strategies.

Substance Cues

Drug-related cues may be more salient in relapse among heroin users than other groups of substance abusers. Heather, Stallard, and Tebbutt (1991) reported that when a sample of heroin users judged the factors precipitating their last relapse, the highest rating was for temptations or urges in the presence of substance cues. Substance cues are capable of eliciting powerful reactions among opioid abusers, including intense craving or desire to use and physiological responses such as withdrawal symptoms. Drug cravings of opioid users may be particularly intense because of the powerful memory of euphoria. Heather et al. (1991) suggest that, in addition to coping skills training, cue exposure techniques be incorporated into RP to combat substance-related urges to use heroin. Methadone maintenance clients who abuse cocaine can benefit from cue exposure treatment to help reduce reactions to cues associated with their cocaine use (Kleber, 1994).

Substance cues include not only the drugs themselves, but also associated cues and situations. One such cue is money. When opioid-dependent clients start opioid replacement therapies such as methadone, the cost and time involved in obtaining illicit opioids is eliminated. This may free up money and energy, which may increase risk of abusing other substances, such as alcohol or cocaine. Receiving large amounts of money, such as lump-sum payments at onset of disability benefits, increases the risk of relapse among methadone maintenance clients (Herbst, Batki, Manfredi, & Jones, 1996). Another substance-related cue is sex. Sexual behavior and drug use are often intricately intertwined; sex may serve as a relapse precipitant. High-risk sexual behavior when using drugs may be difficult to change due to intoxication and disinhibition (e.g., Paul, Stall, & Davis, 1993). Safer-sex skills interventions with in-treatment drug users have lasting effects on sexual behaviors if they involve experiential learning with emotional intensity, like role plays and discussion with peers, and if men and women are in separate sessions (Prendergast, Urada, & Podus, 2001).

CLINICAL INTERVENTIONS TO CONTAIN LAPSES AND RELAPSES

Each lapse or relapse is a rich learning opportunity to understand what led to it, and where the weak parts are in a client's RP plan. Several distinct clinical interventions targeting lapse and relapse to substances can be applied specifically to RP for opioid dependence. Techniques for counselors, therapists, and other health care providers to consider when interacting with opioid abusers are described and numbered in the following section, with an emphasis on harm reduction methods. In addition, empirically studied treatments such as motivational interviewing, cognitive-behavioral therapy, and contingency management are discussed in the context of opioid relapse, along with standard treatment modalities like group therapy and residential programs. Tables 6.1 and 6.2 provide additional resources and Internet sites that may be useful for clinicians.

Clinical Practice Strategies

1. *Remain nonjudgmental with clients.* First and foremost, it is essential to maintain a nonjudgmental stance, so that clients feel safe discussing their drug use honestly with their provider or counselor. This is not easy, as

TABLE 6.1. Additional Resources for Clinical Practice

Topic	Text or manual
Contingency management	Higgins, S. T., & Silverman, K. (1999). *Motivating behavior change among illicit-drug abusers: Research on contingency management.* Washington, DC: American Psychological Association.
Dual diagnosis	Mueser, K. T., Noordsy, D. L., Drake, R. E., & Fox, L. (2003). *Integrated treatment for dual disorders: A guide to effective practice.* New York: Guilford Press.
Group therapy	Velasquez, M. M., Maurer, G. G., Crouch, C., & DiClemente, C. C. (2001). *Group treatment for substance abuse: A stages-of-change therapy manual.* New York: Guilford Press.
Harm reduction	Marlatt, G. A. (Ed.). (1998). *Harm reduction: Pragmatic strategies for managing high-risk behaviors.* New York: Guilford Press.
Motivational interviewing	Miller, W. R., & Rollnick, S. (2002). *Motivational interviewing: Preparing people for change* (2nd ed.). New York: Guilford Press.
Relapse prevention	Gorski, T., & Trundy, A. B. (2001). *Relapse prevention counseling workbook: Managing high-risk situations.* Independence, MO: Herald House.
Safe injection practices	Sorge, R., & Kershnar, S. (1998). *Getting off right: A safety manual for injection drug users.* San Francisco: Harm Reduction Coalition.
Stages of change	Connors, G. J., Donovan, D. M., & DiClemente, C. C. (2001). *Substance abuse treatment and the stages of change: Selecting and planning interventions.* New York: Guilford Press.
Therapeutic community	De Leon, G. (2000). *The therapeutic community: Theory, model and method.* New York: Springer.

Note. Resources provided for informational purposes only and may contain controversial material.

TABLE 6.2. Internet Sites for Clinicians

Topic	Website
Approaches to Drug Abuse Counseling (NIH Publication No. 00-4151)	www.drugabuse.gov/ADAC/ADAC1.html
American Association for the Treatment of Opioid Dependence (AATOD); national organization offering ethical and state guidelines for treatment	www.aatod.org
Breathe: The Overdose Game; a helpful conversation starter and learning tool	www.killpeople.com/breathe
Center for Substance Abuse Treatment (CSAT) publications and Treatment Improvement Protocols (TIPs)	www.csat.samhsa.gov/publications.html
Community-based HIV risk reduction counseling manual for active drug users (NIH Publication No. 00-4812)	www.drugabuse.gov/CBOM/CBOM.html
Drug-user-friendly injection and vein care information	www.erowid.org/chemicals/heroin/heroin.html
Harm Reduction Coalition site with drug information, principles of harm reduction, and brochures/pamphlets for safe injection	www.harmreduction.org
Advocates for the Integration of Recovery and Methadone. Methadone Anonymous mission statement and information	www.afirmfwc.org/methadone-anonymous.htm
Narcotics Anonymous World Services; meeting times and locations	www.na.org
National Institute on Drug Abuse Clinical Toolbox; science-based materials for drug abuse treatment providers	www.drugabuse.gov/TB/Clinical/ClinicalToolbox.html
National Institute on Drug Abuse research reports and factual information on heroin	www.drugabuse.gov/drugpages/heroin.html

Note. Internet sites provided for informational purposes only and may contain controversial material.

it can be extremely frustrating to witness a client's continued drug use and the destructive consequences. It is helpful to remember that in medical care of chronic illness, it is understood that symptoms are often out of control. In the same way, drug-abusing patients will show characteristics of their substance use disorder (e.g., continued use despite problems, inability to control use). Expecting that individuals will present at treatment intake drug-free is unrealistic and a set-up for frustration and shame.

   2. *Encourage clients to return to treatment quickly after lapse or relapse.* To counteract shame and dropping out of treatment, encourage cli-

ents to return to the program as soon as possible after lapsing or relapsing, or as soon as acute intoxication subsides and they can process information. Relapse or periods of return to use should not be equated with treatment failure.

3. *Limit the harm associated with relapse episodes.* Clinicians can help to shorten or reduce the negative impact as well as decrease the emotional and physical damage associated with relapse episodes. Engage clients in maintaining their own safety by discussing ways to limit and reduce harm from their lapse or relapse.

4. *Educate clients on prevention and management of overdose.* One life-saving intervention is to educate clients about increased risk of opioid overdose after opioid detoxification or a period of not using (Seal et al., 2001). Encourage them to use with others rather than alone, to learn life-saving skills such as overdose identification and CPR, and to have a strategy for calling 9-1-1 without getting arrested for illicit drug use (as described in Ochoa, Edney-Meschery, & Moss, 1999).

5. *Discuss safer ways to use drugs.* It is helpful to dialogue about realistic options for using drugs in a safer setting, for example, with friends rather than alone, in a familiar place (in unfamiliar places, use less, as tolerance is reduced), indoors rather than outdoors. Clients can also benefit from discussion of safer drug administration options. Clients may be willing to snort or smoke, rather than inject. If clients inject opioids or other drugs, discuss when and how to use needle exchange and encourage injection hygiene to prevent infections. When discussing safe injection practices, it is important not to be too vivid because it can trigger euphoric recall and strong cravings. Indeed, discussion or demonstration of safer injection practices with in-treatment drug users has not reliably yielded positive effects on injection practices (meta-analysis by Prendergast et al., 2001).

6. *Examine use of drugs other than opioids.* In addition to opioids, other drug use needs to be examined with the client. Among opioid-dependent clients, other drugs are often alcohol or cocaine. Abstinence may be the best choice for nonopioid substances that are abused. Two studies targeting relapse to cocaine among methadone clients showed that an abstinence-reinforcement intervention and abstinence-specific support (i.e., fewer cocaine users in one's social network) are related to lifestyle changes (i.e., avoiding drug users) and cocaine abstinence, respectively (Silverman et al., 1998; Wasserman, Stewart, & Delucchi, 2001). Use of other substances might not need to be altered if they are used without abuse or dependence. For instance, some clients drink consistently within moderation guidelines, and others continue to use marijuana for medicinal purposes or as part of their harm reduction treatment plan (e.g., marijuana maintenance). In order not to "endorse" illegal use, it is helpful to discuss legal harm that can come from use of illicit drugs. However, nonopioid drugs may need to be eliminated if they increase the risk of relapse to prob-

lematic drugs. For example, Henningfield (1984) posited that continued cigarette smoking may be a significant relapse factor for other illicit drug use in patients with substance abuse disorders.

Motivational Interventions

The working assumption of motivational enhancement therapy (MET) is that intrinsic motivation is a necessary and sufficient factor in facilitating change. MET is typically utilized as a structured, four-session intervention that includes a lengthy intake assessment, personalized feedback of test results, and follow-up interviews to facilitate treatment outcome evaluation. MET places emphasis on personal responsibility for change, provides a menu for change options, offers empathy, and facilitates clients' self-efficacy. A clinical research MET manual is available for treating individuals with alcohol abuse and dependence from the Project MATCH study (see Miller, Zweben, DiClemente, & Rychtarik, 1995). While MET has primarily been used to treat problem drinkers, it is highly amenable for targeting abstinence or reduction of opioid use. Motivational Interviewing (MI) is a less standardized version of MET also utilized in the treatment of addictive disorders (Miller & Rollnick, 1991, 2002). MI blends principles of motivational psychology, client-centered therapy, and process of change, and is aimed at reducing harmful behaviors. In one controlled clinical trial, drug abusers attending a methadone clinic were randomly allocated to either a 1-hour brief motivational intervention or an educational control (Saunders et al., 1995). At follow-up, the intervention group demonstrated more favorable outcomes across a variety of measures, including relapsing less quickly, compliance with methadone treatment, fewer opioid-related problems, increased stage of change movement, and more positive outcome expectancies for abstinence, compared to the educational control. Motivational interventions can be utilized as independent, stand-alone interventions; adjunctive treatments; RP or aftercare, and can be integrated with other treatment modalities.

Applying the harm reduction approach to opioid dependence provides information and motivational interventions, but then allows clients to formulate their own treatment plan. The clinician informs the client about the nature of dependence (e.g., if one uses a drug one is addicted to, it tends to escalate out of control), and about treatment options. For example, abstinence requires more radical adjustments, but if attained has positive outcomes. In comparison, continued use requires less change, but also has less predictable outcomes. The client makes the choice, and this choice is respected, no matter what the clinician believes is best. The client tries out and evaluates his or her chosen treatment goal (e.g., maintaining moderate heroin use). The dialogue about treatment goals continues through motivational interventions. Based on the client's experience and dialogue with clinicians, the client may decide to select a different treatment goal (e.g., trial of abstinence). The MI approach normalizes ambivalence by recognizing that both positive and negative factors surrounding opioid abuse serve as the source of ambivalence for changing the behavior.

Cognitive-Behavioral Interventions

Cognitive factors are important to consider in the relapse prevention model for opioid abusers. Marlatt (1985) has described relapse "set-ups" and apparently irrelevant decisions (AIDs). Identifying AIDs and how they set the stage for relapse is critical for opioid abusers. An example scenario of AIDs is provided.

> After picking up his paycheck Jeff decides to walk down a familiar city street to deposit his money—an apparently irrelevant decision (AID). On the way Jeff runs into an old buddy who invites him for coffee; Jeff accepts the invitation–another AID. Outside the coffee shop, Jeff runs right into his drug dealer, who says he just got some "really good dope." Jeff rationalizes the lapse by saying he will use just this one time since the dope is such high quality; he then proceeds to a full-blown relapse. He later feels bad about his lack of will power and justifies the incident by telling his counselor that he could not possibly have avoided the high-risk situation. In the covert planning of this relapse, Jeff made a chain of AIDs to minimize his own guilt and negative reactions from others. He also engaged in the abstinence violation effect (AVE), whereby once he slipped, a full relapse followed. Clients can be taught to recognize how these seemingly unrelated decisions contribute to their behavior. By using self-talk or internal dialogue to highlight the AID as a choice-point, opioid abusers can identify AIDs early in the decision-making process. They can also be educated about the all-or-nothing cognitive distortions of the AVE.

Specific cognitive-behavioral interventions for RP among opioid abusers may include behavioral rehearsal, covert modeling, and cognitive restructuring such as coping imagery or reframing reactions to a slip or lapse. Recognizing cognitive distortions about heroin addiction and identifying one's perceptions of drug use and its consequences is appropriate. Role-playing ways to deal with social pressure, negative affect, and interpersonal situations can be a helpful method to plan or practice learned coping strategies. Having the client describe past relapses and fantasize about future relapse can provide valuable information about the client's affective state and current level of coping skills. Skills training involves learning effective cognitive and behavioral responses to cope with high-risk situations. Lifestyle interventions such as relaxation and exercise help strengthen the client's overall coping capacity. Cue exposure treatment or extinction of conditioned craving is a behavioral intervention to help reduce reactions to cues associated with drug use (e.g., blood, needles, cotton). The client is reintroduced to stimuli initially through mental images, and once strategies for coping have been developed, reentry into the cue-rich environment is facilitated under controlled conditions. For heroin abusers, Marlatt's RP model can be integrated into methadone maintenance treatment as a structured counseling format for clients receiving opioid replacement.

Similarly, in the Center for Applied Sciences (CENAPS) Model of Relapse Prevention Therapy (CMRPT), the relapse process is marked by predictable and identifiable warning signs that come about long before drug use actually occurs. Through directive and supportive (rather than harsh) confrontation, counselors can assist clients to interrupt the relapse progression early and return to recovery. Development of an RP plan early in treatment is key. After a stable recovery plan has been established, focus shifts to core personality and lifestyle problems that can lead to relapse in later recovery. As an applied cognitive-behavioral therapy, CMRPT teaches clients to identify and manage immediate high-risk situations that lead to relapse using seven steps: (1) warning sign review; (2) warning sign analysis; (3) situation mapping; (4) thought management; (5) feeling management; (6) behavior and situation management; and (7) recovery planning (Gorski, 1996). This is accomplished through problem-solving group therapy, individual therapy, and psychoeducation (see Table 6.1 for additional CMRPT resources).

Contingency Management

Based on operant principles, contingency management (CM) uses immediate positive rewards to increase behaviors for which naturally occurring positive consequences are too delayed to change behavior. In clinical practice, it is helpful to first use MI to increase client motivation, then work out a mutually agreed-upon behavioral contract. A behavioral contract specifies what will happen if the client uses or does not use drugs, as measured by urine toxicology screen or other objective measure. Contingent reinforcement of target behaviors, such as drug abstinence and treatment participation, has been shown to lead to favorable behavioral changes in drug abusers. Effective positive consequences for abstinence with opioid-dependent clients include voucher-incentive reinforcements (Silverman et al., 1996) and increased flexibility in methadone-dosing schedules (Brooner & Kidorf, 2002). In contrast, decreasing methadone dose has not been effective, and discharging clients from methadone treatment takes away needed treatment (Kleber, 1994).

The problem of relapse following CM interventions has been a concern of many clinicians because of the limited duration and availability of external incentives. CM does not specifically address intrinsic motivation, and when the voucher is removed, often the client's environment is not able to provide competing reinforcement for drug abstinence. Rapid relapse to illicit substances typically occurs shortly after discontinuation of the reinforcers. Longer duration of CM and lower-cost reinforcement schedules (i.e., nonescalating) may be advantageous in delaying relapse to cocaine or heroin (Preston, Umbricht, & Epstein, 2002). Moreover, transitioning patients to other forms of treatment (e.g., cognitive-behavioral) after the voucher-based reinforcement has achieved its goals may help to sustain long-term abstinence and prevent relapse. A comprehensive text on contingency management procedures for treating substance abuse is available (see Table 6.1).

Gruber, Chutuape, and Stitzer (2000) demonstrated reinforcement-based intensive outpatient treatment (RBT), a novel RP therapy for inner city opioid-dependent individuals. In the study, opioid dependent (non-methadone) patients who were exiting a 3-day detoxification were randomized to either standard aftercare or RBT as an aftercare relapse prevention therapy. RBT involved intensive day treatment, individual counseling, abstinence-contingent access to group therapy (i.e., job seeking and social skills training, AIDS education), and partial abstinence-contingent support for housing, food, and recreational activities. At 1-month follow-up, the RBT group was significantly more likely to be enrolled in outpatient treatment, had longer latency to initial drug use, higher abstinence rates, lower depression severity scores, and higher rates of employment than the control group. These findings suggest the short-term efficacy for RBT as an RP strategy for inner city opioid-dependent individuals. At 3 months the groups were no longer significantly different on most measures, indicating the need for extended treatment interventions. Gruber et al. (2000) report that patients placed in a recovery house stayed in treatment longer and that drug-free housing is a powerful incentive for abstinence.

Group Therapy

Group therapy for opioid abusers can be challenging for counselors because clients are often irritable from painful withdrawal symptoms or heavily sedated from recent methadone dosing. For clients going through detoxification or withdrawal, allowing them to sit back or sit out during group may be beneficial to the group process. Discussion of withdrawal symptoms (e.g., type, duration, severity) particularly their relationship to relapse, can also be incorporated as part of group content. Clients who are nodding or falling asleep should be addressed by the group members and kept engaged with interactive exercises, energetic activities, and periodic stretching or breaks. Methadone "split dosing" may be helpful (i.e., a half dose in the morning and a half dose in the evening) for clients who are unable to stay awake during group. Topics may include risk-behavior management (e.g., sexual behaviors, needle sharing), anger management, mood management or dual diagnosis, and stages of change psychoeducation. McAuliffe (1990) demonstrated the efficacy of a group RP program for opioid-addicted individuals; the program included both professionally facilitated group sessions and peer-led self-help meetings.

Self-help groups are the most common method of aftercare for alcohol and drug abusers. Lifetime abstinence is the primary goal of the Minnesota Model and 12-step facilitation, both based on the philosophy of Alcoholics Anonymous (AA). Group affiliation, frequent meetings with other people in recovery, and changes in daily behaviors are the core agents of change. Narcotics Anonymous (NA) is the largest self-help group available to opioid abusers in the United States. Like AA, NA includes such activities as attending 90 meetings in 90 days, getting a sponsor, and assuming responsibilities within the meeting. Active participation in 12-step fellowships, working the 12 steps, and surrender to a higher power are critical for recovery. Traditionally, clients on methadone were not accepted into NA because of the view that methadone is a drug similar to other illicit substances, regardless of whether it has been prescribed by a doctor. Clients receiving methadone may be stigmatized and viewed as less committed to abstinence and less invested in treatment. Severe opioid abusers and methadone-maintenance clients may not be well suited for traditional self-help group treatment. Nonetheless, "Methadone Anonymous" has been initiated in some communities, on the premise that methadone is a therapeutic tool of recovery that may or may not be discontinued in time, dependent upon the needs of the individual (see Table 6.2).

Residential Programs

Some clients need to enter a controlled environment to prevent or stop a relapse. Although incarceration can provide containment and enforced abstinence, many opioid abusers continue to use drugs while in jail or prison. Residential treatment is preferable, as it provides not only a controlled environment, but also psychosocial support and acculturation into the culture of recovery. Most inpatient facilities embrace an abstinence-oriented approach to recovery. When a client uses alcohol or other drugs while in treatment, he or she is typically asked to leave and regarded as unmotivated for change. In other facilities, the client may be asked to sign a behavioral contract, and the relapse is used as a clinical issue.

Therapeutic communities (TCs) grew out of the self-help movement and are quite different from institutional, clinic, hospital, or traditional drug treatment systems. Therapeutic communities are typically led by people in recovery, involve residential treatment, and promote a drug-free lifestyle. The social environment of the TC is the treatment model: Social organization and communal relationships are aimed at reintegrating the client into society. Services are offered to clients once they understand the TC approach and have become closely involved with their peer community. Specialized services such as child care, parenting/family therapy, mental health counseling, vocational training, and RP training can be integrated into the daily TC schedule. De Leon, Staines, Sacks, Brady, and Melchionda (1997) present a modified therapeutic community model for methadone-maintained clients. Therapeutic communities can be distinguished from other treatment approaches by the use of community as the primary method for facilitating social and psychological change in individuals.

PHARMACOLOGICAL TREATMENT

Medications can have a useful role in preventing relapse to opioid dependence. They can provide a buffer to dampen craving for drugs in high-risk situations and offer a legal alternative to illicit opioid use, and some can even prevent overdose deaths. Medications can provide antagonism to the reinforcing effects of opioid drugs or can provide a stable substitute for illegal drugs (see Hart, McCance-Katz, & Kosten, 2001). Recent research has resulted in the availability of several medications that can be useful in preventing relapse to opioid dependence (see Kranzler, Amin, Modesto-Lowe, & Oncken, 1999; O'Connor & Fiellin, 2000)

Opioid Agonists

Opioid agonists are medications that can be used to replace illegal opioids like heroin. They have many of the same effects as heroin, but they differ in important ways. Because they are taken orally, they do not provide the sudden "rush" that heroin users experience through injection. As previously discussed, injection of opioids also creates a host of medical problems, such as abscesses and cardiovascular difficulties. These problems are avoided by taking replacement medications orally. In addition, these medications last much longer than heroin, so that drug users do not experience the rapid ups and downs that accompany heroin addiction, and instead can lead a relatively stable life. Methadone and LAAM are two opioid agonists approved for treatment of opioid dependence. Pharmacological substitution is a harm or risk reduction technique, used to promote better quality of life and higher functioning overall.

Methadone

Methadone is an opioid agonist that is taken orally once per day. It is usually given in the morning, in dosages at or above 60 mg. In the United

States over 170,000 patients receive methadone, and it accounts for 97% of clients who receive opioid-replacement medications (Substance Abuse and Mental Health Services Administration, 2002a). Maintenance is the most common venue for delivering methadone. It involves daily outpatient dosing, coupled with individual or group counseling. Methadone maintenance is the most carefully studied of drug treatment modalities, and the research clearly demonstrates its effectiveness in reducing the use of heroin and associated criminal behaviors. Methadone is not a treatment for nonopioid substances such as cocaine or alcohol, although some studies have shown that methadone maintenance treatment can help heroin- and cocaine-dependent patients reduce their cocaine use (Magura, Rosenblum, Fong, Villano, & Richman, 2002).

Methadone has been a Food and Drug Administration (FDA) approved treatment for opioid use for over 30 years. Methadone maintenance can be a powerful tool in preventing relapse for a number of reasons. Methadone has the same effect as heroin on opiate receptors, so patients will be much less likely to feel a need for heroin when they are in high-risk situations. In addition, the counseling they participate in gives clients more chance to build refusal skills and alternatives to drug use.

Detoxification with methadone, lasting from 21 days to 6 months, is another treatment modality. Detoxification with methadone involves gradual tapering of methadone over the treatment period, usually as an outpatient. Although methadone detoxification has short-term advantages of getting patients off of drugs and possibly connected with medical treatments, research has not shown much long-term benefit. Vaillant (1988) suggests that the goal of treatment should be long-term prevention of relapse, rather than detoxification.

LAAM

Levo-alpha-acetylmethadol (LAAM) is an alternative to methadone that has been approved as a maintenance medication for opioid use disorders since 1993. LAAM is similar to methadone, but its metabolites accumulate after the initial dose and plasma levels reach a relatively stable state after about 2 weeks of treatment. Thus, patients can take LAAM about 3 times per week rather than needing to come to the clinic daily. In 2001 the FDA restricted the use of LAAM in the United States due to cases of life-threatening cardiac arrhythmias, so currently it is used as a second-line treatment for opioid dependence.

Narcotic Antagonists

An antagonist is a medication that counteracts the effects of a drug. Naltrexone is a long-acting, orally administered opioid antagonist that counteracts the medical effects of heroin. When an individual takes naltrexone it occupies the brain's opioid receptor sites. If that individual then uses heroin, the heroin will not be able to displace naltrexone, and the heroin will not have any effect. From the viewpoint of the patient, using heroin has no effect. In this way naltrexone provides psychological insurance against the use of heroin, and naltrexone treatment can be a formidable barrier to relapse

If the individual takes an initial dose of heroin while on naltrexone and does not experience an effect he or she might "shoot up" again searching for the effect. If the dosage has been set adequately, a heroin overdose is extremely unlikely, yet there are cases where overdose has occurred during treatment (Mioto, McCann, Rawson, Frosch, & Ling, 1997). However, the risk of heroin overdose is elevated after naltrexone treatment (Ritter, 2001), as a result of the individual's reduced tolerance for opioids.

Most heroin users have been unwilling to take naltrexone. Some are hesitant because it has no psychoactive effects for them, others are afraid of experiencing opioid withdrawal when they begin the treatment. Naltrexone has been available as a narcotic treatment since 1984, but it has not made a noticeable dent as a treatment modality.

Naloxone (brand name Narcan) is a short-acting narcotic antagonist that is usually administered by intravenous injection. Its most common use is in medical emergency treatment to reverse the effects of heroin overdose. Naloxone plays a crucial role in preventing heroin-related overdose deaths through its use in ambulances and hospital emergency rooms. Some are experimenting with making naloxone available to police officers and to narcotic users as a way to treat overdoses before medical services have arrived (Sporer, 2003).

Buprenorphine: Recently Approved Mixed Agonist–Antagonist

The most recently available treatment for heroin dependence, receiving FDA approval in 2002, is an opioid partial agonist. That is, while buprenorphine is an opioid and thus can act like an opioid agonist, its effects and side effects are less than those of full agonists like methadone, LAAM, or heroin. When the dose is low, buprenorphine has enough agonist effect to help opioid-dependent individuals stop using heroin without withdrawal symptoms. But at moderate doses the agonist properties reach a ceiling. Thus, buprenorphine has a lower risk of abuse and side effects compared to full opioid agonists. Buprenorphine is taken as a tablet, under the tongue. Research has shown that buprenorphine is about as effective as methadone or LAAM in dealing with opioid use. As a medication to prevent relapse, buprenorphine has the possibility of being more widely available than methadone because it will be prescribed by physicians in their offices, rather than in highly regulated clinics, the way methadone and

LAAM maintenance programs operate. Note that the FDA approved two buprenorphine medications for use in addiction. One is simply buprenorphine (brand name Subutex), while the other is a buprenorphine–naloxone combination (brand name Suboxone), developed with the thought that the combination medication is less likely to be diverted from clinics and has less abuse potential. Patients may be prescribed Subutex during a short induction period, which will be closely supervised by their physician, before being switched to Suboxone.

Medications in Context

A number of other medications are available to treat opioid use. Clonidine, for example, is a nonaddictive agent that can counteract opioid withdrawal symptoms. As with cocaine dependence (see Carroll & Rawson, Chapter 5, this volume), many more medications have been tried than have been successful.

From the viewpoint of RP, medications are most useful in conjunction with psychosocial and behavioral treatments. Carroll (1997) points out that these medications tend to affect the symptoms of substance abuse, but they have little influence on the long-lasting behavioral correlates of drug dependence. With supportive counseling, high-risk situations can be identified, coping skills and avoidance strategies can be rehearsed, and a general plan can be devised for dealing with lapses and building on the patient's strengths. Medications can be helpful in strengthening a patient's ability to remain abstinent, or providing an alternative to illegal drugs, but recovery from opioid addiction is a process in which key elements are individual motivation and supportive human services to help drug users achieve a more rewarding lifestyle.

ALTERNATIVE THERAPIES

Because of the diversity in client characteristics and available resources, it is important to offer a description of alternative therapies that have potential application for opioid dependence. Although not empirically established like the previously described treatments, the use of acupuncture and spiritual interventions may offer clinicians complementary and supplementary RP tools.

Acupuncture

Acupuncture is a nontraditional method used to treat a variety of conditions, including substance abuse. In Chinese medicine, disease is regarded as an imbalance of chi, or energy; acupuncture is used to influence and harmonize the body's flow of chi. Stimulation of specific external body locations (or acupuncture points) by needle insertion is believed to effect meridian pathways (energy channels) and have analgesic effects on internal organs. For RP, acupuncture has been employed to promote relaxation and relieve or prevent drug craving (McLellan, Grossman, Blaine, & Haaverkos, 1993). Acupuncture is an available service in 5% of drug treatment programs across the United States (Substance Abuse and Mental Health Services Administration, 2000). Several studies have suggested that the mechanism of acupuncture's action on opioid withdrawal is related to increased production of endogenous opioid peptides such as beta-endorphins and enkephalins. Efficacy research on the use of acupuncture for opioid treatment is lacking in the literature, with most studies using nonrandomized, nonblind designs, and having high attrition rates (see review Moner, 1996).

Washburn and colleagues (1993) conducted a single-blind design with 100 heroin abusers in San Francisco, comparing standard acupuncture with a placebo "sham" treatment for 21 days. They found that subjects receiving acupuncture compared to the sham condition were more likely to return to treatment; "light" heroin users (i.e., once daily or less) in the acupuncture group self-reported decreased heroin use and had less incidence of positive drug screens than controls. Although the effects were modest, the authors suggest that acupuncture may be a feasible, drug-free treatment for less severe heroin users or those who have not opted for opioid replacement therapy. Auricular (ear) acupuncture is being used to help with both detoxification and ongoing stress reduction across the United States, using a model that was developed at Lincoln Hospital in New York City. Clinical experience suggests acupuncture has potential as a safe, adjunctive treatment and an RP strategy for opioid abuse.

Spiritual Interventions

There is a need for alternative RP treatments that are cost-effective, innovative, and comprehensive. Spiritually based interventions for opioid dependence have promise to fill this gap. As a multidimensional concept, spirituality involves a personal search for meaning and fulfillment in life, offering inner harmony and interconnectedness at all levels of existence. Spirituality can also be defined as a healthy relationship with the things and people who are valued. By helping the client improve his or her relationships, spirituality becomes a primary agent of change. Addiction is viewed as a negative habit arising from incomplete understanding of the relationship between mind, body, and environment. From this perspective, an illness such as addiction can provide opportunity for growth and serve as a signal for change. Religion is an organized system of beliefs and worship to develop spiritual awareness, providing a framework, structure, and discipline. Both spirituality and religion may be important protective factors in preventing relapse to opioids by offering an effective coping strategy and stress buffer. Avants, Warburton, and Margolin (2001) reported that methadone-maintenance patients with high rates of perceived spiritual or religious support were abstinent from illicit drugs significantly longer during the first 6 months of treatment than patients with lower ratings. In addition, strength of spiritual or religious support was a significant independent predictor of abstinence, controlling for other factors.

Several addiction treatments incorporate spiritual or religious components. AA is based in spiritual principles of surrender to a higher power; long-term recovery is considered a process of spiritual renewal. Transcendental Meditation (TM) is a spiritual technique widely employed to reduce stress and is increasingly used in RP for alcohol and substance abuse (e.g., O'Connell, 1991). TM is a simple mental exercise of allowing one's mind to settle into deeper, more subtle levels of consciousness. It is practiced 20 minutes a day, requiring no change in beliefs or lifestyle, appropriate for diverse populations, and predicted to benefit all levels of functioning. In a meta-analysis, Alexander, Robinson, and Rainforth (1994) found a large effect size for TM reduction of illicit substance use, compared to controls. Because TM is purported to increase benefits to the client over time, it has implications for RP and a viable aftercare treatment. In addition, Margolin and Avants (2002) have developed a treatment manual for Spiritual Self-Schema Therapy (3-S), a cognitive therapy informed by Buddhist psychology for helping drug abusers activate a spiritual self-schema that fosters drug abstinence and reduction of HIV risk-behavior.

CONCLUSIONS

In 1977 William S. Burroughs published a book about his experience with heroin addiction entitled *Junky*. He declared:

> I knew that I did not want to go on taking junk. If I could have made a single decision, I would have decided no more junk ever. But when it came to the process of quitting, I did not have the drive. It gave me a terrible feeling of helplessness to watch myself break every schedule I set up as though I did not have control over my actions. (p. 125)

Fortunately today, the struggle of opioid dependence can be fought and in many cases overcome with empirically supported treatments, both pharmacological and psychosocial/behavioral. Harm reduction techniques play a major role in attenuating uncomfortable physiological symptoms, lessening psychological distress, and decreasing high-risk behaviors. Regardless of treatment modality, relapse is high among opioid-dependent individuals.

Lapse and relapse to "junk" is expected on the road to recovery and can be accepted by clinicians without judgment. Tremendous scientific advancements in the field of opioid addiction render the healing process less painful and remarkably hopeful.

ACKNOWLEDGMENTS

The writing of this chapter was partially supported by the National Institutes of Health Grant Nos. P50 DA09253, U10DA15815, and R01DA14922. We are sincerely grateful to the clinical and research staff at the San Francisco General Hospital, Opiate Treatment Outpatient Program, and Division of Substance Abuse and Addiction Medicine for their time, concern for patients, and enthusiasm.

REFERENCES

Abrams, B., Sklaver, A., Hoffman, T., & Greenman, R. (1979). Single or combination therapy of staphylococcal endocarditis in intravenous drug users. *Annals of Internal Medicine, 90*, 1106–1107.

Alexander, C. N., Robinson, P., & Rainforth, M. (1994). Treating and preventing alcohol, nicotine, and drug abuse through Transcendental Meditation: A review and statistical meta-analysis. *Alcoholism Treatment Quarterly, 11*, 13–87.

American Psychiatric Association. (1994). *Diagnostic and statistical manual of mental disorders* (4th ed.). Washington, DC: Author.

Avants, S. K., Warburton, L. A., & Margolin, A. (2001). Spiritual and religious support in recovery from addiction among HIV-positive injection drug users. *Journal of Psychoactive Drugs, 33*, 39–45.

Biderman, P., & Hiatt, J. R. (1987). Management of soft-tissue infections of the upper extremity in parenteral drug abusers. *American Journal of Surgery, 145*, 526–528.

Bodenheimer, T., Wagner, E. H., & Grumbach, K. (2002). Improving primary care for patients with chronic illness. *Journal of the American Medical Association, 14*, 1775–1779.

Bradley, B. P., Phillips, G., Green, L., & Gossop, M. (1989). Circumstances surrounding the initial lapse to opiate use following detoxification. *British Journal of Psychiatry, 154*, 354–359.

Brooner, R. K., & Kidorf, M. (2002). Using behavioral reinforcement to improve methadone treatment participation. *Science and Practice Perspectives, 1*, 38–48.

Brooner, R. K., King, V. L., Kidorf, M., Schmidt, C. W., Jr., & Bigelow, G. E. (1997). Psychiatric and substance use comorbidity among treatment seeking opioid abusers. *Archives of General Psychiatry, 54*, 71–80.

Burroughs, W. S. (1977). *Junky.* New York: Penguin.

Carroll, K. M. (1997). Integrating psychotherapy and pharmacotherapy to improve drug abuse outcomes. *Addictive Behaviors, 22*(2), 233–245.

Cecero, J. J., Ball, S. A., Tennen, H., Kranzler, H. R., & Rounsaville, B. J. (1999).

Concurrent and predictive validity of antisocial personality disorder subtyping among substance abusers. *Journal of Nervous and Mental Disease, 187*, 478–486.

Cherubin, C. E., & Sapira, J. D. (1993). The medical complications of drug addiction and the medical assessment of the intravenous drug user: 25 years later. *Annals of Internal Medicine, 119*, 1017–1028.

De Leon, G., Staines, G. L., Sacks, S., Brady, R., & Melchionda, R. (1997). Passages: A modified therapeutic community for methadone maintained clients. In G. De Leon (Ed.), *Community as method: Therapeutic communities for special populations and special settings* (pp. 225–246). Westport, CT: Greenwood.

Des Jarlais, D. C., Marmor, M., Paone, D., Titus, S., Shi, Q., Perlis, T., Jose, B., & Friedman, S. R. (1996). HIV incidence among injecting drug users in New York City syringe-exchange programs. *Lancet, 12*, 987–991.

DiClemente, C. C., & Prochaska, J. O. (1998). Toward a comprehensive Transtheoretical model of change: Stages of change and addictive behaviors. In W. Miller & N. Heather (Eds.), *Treating addictive behaviors* (2nd ed., pp. 3–24). New York: Plenum.

Edlin, B. R., Seal, K. H., Lorvick, J., Kral, A. H., Ciccarone, D. H., Moore, L. D., & Lo, B. (2001). Is it justifiable to withhold treatment for hepatitis C from illicit-drug users? *New England Journal of Medicine, 345*, 211–214.

Goldfried, M. (1980). Psychotherapy as coping skills training. In M. Mahoney (Ed.), *Psychotherapy process* (pp. 89–119). New York: Plenum.

Gorski, T. T. (1996, June). The high cost of relapse. *Professional Counselor, xvi*, 29–30.

Gossop, M., Green, L., Phillips, G., & Bradley, B. P. (1989). Lapse, relapse, and survival among opiate addicts after treatment: A prospective follow-up study. *British Journal of Psychiatry, 154*, 348–353.

Gossop, M., Stewart, D., Brown, N., & Marsden, J. (2002). Factors associated with abstinence, lapse or relapse to heroin use after residential treatment: Protective effect of coping responses. *Addiction, 97*, 1259–1267.

Gruber, K., Chutuape, M. A., & Stitzer, M. L. (2000). Reinforcement-based intensive outpatient treatment for inner city opiate abusers: A short-term evaluation. *Drug and Alcohol Dependence, 57*, 211–223.

Hart, C., McCance-Katz, E. F., & Kosten, T. R. (2001). Pharmacotherapies used in common substance use disorders. In F. M. Tims, C. G. Leukefeld, et al. (Eds.), *Relapse and recovery in addictions* (pp. 303–333). New Haven, CT: Yale University Press.

Heather, N., Stallard, A., & Tebbutt, J. (1991). Importance of substance cues in relapse among heroin users: Comparison of two methods of investigation. *Addictive Behaviors, 16*, 41–49.

Heinssen, R. K., Levendusky, P. G., & Hunter, R. H. (1995). Client as colleague: Therapeutic contracting with seriously mentally ill. *American Psychologist, 50*, 522–532.

Henningfield, J. E. (1984). Pharmacological basis and treatment of cigarette smoking. *Journal of Clinical Pharmacology, 45*, 24–34.

Herbst, M. D., Batki, S. L., Manfredi, L. B., & Jones, T. (1996). Treatment outcomes for methadone clients receiving lump-sum payments at initiation of disability benefits. *Psychiatric Services, 47*, 119–120.

Hser, Y., Hoffman, V., Grella, C. E., & Anglin, M. D. (2001). A 33-year follow-up of narcotics addicts. *Archives of General Psychiatry, 58,* 503–508.

Johnston, L. D., O'Malley, P. M., & Bachman, J. G. (2002). *Ecstasy use among American teens drops for the first time in recent years, and overall drug and alcohol use also decline in the year after 9/11.* Ann Arbor, MI: University of Michigan News and Information Services.

Kleber, H. D. (1994). Assessment and treatment of cocaine-abusing methadone-maintained patients. *Treatment Improvement Protocol Series, 10* (DHHS Publication No. 94-3003). Rockville, MD: Department of Health and Human Services.

Kranzler, H. R., Amin, H., Modesto-Lowe, V., & Oncken, C. (1999). Pharmacologic treatments for drug and alcohol dependence. *Addictive Disorders, 22,* 401–423.

MacCoun, R. J. (1998). Toward a psychology of harm reduction. *American Psychologist, 53,* 1199–1208.

Magura, S., Rosenblum, A., Fong, C., Villano, C., & Richman, B. (2002). Treating cocaine-using methadone patients: Predictors of outcome in a psychosocial clinical trial. *Substance Use and Misuse, 37*(14), 1927–1953.

Margolin, A., & Avants, S. K. (2002). *Spiritual Self-Schema Therapy (3-S) for reducing the transmission of HIV and other infections among inner-city drug users* [Treatment manual and proposed assessment battery]. Manuscript in preparation. Copyright Yale University.

Marlatt, G. A. (1985). Determinants of relapse and skill-training interventions. In G. A. Marlatt & J. R. Gordon (Eds.), *Relapse prevention: Maintenance strategies in the treatment of addictive behaviors* (1st ed.). New York: Guilford Press.

Marlatt, G. A., Blume, A. W., & Parks, G. A. (2001). Integrating harm reduction therapy and traditional substance abuse treatment. *Journal of Psychoactive Drugs, 33,* 13–21.

McAuliffe, W. E. (1990). A randomized controlled trial of recovery training and self-help for opioid addicts in New England and Hong Kong. *Journal of Psychoactive Drugs, 22,* 197–209.

McCarthy, J. J., & Flynn, N. (2001). Hepatitis C in methadone maintenance patients: Prevalence and public policy implications. *Journal of Addictive Diseases, 20,* 19–31.

McLellan, A. T., Grossman, D. S., Blaine, J. D., & Haaverkos, H. W. (1993). Acupuncture treatment for drug abuse: A technical review. *Journal of Substance Abuse Treatment, 10,* 568–576.

Meichenbaum, D., & Turk, D. C. (1987). *Facilitating treatment adherence.* New York: Plenum.

Miller, W. R., & Rollnick, S. (1991). *Motivational interviewing: Preparing people to change addictive behavior.* New York: Guilford Press.

Miller, W. R., & Rollnick, S. (2002). *Motivational interviewing: Preparing people for change* (2nd ed.). New York: Guilford Press.

Miller, W. R., Zweben, A., DiClemente, C. C., & Rychtarik, R. G. (1995). *Motivational enhancement therapy manual: A clinical research guide for therapists treating individuals with alcohol and drug dependence* (NIAAA Project MATCH Monograph Series, 2; US DHHS Publication 94-3723). Washington, DC: U.S. Government Printing Office.

Mioto, K., McCann, M. J., Rawson, R. A., Frosch, D., & Ling, W. (1997). Overdose, suicide attempts and death among a cohort of naltrexone-treated opioid addicts. *Drug and Alcohol Dependence, 45*, 131–144.

Moner, S. E. (1996). Acupuncture and addiction treatment. *Journal of Addictive Diseases, 15*, 79–100.

National Institute on Drug Abuse. (1997). *Heroin abuse and addiction. Research Report Series.* (NIH Publication No. 00-4165). Washington, DC: U. S. Government Printing Office.

National Institute on Drug Abuse. (2000). *Epidemiologic Trends in Drug Abuse: Vol. 1. Highlights and Executive Summary, Community Epidemiology Work Group.* (NIH Publication No. 00-4739). Washington, DC: U.S. Government Printing Office.

Ochoa, K., Edney-Meschery, H., & Moss, A. (1999). Understanding heroin overdose. *Harm Reduction Communication, 9*, 10–12.

O'Connell, D. F. (1991). The use of Transcendental Meditation in relapse prevention counseling. *Alcoholism Treatment Quarterly, 8*, 53–68.

O'Connor, P. G., & Fiellin, D. A. (2000). Pharmacologic treatment of heroin-dependent patients. *Annals of Internal Medicine, 133*(1), 40–54.

O'Connor, P. G., & Selwyn, P. A. (1997). Medical issues in the care of opioid-dependent patients. In T. R. Kosten & S. M. Stine (Eds.), New treatments for opiate dependence (pp. 199–227). New York: Guilford Press.

Paul, J. P., Stall, R., & Davis, F. (1993). Sexual risk for HIV transmission among gay/bisexual men in substance abuse treatment. *AIDS Education and Prevention, 5*, 11–24.

Prendergast, M. L., Urada, D., & Podus, D. (2001). Meta-analysis of HIV risk-reduction interventions within drug abuse treatment programs. *Journal of Consulting and Clinical Psychology, 69*, 389–405.

Preston, K. L., Umbricht, A., & Epstein, D. H. (2002). Abstinence reinforcement maintenenace contingency and on-year follow-up. *Drug and Alcohol Dependence, 67*, 125–137.

Prochaska, J. O., Velicer, W. F., DiClemente, C. C., & Fava, J. (1988). Measuring processes of change: Applications to the cessation of smoking. *Journal of Consulting and Clinical Psychology, 56*, 520–528.

Ritter, A. J. (2001). Naltrexone in the treatment of heroin dependence: Relationship with depression and risk of overdose. *Australian and New Zealand Journal of Psychiatry, 36*, 224–228.

Rosen, M. I., Rigsby, M. O., Dieckhaus, K. D., & Cramer, J. A. (2003). Effects of illicit drug use on adherence to prescribed antiretroviral medication. *American Journal on Addictions, 12*, 455–458.

Rounsaville, B. J., Kranzler, H. R., Ball, S., Tennen, H., Poling, J., & Triffleman, E. (1998). Personality disorders in substance abusers: Relation to substance use. *Journal of Nervous and Mental Disorders, 186*, 87–95.

Rounsaville, B. J., Weissnam, M. M., Kleber, H., & Wilber, C. (1982). Heterogeneity of psychiatric diagnosis in treated opiate addicts. *Archives of General Psychiatry, 39*, 161–166.

Samet, J. H., Libman, H., Steger, K. A., Dhawan, R., Chen, J., Schits, A. H., Dewees-Dunk, R., Levinson, S., Kufe, D., & Craven, D. E. (1992). Compliance with zidovudine therapy in patients infected with human immunodeficiency virus, Type 1: A cross-sectional study in a municipal hospital clinic. *American Journal of Medicine, 92*, 495–502.

Saunders, W., Wilkinson, C., & Phillips, M. (1995). The impact of a brief motivational intervention with opiate users attending a methadone programme. *Addiction, 90*, 415–422.

Seal, K. H., Kral, A. H., Gee, L., Moore, L. D., Bluthenthal, R. N., Lorvick, J., & Edlin, B. R. (2001). Predictors and prevention of nonfatal overdose among street-recruited injection heroin users in the San Francisco Bay Area, 1998–1999. *American Journal of Public Health, 91*, 1842–1846.

Silverman, K., Higgins, S. T., Brooner, R. K., Montoya, I. D., Cone, E. J., Schuster, C. R., & Preston, K. L. (1996). Sustained cocaine abstinence in methadone maintenance patients through voucher-based reinforcement therapy. *Archives of General Psychiatry, 53*, 409–415.

Silverman, K., Wong, C. J., Umbricht-Schneiter, A., Montoya, I. D., Schuster, C. R., & Preston, K. L. (1998). Broad beneficial effects of cocaine abstinence reinforcement among methadone patients. *Journal of Consulting and Clinical Psychology, 66*, 811–824.

Sorensen, J. L., Deitch, D. A., & Acampora, A. (1984). Treatment collaboration of methadone maintenance programs and therapeutic communities. *Journal of Psychoactive Drugs, 10*, 347–359.

Sporer, K. A. (2003). Strategies for preventing heroin overdose. *British Medical Journal, 326*, 442–444.

Substance Abuse and Mental Health Services Administration. (2000). *National survey of substance abuse treatment services (N-SSATS)*. Rockville, MD: Author.

Substance Abuse and Mental Health Services Administration. (2001, July 20). Heroin—Changes in how it is used. *DASIS Report.*

Substance Abuse and Mental Health Services Administration. (2002a, December 6). Facilities providing methadone/LAAM treatment to clients with opiate addiction. *DASIS Report.*

Substance Abuse and Mental Health Services Administration. (2002b, June 14). Heroin treatment admissions in urban and rural areas. *DASIS Report.*

Substance Abuse and Mental Health Services Administration. (2004, September). Narcotic analgesics, 2002 Update. In *The DAWN report*. Rockville, MD: Author.

Unnithan, S., Gossop, M., & Strang, J. (1992). Factors associated with relapse among opiate addicts in an out-patient detoxification programmme. *British Journal of Psychiatry, 161*, 654–657.

Valliant, G. E. (1988). What can long-term follow-up teach us about relapse and prevention of relapse in addictions? *British Journal of Addiction, 83*, 1147–1157.

Wall, T. L., Sorensen, J. L., Batki, S. L., Delucchi, K. L., London, J. A., & Chesney, M. A. (1995). Adherence to zidovudine (AZT) among HIV-infected methadone patients: A pilot study of supervised therapy and dispensing compared to usual care. *Drug and Alcohol Dependence, 37*, 261–269.

Washburn, A. M., Fullilove, R. E., Fullilove, M. T., Keenan, P. A., McGee, B., Morris, K. A., Sorensen, J. L., & Clark, W. W. (1993). Acupuncture heroin detoxification: A single-blind clinical trial. *Journal of Substance Abuse Treatment, 10*, 345–351.

Wasserman, D. A., Stewart, A. L., & Delucchi, K. L. (2001). Social support and abstinence from opiates and cocaine during opioid maintenance treatment. *Drug and Alcohol Dependence, 65*, 65–75.

Wasserman, D. A., Weinstein, M. G., Havassy, B. E., & Hall, S. M. (1998). Factors associated with lapses to heroin use during methadone treatment. *Drug and Alcohol Dependence, 52,* 183–192.

Westermeyer, J. (1989). Nontreatment factors affecting treatment outcome in substance abuse. *American Journal of Drug and Alcohol Abuse, 15,* 13–29.

Williams, I. (1999). Epidemiology of hepatitis C in the United States. *American Journal of Medicine, 107,* 2S–9S.

Zweben, J. E. (1991). Counseling issues in methadone maintenance treatment. *Journal of Psychoactive Drugs, 23,* 177–190.

CHAPTER 7

Relapse Prevention for Cannabis Abuse and Dependence

Roger A. Roffman
Robert S. Stephens

EPIDEMIOLOGY OF CANNABIS USE AND DEPENDENCE

Self-report of illegal behavior may lead to inaccuracies in estimation, most likely with an underreporting bias, of the incidence and prevalence of cannabis use and associated consequences. That caveat notwithstanding, it is estimated that 5,800 individuals start using cannabis every day in the United States, with as many as 2,500,000 first having used it in 1999 (Gfroerer, Wu, & Penne, 2002). According to the 2002 National Household Survey on Drug Abuse, more than 95 million Americans age 12 and older have tried marijuana at least once (Substance Abuse and Mental Health Services Administration [SAMHSA], 2003).

There are an estimated 14.6 million current users in the United States, with current use being defined as one or more occasions of use in the month prior to being surveyed (SAMHSA, 2003). Of these individuals, about one-third (4.8 million persons) used marijuana on 20 or more days in the past month.

It is estimated that 11–16% of current users (1.6–2.3 million individuals) qualify for the diagnosis of cannabis dependence. In 2001, 3.5 million people met criteria for past-year cannabis abuse or dependence. In the decade spanning 1991–1992 to 2001–2002, data from two national surveys indicate that while the prevalence of cannabis use remained stable among adults, the prevalence of cannabis abuse or dependence, as defined by the *Diagnostic and Statistical Manual of Mental Disorders*, fourth edition (DSM-IV; American Psychiatric Association, 1994), increased significantly, with the greatest increases among young African American men and women and young Hispanic men (Compton, Grant, Colliver, Glantz, & Stinson, 2004). Treatment for cannabis disorders was provided to 974,000 individuals in 2002, and there is evidence of a steadily increasing demand for treatment.

One can estimate the prevalence of problems associated with cannabis use by looking at two subgroups: those who have used it at least once in the past year and those who have used it at least once in the past month. Among those who have used cannabis one or more times in the previous year, two fairly large longitudinal studies offer estimations. Measuring indicators of abuse and dependence, one study found that 6% qualified for a diagnosis of cannabis dependence and 23% qualified for a diagnosis of abuse (Grant & Pickering, 1998). Another study focused on self-report of problems attributed to cannabis by respondents (e.g., health, psychological, social functioning). These researchers found that 85% reported no problems, 15% reported one, 8% reported at least two, and 4% reported at least three (National Institute on Drug Abuse [NIDA], 1991). When current users (i.e., used cannabis at least once in the prior month) are considered, roughly 11–16% (1.6–2.3 million individuals) qualify for the diagnosis of cannabis dependence. In summary, the risk for the occurrence of three or more problems (a proxy indicator for dependence) among those who have used cannabis at least once in the past year appears to be roughly 4–6%, and it is 11–16% for those who have used it at least once in the past month.

Another approach to estimating problematic consequences involves time frame from initial use. Epidemiologists estimate that almost 2% of users develop cannabis dependence within the first 2 years of initiating use. Based on the estimate that 2.5 million individuals first used cannabis in 1999, it would be expected that 50,000 of them would have experienced cannabis dependence within 2 years of initial use. Within roughly 10 years after first use of cannabis, an estimated 10% of cannabis users develop the cannabis dependence syndrome (Anthony, Warner, & Kessler, 1994; Wagner & Anthony, 2002).

Finally, the relative risk of becoming cannabis dependent if one uses this drug at least once can be examined in the context of risk levels for those who have used other substances at least once. Anthony and his colleagues (1994) identify the following relative risk levels for dependence: tobacco (31.9%), heroin (23.1%), cocaine (16.7%), alcohol (15.4%), stimulants (11.2%), and cannabis (9.1%).

CO-OCCURRING DISORDERS

There is some evidence of an elevated risk of co-occurring psychological problems among various subgroups of cannabis users. For example, among adolescents receiving outpatient treatment for cannabis abuse or dependence, 75% were found to have at least one comorbid psychological problem (Tims et al., 2002). Conduct disorders (53%) were most common, followed by attention-deficit/hyperactivity disorder (38%). Similarly, adults being treated for cannabis dependence evidenced a high comorbidity for psychological distress in two controlled trials (Copeland, Swift, & Rees, 2001; Stephens, Roffman, & Simpson, 1993). Finally, data from an Australian national survey of adults pointed to a positive correlation between cannabis use and DSM-IV affective and anxiety disorders (Degenhardt, Hall, & Lynskey, 2001).

EVIDENCE OF A CANNABIS DEPENDENCE SYNDROME

The concept of cannabis dependence is controversial, and a full discussion of the many involved issues goes beyond the scope of this chapter. Earleywine's (2002) *Understanding Marijuana* offers a thoughtful and extended analysis of the contributing factors to the controversy. Babor (in press) presents a historical perspective of the nosology and diagnosis of cannabis disorders. Finally, Stephens and Roffman (2005) offer an in-depth discussion of measurement tools and challenges related to cannabis use behaviors.

One factor in the controversy arises from the political arena, with some arguing that cannabis dependence is a phenomenon that has been socially constructed to meet ideological purposes. This position sees the invention and definition of a cannabis dependence disorder as intended to convey and reinforce the prevailing values of a certain historical era. The early 21st century in the United States, as well as in a number of other nations, is witnessing considerable advocacy favoring and opposing sanctions concerning both the medical and nonmedical uses of cannabis. In these debates, stakeholders may choose to either promote or minimize the existence and severity of cannabis dependence.

A second important factor pertains to the evolution of the concept of dependence and its distinction from the more physiologically oriented concept of addiction. In the mid-1960s, an expert committee of the World Health Organization endorsed a more behaviorally oriented concept of drug dependence that incorporates a cluster of physiological, behavioral, and cognitive phenomena (World Health Organization, 1964). Support for the existence of a cannabis dependence syndrome has been based partly on this conceptual shift and from nonhuman and human studies that demonstrate cannabis withdrawal (Budney, Novy, & Hughes, 1999; Crowley, Macdonald, Whitmore, & Mikulich, 1998; Haney, Ward, Comer, Foltin, & Fischman, 1999; Weisbeck, Schuckit, Kalmijn, Tipp, Bucholz, & Smith, 1996).

Finally, considerable evidence for a biological basis to cannabis dependence has accumulated since the identification of specific cannabinoid receptors in the brain (Devane, Dysarz, Johnson, Melvin, & Howlett, 1988) and the discovery of the endogenous cannabinoid anandamide, a compound that binds to and activates the same receptor sites in the brain as delta-9-tetrahydrocannabinol (THC), the active ingredient in cannabis (Devane et al., 1992). Subsequently, researchers discovered a cannabinoid antagonist, a compound that blocks anandamide action in the brain (Rinaldi-Carmona et al., 1994). Taken together, these discoveries have made it possible to systematically study the effects of chronic exposure to cannabis, thus enhancing our understanding of the cannabinoid neuro-chemical system's physiology and some of the mechanisms involved in the etiology of cannabis dependence.

QUANDARIES, POLITICS, AND CLINICAL CHALLENGES: THE CONTEXT OF CANNABIS INTERVENTIONS

Before reviewing the trials in which RP interventions have been tested with cannabis-dependent individuals, a few comments about challenges commonly encountered by clinicians when working with this population might be helpful. These challenges include attitudes concerning cannabis legalization, grievances concerning the fairness of using urinalysis data vis-à-vis employment sanctions, ambivalence about the existence and severity of adverse effects, abstinence versus moderation as outcome goals, dealing with problematic use in the context of medical necessity, and emerging knowledge concerning cannabis withdrawal and its amelioration.

Client Attitudes Concerning Cannabis Legalization

Whether treatment has been entered voluntarily or through coercion, it is very common for clients to strongly express opposition to cannabis prohibition. Indeed, many argue that their sole difficulty with cannabis is due to its illegal status, with either the occurrence of an arrest or pressure from a concerned family member or friend about this possibility having prompted treatment entry. It is likely that some clinicians also will favor cannabis legalization. A clinical challenge is to not let this issue obfuscate the assessment process. As therapist and client candidly and thoroughly assess the impact that cannabis use is having in the client's life, the clinician needs to be open to the possibility that the drug's illegality may be the only cause of his or her problems. He or she must also be attuned to the occurrence of adverse impacts in other domains of the client's functioning. It is worth noting that the primary concerns of those voluntarily seeking treatment for cannabis use are self-control and health, rather than social or legal pressures (McBride et al., 1994; Stephens, Babor, Kadden, Miller, & the Marijuana Treatment Project Research Group, 2002).

Grievances Concerning the Fairness of Using Urinalysis Data vis-à-vis Employment Sanctions

As an alternative to dismissal, some employers require treatment of employees whose urine tests indicate cannabis use. Because cannabis metabolites are slowly excreted from the body, the employee who gets high only when not at work will nonetheless be vulnerable to sanctions. The client may argue that what one does during nonwork hours is not the employer's business. As with the legalization issue, the challenge to the clinician is to maintain an empathic stance while also conducting a wider assessment of the client's experiences with cannabis.

Ambivalence about the Existence and Severity of Adverse Effects

While some clients enter treatment with a strong and sustained motivation to quit or reduce cannabis use, many others struggle with mixed and competing views concerning their goals. It is likely that claims made by proponents and opponents of legalization, in terms of risks and benefits associated with use, contribute to the individual's quandary in self-assessment of cannabis effects. It is also likely that the adverse effects that the client is experiencing, when compared with those associated with other drugs, are of sufficient subtlety so as to warrant concern at times and, at other times, a belief that the benefits outweigh any costs. Not uncommonly, in seeking a resolution of his or her ambivalence, a client will ask, "Isn't there something really harmful about cannabis you can tell me so that I'll get motivated?"

Abstinence versus Moderation as Outcome Goals

Very commonly clients will shift between abstinence and moderation outcome goals. While this is not unique to cannabis-using populations, it may be particularly a challenge for those users who remain employed, have not experienced major problems in functioning or health, and find themselves grappling with the subtlety of negative effects commented on in the preceding paragraph.

Although published protocols for moderation in cannabis use have not yet appeared, clinicians might consider incorporating into counseling the reading of self-help books that have been written to assist drinkers achieve and maintain moderate use.

Dealing with Problematic Use in the Context of Medical Necessity

The client who both recognizes that his or her cannabis use has become excessive and is partly using cannabis for its medical benefits is likely to bring a number of challenges to counseling. The individual's ability to self-appraise the consequences associated with nonmedical use may be clouded by both resentment of the illegality of usage for medical purposes and the absence of clear protocols to guide the medical-use dosage regimen.

Emerging Knowledge Concerning Cannabis Withdrawal

Although DSM-IV noted that withdrawal in cannabis-dependent individuals had "not yet been reliably shown to be clinically significant," an emerging empirical literature has documented that cessation of use by chronic heavy users may produce a withdrawal syndrome broadly characterized by anger/aggression, decreased appetite or weight loss, irritability, nervousness/anxiety, restlessness, and sleep difficulty or unusual dreaming. Less commonly observed withdrawal symptoms include chills, depressed mood, stomach pain, shakiness, and sweating. (Budney et al., 1999; Crowley et al., 1998; Haney et al., 1999; Jones et al., 1981; Weisbeck et al., 1996).

It is likely that future studies will further explicate withdrawal phenomena in this population and test biomedical and behavioral interventions to ameliorate cannabis withdrawal symptoms. At the present time, however, clinicians need to be prepared to offer cognitive-behavioral skills training as a first-order approach to preparing the client to deal with withdrawal symptoms, and consider short-term medication for clients whose withdrawal experiences are more intense.

INTERVENTION TRIALS WITH TREATMENT-SEEKING ADULTS

The remainder of this chapter reviews intervention trials with cannabis-using adults and adolescents. This review, however, is limited to those studies in which cognitive-behavioral strategies focusing on RP were evaluated. Thus, the following studies are omitted: Morakinyo's (1983) uncontrolled trial in Nigeria in which nine heavy-cannabis-using male adults were treated with aversion therapy (intramuscular emetine to induce nausea), and the supportive–expressive dynamic therapy intervention developed by Grenyer and Solowij (in press).

A second caveat pertains to the multicomponent character of most of the RP interventions tested to date. That is, many of these treatment studies have embedded RP strategies in more broadly encompassing cognitive-behavioral skills training (e.g., relaxation training, boredom management, increasing pleasant activities, self-talk, problem-solving skills). Additionally, motivational enhancement therapy (MET) protocols tested with cannabis-dependent clients have typically included RP modules that are either universally delivered or selectively offered to clients who are motivated to change. Finally, investigators have sometimes tested interventions that combine RP and cognitive-behavioral therapy with contingency management, case management, or something else. In the absence of dismantling studies, at this point only in their infancy in this area of study, it is impossible to know the contribution of each interventive component.

Three-Session Group Cognitive-Behavioral Therapy Intervention Following a 5-Day Course of Aversion Therapy

Smith, Schmeling, and Knowles (1988) reported the results of a single group pretest–posttest design study of 22 adult cannabis smokers who were treated with aversion therapy augmented by cognitive-behavioral skills training. The study participants, who had responded to advertisements placed in local newspapers, had a mean age of 29.8 years (range: 24–40), had been smoking for an average of 13.7 years (range: 7–22), and had smoked an average of 3.4 joints per day (range: 1–8). Treatment began with 5 consecutive days of aversion therapy (mild electric shock, rapid smoking, and quick puffing), with two periods of aversion each day. NIDA-supplied THC-free cigarettes were utilized, with the faradic stimulus being administered while the participant was rolling a joint or smoking it. A portion of each of the 5 aversion treatment days was devoted to self-management counseling, and this counseling continued over the following 3 weeks with weekly group-counseling meetings. The self-management topics included identifying alternatives to cannabis smoking, identifying situations in which temptation to smoke cannabis would be likely and ways of coping with the temptation, listing negative consequences of continued cannabis use, listing anticipated positive consequences from quitting cannabis, establishing balanced diet and regular exercise regimens, and discussing strategies to maintain abstinence (e.g., forming new lifestyle habits, using techniques of stress management, and coping with negative emotional states).

The researchers reported the following rates of self-reported abstinence (defined as no cannabis use since the most recent treatment): conclusion of the 1-month treatment (90.5%), 6 months posttreatment (75.0%), and 12 months posttreatment (84.2%). The researchers concluded that their results, although derived from an uncontrolled trial, indicated the potential efficacy of this treatment approach and recommended that a replication be conducted with a larger sample.

Ten-Session Group Cognitive-Behavioral Therapy Intervention

A 1986–1989 study funded by NIDA compared the effectiveness of a 10-session RP group intervention with a 10-session social support group discussion condition (Stephens, Roffman, & Simpson, 1994).

The RP treatment closely followed the suggested treatment techniques articulated in the first edition of *Relapse Prevention: Maintenance Strategies in the Treatment of Addictive Behaviors* (Marlatt & Gordon, 1985). It focused on strengthening the participant's skills in effectively coping with relapse vulnerabilities. Early treatment elements were designed to enhance motivation for change through identifying the participant's reasons for quitting, offering education about cannabis and its effects, listening to participant's recounting of his or her history of use, and reviewing self-monitoring data in order to identify high-risk situations for relapse. A quit ceremony in the fourth session involved the discarding of paraphernalia and the signing of a contract to formalize commitment. Subsequent sessions involved debriefing recent high-risk situations, noting the successful use of coping strategies, and role-playing ways in which difficult situations could be handled effectively. Exercises, modeling by therapists, homework assignments, and handouts further reinforced key cannabis-cessation skills (e.g., assertion and relaxation). Participants were encouraged to seek support from others in their social network, and lifestyle balance was discussed in the context of how initial changes can be maintained. Participants self-monitored daily activities, and these were debriefed with attention given to seeking a balance between "shoulds" and "wants." Likely cognitive and affective responses to slips were countered with cognitive restructuring that reframed slips as signals of the need for more practice with coping strategies rather than as indications of failure. Participants anticipated seemingly irrelevant decisions that might lead to slips by preparing hypothetical relapse road maps and generating coping alternatives.

The social support treatment emphasized the use of group support for change. Therapists initiated discussions of such topics as getting and giving support, dealing with mood swings, faltering in motivation, identifying and dealing with denial, and relating to peers who continued to use cannabis. While there was some overlap in topics covered in both treatment conditions, the social support treatment did not involve modeling, skills training, or role plays.

The participants were 212 marijuana smokers who averaged over 10 years of near-daily marijuana use. Following the completion of treatment and for the next 2.5 years, during which participants were periodically reassessed, there were no significant differences between conditions in terms of outcomes (abstinence rates, days of marijuana use, problems related to use). During the final 2 weeks of counseling, 63% of the total sample reported being abstinent. While only 14% were continuously abstinent after 1 year, 36% had achieved improvement at that point (i.e., either abstinence or reduction to 50% or less of the baseline use level and no reported marijuana-related problems). At 30 months posttreatment, 28% reported abstinence for the past 90 days. Thus, both counseling approaches were modestly effective in helping a significant percentage of participants achieve either abstinence or improvement.

Fourteen-Session Group Cognitive-Behavioral Therapy

In a second NIDA-funded study (1989–1994), a three-group design with 291 adult daily marijuana smokers permitted the comparison of two active treatments with a delayed-treatment control condition (Stephens, Roffman, & Curtin, 2000). One of the active treatments involved 14 cognitive-behavioral skills training group sessions over a 4-month period, emphasizing both the enhancement of coping capacities in dealing with situations presenting high risk of relapse and the provision of additional time for the building of group cohesion and mutual support. The second active treatment involved two individual MET counseling sessions delivered over a 1-month period. The latter approach appeared promising, inasmuch as a growing literature in the addiction treatment field was supporting the effectiveness of short-term interventions (Bien, Miller, & Tonigan, 1993) utilizing motivational interviewing strategies (Miller & Rollnick, 1991) that are designed to strengthen the individual's readiness to change (e.g., providing participants with normative comparison data concerning their marijuana use patterns). The first session in this condition involved the counselor reviewing with the participant a written Personal Feedback Report generated from data collected during the study's baseline assessments. The counselor used this review as an opportunity to seek elaboration from the participant when expressions of motivation were elicited, to reinforce and strengthen efficacy for change, and to offer support in goal setting and selecting strategies for behavior change. One month later, the second session afforded the opportunity to review efforts and coping skills utilized in the interim period. In both conditions, participants had the option of involving a supporter.

Following treatment, there was no evidence of significant differences between the two active treatments in terms of abstinence rates, days of marijuana use, severity of problems, or number of dependence symptoms. At the 16-month assessment, 29% of group counseling participants and 28% of individual counseling participants reported having been abstinent for the past 90 days. Both active treatments produced substantial reductions in marijuana use, dependence symptoms, and negative consequences relative to the delayed-treatment control participants, who waited 4 months for treatment. The results of this study suggest that minimal interventions may be more cost-effective than extended group counseling efforts for this population.

Six-Session and One-Session Individual Cognitive-Behavioral Therapy

In this Australian study conducted between 1996 and 1998, 229 participants who expressed a desire to quit the use of cannabis were randomly assigned to either a six-session cognitive-behavioral therapy (CBT) treatment, a one-session CBT treatment, or to a delayed-treatment controlled condition (Copeland, Swift, Roffman, & Stephens, 2001).

Both active treatments began with a MET component involving review and discussion of a document ("Your Cannabis Use in Profile") that included feedback from the participant's pretreatment assessment. CBT elements in the six-session condition included behavioral self-monitoring, urge monitoring and management strategies, cannabis withdrawal and its management, social support, drug-refusal skills, cognitive restructuring, identifying and responding to negative thinking, "seemingly irrelevant decisions" that can precede a slip, relaxation training, coping with sleep difficulties, assertiveness, communication and anger management skills, and lifestyle balance to enhance behavior change maintenance. Individuals in the one-session condition received a handbook and worksheets that covered CBT content from the extended treatment.

The participants were predominantly male (69.4%), had a mean age of 32.3 years (range: 18–59), and had been using cannabis at least weekly for a mean of 13.9 years (range: 1–34). The majority were daily or near-daily users, and 96.4% met DSM-IV criteria for cannabis dependence.

Participants were reassessed 24 weeks following treatment completion, with urine-screen data collected to corroborate self-report. Continuous abstinence since treatment completion was reported by 6.5% of the sample (six-session: 15.1%; one-session: 4.9%; delayed-treatment control condition: 0%). The mean percentage of days abstinent reported at follow-up was 37.0% (six-session: 35.9%; one-session: 44.8%; delayed-treatment control condition: 29.7%). There was a marginally significant effect of treatment on complete abstinence in the month prior to follow-up, with those in the active treatments more likely to report abstinence during this period than those in the delayed-treatment control condition (six-session: 20.8%; one-session: 17.2%; delayed-treatment control condition: 3.6%).

Fourteen-Session Individual Cognitive-Behavioral Therapy

In a study funded by NIDA, Budney and colleagues randomly assigned 60 cannabis-dependent adults to one of three 14-week treatments: MET, MET plus coping skills training, or MET plus coping skills training plus voucher-based incentives (Budney, Higgins, Radonovich, & Novy, 2000). In the latter condition, participants who were drug abstinent—documented with twice-weekly urinalysis screening—received vouchers that were exchangeable for retail items (e.g., movie passes, sporting equipment, educational classes, etc.). The value of each voucher increased with consecutively negative specimens. Conversely, the occurrence of a cannabinoid-positive urine specimen or failure to submit a sample was not reinforced and led to a reduction of the next potential voucher's value to its initial level.

The participants were primarily Caucasian (95%) and male (83%), and had a mean age of 32 years (range: 18–48). They reported a 15-year average history of regular cannabis use and had used it an average of 22.5 days per month when enrolled.

Participants in the voucher-based incentive condition were more likely to achieve periods of documented continuous abstinence from cannabis during treatment than were participants in the other two conditions. Additionally, a greater percentage of participants in the voucher-based condition (35%) were abstinent at the end of treatment than was the case in the skills training (10%) or MET (5%) conditions. The absence of long-term posttreatment assessment data limits comparisons of this study's outcomes with those from the other trials discussed earlier. However, based on their earlier research with voucher-based incentives in treating cocaine dependency, the authors were hopeful that future studies would demonstrate successful long-term outcomes in cannabis-dependent participants who achieve and maintain abstinence during treatment.

Nine-Session Individual Cognitive-Behavioral Therapy

A multisite Center for Substance Abuse Treatment-funded trial (1996–2000) employed a three-group design with a delayed-treatment control condition (MTP Research Group, 2004). One of the active treatments involved nine individual counseling sessions delivered over a 12-week period, with the initial sessions focusing on MET and the later content emphasizing cognitive-behavioral skills training and, as needed, case management. The other active treatment involved two individual MET sessions delivered over a 1-month period. (This condition replicated the brief intervention in the previously mentioned 1989–1994 study conducted by Stephens and Roffman). Steinberg and colleagues (2002) offer a detailed discussion of the intervention protocols.

The nine-session multicomponent therapy was designed to permit a tailoring of content and emphasis to meet the needs of a diverse sample. Following the intake assessment, each participant received MET at Weeks 1 and 2. However, the MET protocol offered guidelines for the counselor concerning how, throughout the nine sessions, he or she might acknowledge the client's current stage of change (Prochaska & DiClemente, 1992) (e.g., fully committed to quitting; not motivated to quit, but wishing to become moderate in cannabis use; ambivalent about initiating any change) and assist the participant in how to make use of the upcoming sessions given their outcome goal and current motivational level.

The protocol for case management also permitted tailoring to the needs of individual clients. This module was intended to provide a standardized means of addressing nonsubstance problems that could pose obstacles to the participant's successful achievement of his or her cannabis outcome goals, for example, legal, housing, support, vocational, psychiatric, transportation, parenting, and medical problems. Based on data from the pretreatment assessment battery (and particularly the Addiction Severity Index), as well as the participant's self-report and stated goals, the counselor helped the participant identify problems that would be barriers to abstinence. They subsequently worked together in goal setting, resource identification, the development of a plan to address each target problem, and monitoring progress in goal attainment. For each target problem, the counselor followed up with the participant at every session on the progress he or she had made. Difficulties and obstacles were discussed and revisions of the plan were made as needed. Counselors used motivational strategies as needed to bolster the participant's commitment to working on the target problems. Because clients differed considerably in their needs for case management, counselors were guided by the protocol in devoting more or less time in the nine sessions to this treatment component.

The cognitive-behavioral skills training component of the treatment protocol offered the third opportunity for tailoring to the needs of a diverse clientele. The protocol included five core and five elective CBT modules, and counselors were given latitude in deciding along with the client whether to cover all CBT modules, modify the order in which they were covered, and/or substitute certain electives for core modules. During this phase of the treatment, the counselor guided the client in learning cognitive and behavioral strategies that could be useful both for initiating and maintaining changes in cannabis use. The core sessions were as follows: (1) Understanding Marijuana Use Patterns, (2) Coping with Cravings and Urges to Use, (3) Managing Thoughts about Restarting Marijuana Use, (4) Problem Solving, and (5) Marijuana-Refusal Skills. Five elective modules covered the following areas: (1) Planning for Emergencies/Coping with a Lapse, (2) Seemingly Irrelevant Decisions, (3) Managing Negative Moods and Depression, (4) Assertiveness, and (5) Anger Management.

In the nine-session intervention, up to two sessions could involve the participation of a supportive family member or friend (i.e., significant other). The first session oriented the significant other to the treatment and sought to foster the client's motivation by encouraging the significant other and the participant to discuss the impact of the participant's cannabis use on the relationship or family. The counselor helped the significant other and client formulate a change plan that involved identifying areas where the former could help the participant with treatment goals. The second session debriefed how the significant other and the client had worked with one another, permitted a focus on enhancing their communication skills, and considered how future support for the achievement and maintenance of behavior change could be accomplished.

The 450 participants were primarily male (68%), Caucasian (69%), and employed full-time (69%). Their mean age was 36 and their average number of years of education was 14. On average, participants at enrollment reported using cannabis on 82 of the past 90 days, smoking 3.7 times a day, and being high more than 6 hours a day.

At the 9-month follow-up, both active treatments produced outcomes superior to the 4-month delayed treatment control condition. Further, the nine-session intervention produced significantly greater reductions in cannabis use and associated negative consequences compared to the two-session intervention. Abstinence rates at the 4- and 9-month follow-ups for the nine-session intervention were 23% and 13%, respectively. These differences between the two active treatments were apparent as early as 4 weeks into the treatment period and were sustained throughout the first 9 months of follow-up.

Single Cognitive-Behavioral Therapy Session

In 1997–1998, researchers on the staff of Turning Point, an Australian drug treatment agency in Melbourne, developed and evaluated a single-session intervention (Integrated Brief Intervention) for cannabis users (Lang, Engelander, & Brooke, 2000). Participants were recruited by physicians, health clinics, substance abuse agencies, a telephone information and referral service, and news coverage in local media. Eligibility criteria included self-defined problematic cannabis use, age 16 or older, and absence of a concurrent psychiatric illness or other drug dependence.

The first step for participants was receiving a mailed "pot pack" that included a cannabis use diary in which individuals were encouraged to record their daily goals concerning use and the circumstances related to how, when, where, with whom, and the mood state associated with each use occasion. Then, the 2.5-hour session began with a clinical assessment in which the diary was reviewed and the participant was queried concerning his or her present and future goals and what he or she hoped to achieve from the session. The rest of the session focused on (1) education about psychological and physiological effects of cannabis use; (2) factors, including relationships, that influenced and were affected by the individual's use pattern; and (3) skills and coping strategies, with an emphasis on RP, harm reduction, steps in achieving abstinence or controlled use, and lifestyle changes that would support modifications in the participant's cannabis use. A self-help booklet focusing on cognitive-behavioral strategies was given to the participant to take home.

Data were reported concerning 30 participants who enrolled in this pretest–posttest single-group design study. The participants were primarily male (63%), employed (73%), and single (60%). Their mean age was 29 years (range: 20–34). The majority (73%) had first smoked cannabis prior to the age of 16, and 73% had been using it for 10 or more years. Most (73%) were smoking daily or near-daily prior to the trial.

Follow-up interviews were conducted at 1 and 3 months following treatment. Participants' maximum daily consumption was categorized as 0–10, 11–20, and 21+ "bongs," with three bongs being equivalent to one joint. In contrast with the month prior to treatment, when 70% reported a maximum daily consumption of 21 or more bongs, 24% and 20% reported use at that level when assessed at 1 and 3 months following treatment, respectively. The percentages reporting the lowest maximum daily use levels (0–10 bongs) were 6.7% (pretreatment), 58.6% (1 month posttreatment), and 60% (3 months posttreatment). Paralleling the reduced consumption levels were indications of improved health and social functioning.

Four Individual versus Four Group Motivational Enhancement/Cognitive-Behavioral Therapy Sessions

Individual and group versions of MET and cognitive-behavioral skills training intervention termed "Guided Self-Change" were evaluated in a randomized controlled trial conducted at the Addiction Research Foundation (Sobell, Sobell, Wagner, Agrawal, & Ellingstad, in press). Following a 2-hour individual assessment, participants were randomized to either the individual or group version, received four weekly sessions, were contacted by telephone by counselors at 1 and 3 months posttreatment for aftercare check-ins, and were reassessed at 6 and 12 months following treatment.

The intervention acknowledged that participants might vary in their behavior change goals, that is, some would choose abstinence while others would seek to become moderate users. Components of both the individual and group versions of the intervention included feedback of assessment findings (e.g., extent of use, problem severity), a decisional balance exercise concerning the pros and cons of changing, treatment goal advice and client-directed goal setting, motivational strategies, self-monitoring of use during treatment, readings and homework assignments focusing on identifying high-risk situations and the selection of problem-solving strategies, and a cognitive perspective on relapse management.

Seventeen participants with a cannabis problem were studied. Most were male; their mean age was 30.4 years; they had had some experience in higher education (mean = 13.8 years); and most were employed (mean = 82.4%). These participants perceived their cannabis problem as having been long-standing (mean = 8.4 years), and they were currently daily or near-daily users. Nearly two-thirds (64.7%) chose a moderation outcome goal.

At baseline, treatment completion, and the 12-month follow-up, these participants reported their mean percentage of abstinence days as 10.7%, 54.5%, and 39.6%, respectively.

INTERVENTION TRIALS WITH TREATMENT-SEEKING ADOLESCENTS

Five-Session and 12-Session Individual Motivational Enhancement/Cognitive-Behavioral Therapy

The Cannabis Youth Treatment (CYT) project was a multisite randomized intervention study funded by the Center for Substance Abuse Treatment to test the relative treatment- and cost-effectiveness of five cannabis interventions for adolescents. The interventions included (1) 5-session motivational and cognitive-behavioral therapy (MET/CBT), (2) 12-session motivational and cognitive-behavioral therapy, (3) family support network plus the 12-session motivational and cognitive-behavioral therapy, (4) adolescent community reinforcement approach, and (5) multidimensional family therapy. Participants were reassessed at 3, 6, 9, and 12 months after treatment.

The CYT project recruited 600 adolescent participants between the ages of 12 and 18 who reported smoking marijuana in the past 90 days, reported problems related to marijuana abuse or dependence, and met placement criteria for outpatient substance abuse treatment. The participating adolescents were predominantly male (83%), Caucasian (62%), age 15 or 16 (55%), and attending school (87%). Many also smoked tobacco (80%) and drank alcohol (72%). Over 71% used marijuana weekly and 96% met criteria for abuse or dependence. At the time of admission, 74% had no history of substance abuse treatment and 80% did not believe they had a drug or alcohol problem (Dennis et al., 2004).

Preliminary outcome data support the overall effectiveness of these interventions and compare favorably with findings from prior studies. From intake to 6 months, the percentage of adolescents who reported abstinence increased from 4 to 34%. Evidence of marijuana metabolites in urine decreased from 31 to 25% and the presence of symptoms of marijuana abuse or dependence in the past month decreased from 61 to 19%. Decreases in a range of other behavior problems (e.g., truancy, criminal justice involvement, school problems, family problems, and violence) at 6 months after intake also were evident. Approximately 21% of participants continued to obtain additional treatment in the 3 months following their CYT treatment. There was some evidence for differential effectiveness of the five treatments by problem severity. For example, at 3 months, the five-session MET/CBT treatment was more effective than other treatments in symptom reduction with low-severity adolescents, while family support network was more effective with high-severity adolescents. The CYT provides valuable information regarding the relative effectiveness of five interventions with adolescent marijuana users, most of whom are nonvoluntary, and offers a menu of treatments depending on the severity of substance use problems. Although the CYT identifies effective treatments, the results may apply primarily to adolescents coerced into treatment. Interventions tailored to at-

194

tract voluntary, self-referred adolescents to treatment have not been developed or studied systematically.

Three-Session Individual Motivational Enhancement versus Three-Session Individual Motivational Enhancement/Contingency Management

In study focusing on young probation-referred cannabis abusers, 65 participants (ages 18–25) were randomly assigned to two alternate three-session interventions (Carroll, Sinha, & Easton, in press). All had been referred for evaluation and treatment by the adult probation departments in the Greater New Haven area. All met criteria for cannabis abuse (25%) or dependence (75%).

One condition involved MET while the other augmented MET with contingency management (CM), with vouchers being given for treatment attendance. Elements of the MET intervention included rapport building, providing feedback to participants regarding the effects of marijuana use on their functioning, preparation of a quit contract, involving a significant other in a session in order to enhance social support, formulating a change plan, identifying alternatives to smoking cannabis and ways to avoid high-risk situations, debriefing recent high-risk situations, and skills training in ways of coping with cravings and slips. The contingency management intervention involved the issuance of vouchers of escalating value for prompt session attendance (first session: $25; second session: $35; third session: $45; promptness bonus for each session: $5).

Participants were assessed at baseline, weekly during treatment, at a posttreatment (28-day) interview, and at a 1-month follow-up. Both treatment engagement and self-report of cannabis use were primary outcomes. With reference to engagement, a significantly higher number of participants in the MET/CM condition completed treatment in 28 days. While there were substantial improvements in cannabis use, severity of legal problems, and readiness for change for participants as a whole, there were no significant differences between conditions on the frequency of cannabis use at follow-up.

INTERVENTION TRIALS WITH NON-TREATMENT-SEEKING ADULTS

Adapting Miller's "Drinker's Check-Up" for an adult population of non-treatment-seeking cannabis users, we obtained NIDA funding to evaluate a brief motivational enhancement intervention called "The Marijuana Check-Up" (MCU). For a 1-year period beginning in March 1998, a variety of recruitment strategies targeted adults over the age of 18 who used cannabis and wanted information. These strategies highlighted the objective, nonjudgmental, and confidential approach of the study. All announcements emphasized that the MCU was not a treatment program but rather an opportunity to take stock of one's use.

In a 3(groups) × 4(assessment points) fully randomized clinical trial, 188 participants were randomly assigned to receive (1) personalized feedback (PF; $n = 62$), (2) multimedia feedback (MMF; i.e., information-only condition; $n = 62$), or (3) delayed feedback (DF; $n = 64$). The enrolled sample was composed primarily of individuals who were not considering changing their cannabis use (39%) or who were highly ambivalent about doing so in the near future (30%). Thus, recruitment was successful in capturing the target population of cannabis smokers who were not considering change and who would not be likely to approach formal drug abuse treatment.

Of the 188 participants randomized to treatment, 74% were male and 87% were white. Their mean age was 31.83; they reported using cannabis on an average of 25.47 days per month during the past 90 days; and they smoked cannabis during 2.08 quadrants of the days on which they smoked. Based on Structured Clinical Interview for DSM-IV interviews, 64% met diagnostic criteria for cannabis dependence and, of those who did not meet dependence criteria, 89.4% met criteria for cannabis abuse (American Psychiatric Association, 1994).

The PF feedback session was approximately 90 minutes in length. The interviewer provided the participant with a Personal Feedback Report (PFR) based on his or her initial assessment data. The feedback report consisted of five sections: Your Cannabis Use, Risk Factors, Consequences of Use, Anticipated Consequences of Reducing Use, and Confidence in Avoiding Cannabis Use. Each section presented summaries of the participant's responses that were compared to cannabis users who had sought treatment and completed similar measures in the investigators' previous studies. An accompanying document, "Understanding Your Personal Feedback Report," explained the meaning of the scores in each section and was given to the participant to take home after the feedback session. During the feedback session, the focus was on encouraging the participant to explore the meaning of the information in a nonjudgmental fashion. Any self-motivational statements were reinforced via reflective listening, and resistance was avoided by giving equal attention to any expressed ambivalence about change. When participants clearly expressed a desire to change their cannabis use, counselors supported their efficacy by discussing various change options, including self-assisted change or contacting one of several drug treatment providers in the area. A brief pamphlet on cognitive-behavioral strategies to reduce cannabis use developed in the investigators' treatment research was made available to participants in this condition upon request, and 38% accepted this offer.

The MMF condition was approximately 90 minutes in length. As an information-only control condition, it was intended to be comparable to PF in duration and in contact with a counselor who could provide information on the health and psychological effects of cannabis use. In contrast to the PF condition, the primary focus of the MMF was to inform the client of current scientific information about cannabis. Participants in the MMF condition were met by a counselor who introduced a 30-minute videotaped television documentary titled, "Marijuana: What's Your Poison?" (Bell, 1997). This video was chosen because of its focus on key issues in the study of cannabis effects, its high-quality production, and its even-handedness in discussing the evidence for and against potential beneficial and harmful effects of cannabis use. Originally produced for Australian television, the video offered current scientific knowledge on cannabis via interviews with noted experts in Australia, interspersed with more positive testimonials from actual cannabis users. After the video ended, the counselor returned and led the participant through a more in-depth presentation of empirical findings on cannabis using computerized slides created and presented with Microsoft PowerPoint software. Participants could ask questions at any time, and the counselors attempted to answer the questions factually when they were aware of relevant research. General linear model (GLM) analyses, with treatment condition as the between-subjects factor and time (baseline vs. 7-week follow-up) as the within-subjects factor, revealed a significant condition by time effect on quadrants per smoking day when covarying for stage of change at baseline. Within-group analyses revealed that only participants in the PF condition made significant reductions in days of cannabis use and quadrants of use per day. A time by randomization effect on the proportion of days smoked during a typical week approached statistical significance.

At the 6-month follow-up, 19.6% of those in the PF condition and 10.6% of those in the MMF condition reported having sought treatment for drug use. Although significant between-condition effects were not detected, PF participants appeared somewhat more likely to enter treatment.

The results of this study indicate that the MCU attracted heavy, chronic cannabis users who were ambivalent about reducing their cannabis use. Almost 40% were characterized as precontemplators (i.e., not considering change) and another 30% were characterized as contemplators regarding their current cannabis use. Therefore, they would not have been likely to approach treatment or self-initiate change in the near future. Baseline assessment data showed them to be using cannabis on more than 80% of the days prior to the interventions and typically using it during two or more quadrants of each day. Most participants (64%) met criteria for a diagnosis of cannabis dependence, and they reported an average of four adverse consequences associated with their use. Thus, the MCU was successful in reaching a population of cannabis users who were exhibiting clinically significant impairments.

Outcome analyses indicated that the PF condition produced greater reductions in the amount of cannabis use per day at the 7-week follow-up compared to the MMF and DF control conditions. There was a similar, nearly significant, reduction in the number of days of cannabis use for the PF condition as well. The MMF and DF conditions did not change significantly during this period, further indicating that the population attracted to the MCU was highly ambivalent about change. Unfortunately, the amount of change was modest and not likely to be clinically meaningful. PF participants reduced their use by about 1 day per week and by 0.40 quadrants on the days when they used it. Even these small reductions in use seem to have largely disappeared by the 6-month follow-up, based on our preliminary analyses. Very few participants engaged in any additional efforts to seek treatment or support for change, and there was little evidence that PF participants were any more likely to do so than those in the control conditions.

INTERVENTION TRIALS WITH NON-TREATMENT-SEEKING ADOLESCENTS

Two-Session In-School Motivational Enhancement/Cognitive-Behavioral Therapy

Funded by NIDA, Roffman, Stephens, and Berghuis (Roffman, 2001) completed a single-group, pre–post design study of an ME intervention ("The Teen Marijuana Check-Up" [TMCU]) with adolescent cannabis smokers. The intervention was tailored to be delivered in high schools and to attract adolescents in the precontemplation or contemplation stages of change (Prochaska & DiClemente, 1992). Institutional review board approval was granted for waiving parental consent for participants ages 14 and older.

Marketing and recruitment for the project began in September 1999 and was completed by early April 2000, with most participants learning about the project through presentations given by project staff about cannabis in high school classes such as health education. Other enrollments resulted from referrals by high school counselors, teachers, or concerned parents or friends. Family members or friends who contacted the project received advice on how to communicate their concerns to the adolescent.

The TMCU involved two sessions: an assessment interview and a subsequent feedback session held 1 week later. The individualized baseline assessment session lasted 60–90 minutes. Participants were interviewed regarding their cannabis, alcohol, and other drug use in the past 90 days using time-line follow-back procedures, recent treatment, important personal referents (e.g., family, friends) and these individuals' knowledge of and feelings about the participant's cannabis use, their life goals for the next few years, and how their cannabis use fit with these goals. Self-report questionnaires also were administered regarding the positive and negative effects of smoking cannabis, expected costs and benefits of reducing use, stage of change, depressive symptoms, and immediate goals regarding cannabis.

The PF session was scheduled 1 week after the assessment session and was approximately 60 minutes in length. Each PF session was conducted by the same health educator who administered the participant's baseline assessment, in order to facilitate rapport building. The health educator reviewed with the participant a Personalized Feedback Report regarding his or her use. The report consisted of sections reviewing expected (positive and negative) cannabis effects; personal cannabis, alcohol, and other drug use; anticipated consequences of changing cannabis use; the attitudes of personal referents regarding the participant's cannabis use; and general life and cannabis-related goals. The substance use sections also provided normative comparisons using pie charts to show how participants' levels of substance use compared with other age- and gender-matched adolescents in Washington State. An accompanying document, "Understanding your Personal Feedback Report," explained the meaning of the scores in each section and was given to the participant to take home after the feedback session. While presenting each piece of information, the health educator used motivational interviewing strategies to encourage the participant to explore the meaning of the information in an objective fashion. Any self-motivational statements were reinforced via reflective listening, and resistance was avoided by giving equal attention to ambivalence about change. When participants clearly expressed a desire to change their cannabis use, the health educator supported their efficacy by discussing various change options, including self-assisted change or contacting one of several drug treatment providers in the area. The health educator also facilitated a process of goal setting and strategizing, including review and completion of a change plan worksheet the participant could take home. A brief pamphlet on coping strategies to reduce cannabis use was provided to participants upon request. One additional session was offered, as needed.

Eligibility criteria required participants to be 14–18 years of age, to have smoked cannabis at least once in the past 30 days, to be literate English speakers, and not to have evidence of significant psychiatric impairment that would diminish their ability to participate in the project. Participants were given two $15 gift certificates (one at the beginning of the feedback session and one at the time of the follow-up assessment session). All were reassessed at a 3-month follow-up session by a health educator who had not delivered the baseline assessment or feedback session to this individual, in order to reduce demand characteristics.

Fifty-four participants completed the assessment, feedback, and 3-month follow-up sessions and were included in the analyses. The typical participant was a 15-year-old white male who lived with his parents. On average, participants reported smoking cannabis on 10 of the last 30 days (range = 1–30). Due to the wide range in frequency of smoking, the sample was divided into lighter (8 days or less in last 30 days; n = 27) and heavier (9+ days in last 30 days; n = 27) smoker comparison groups. This cutoff was chosen because it hypothetically distinguished between participants who smoked primarily on weekends (on average 2 or fewer days per week) from those who smoked more frequently (over 2 days per week on average). Heavier smokers reported greater importance of continuing their current level of smoking than lighter smokers and anticipated a greater number of adverse consequences if they were to reduce or cease their use. While a majority of participants had attempted on multiple occasions to voluntarily reduce (56%) or stop (80%) their cannabis use, more than half of the heavier users were not currently committed to change.

Reductions in cannabis use were found at the 3-month follow-up, specifically among heavier smokers. Forty-four percent of participants (n = 24) reported having made voluntary reductions in their cannabis use since the intervention, and almost 15% (n = 8) reported abstinence from cannabis in the 30 days prior to their follow-up session. Marginally significant increases in alcohol use also were evident at follow-up among heavier users, suggesting that these participants may have increased their alcohol use while reducing their cannabis use. In terms of stage of change, reductions in the ambivalence and problem-recognition subscales of the Stages of Change Rates (SOCRATES; Hewes & Janikowski, 1998) were evident at follow-up. Non-white ethnicity and being a heavier smoker at baseline were associated with reductions in cannabis use.

The findings from this exploratory research indicate that the TMCU was able to effectively recruit and retain voluntary non-treatment-seeking adolescent cannabis smokers, nearly half of whom were in the precontemplation or contemplation stages of change. The follow-up interviews offered evidence for reductions in cannabis use following the intervention, particularly among the heavier smokers and persons of color. Alcohol use may need to be addressed further in future interventions to discourage potential increased use of alcohol in correspondence to reduced use of cannabis (i.e., substance substitution).

SUMMARY OF CANNABIS OUTCOME STUDIES WITH RELAPSE PREVENTION INTERVENTIONS

The empirical literature on tested cannabis interventions has grown considerably since the late 1980s. RP strategies have been incorporated in all of the 12 trials considered, sometimes augmented by treatment components focusing on aversion training, motivational enhancement, contingency reinforcement, and case management. In this chapter we have briefly discussed 10 outcome studies, 8 of which were controlled, in which RP interventions were evaluated with treatment-seeking adults or adolescents. Two other RP trials, one of which was controlled, evaluated tailored motivational enhancement therapy approaches for non-treatment-seeking adults and adolescents, respectively, who smoked marijuana and were at early stages of readiness of change.

In some respects, intervention research focusing on cannabis abuse and dependence remains in its infancy. Very few efforts to replicate earlier findings have been made, and little can be said about the generalizability of outcomes to diverse populations. The variety of outcome measures and follow-up assessment time frames utilized make synthesis difficult, and the extent to which these treatments led to the achievement of either durable cannabis cessation or reduced use to a nonproblem level is quite modest. Nonetheless, this body of empirical work represents a solid beginning in understanding how to reach and effectively support individuals whose cannabis use is causing harm. Increased knowledge concerning the efficacy of behavioral interventions has paralleled the emergence of important findings concerning the biological bases for cannabis dependence. Given the epidemiological data concerning cannabis abuse and dependence presented at the beginning of this chapter, the public health will be served by greater attention devoted to designing and testing cannabis interventions based on both behavioral and biological knowledge.

CANNABIS OUTCOME STUDIES AND RELAPSE PREVENTION THEORY

In the following section we discuss data from cannabis outcome trials that speak to theory concerning relapse and RP.

Relapse Situations

RP theory predicts that slips back into substance use after successful treatment are more likely to occur when former users encounter high-risk situations. The identification of high-risk situations is an early strategy in the RP treatment approach and sets the stage for the training of coping skills to reduce the probability of using the substance in those situations. These high-risk situations are assumed to be idiographic, but prior research has shown there to be surprising commonalities in the types of situations that precipitate slips and ultimately relapses. Negative emotional states, interpersonal conflict, and direct social pressure to use are the most common precipitating situations across samples of alcohol abusers, cigarette smokers, and heroin addicts (Marlatt & Gordon, 1985).

High-risk situations for relapse were investigated in a sample of adult marijuana users following either RP or group discussion treatment (Stephens,

Roffman, & Simpson, 1994). Questionnaire data collected from 103 participants who had become abstinent for at least 7 days revealed that the most common precipitating situations for a slip were negative emotional states (33%), direct social pressure (24%), and positive emotional states (22%). The larger role of positive emotional states in precipitating a return to marijuana use compared to other drugs suggests that some heavy marijuana users frequently use the drug to enhance already positive emotions. Thus, treatment needs to identify this function of marijuana use in order to develop alternative strategies.

Self-Efficacy and Coping Skills

Key tenets of the RP approach include the development of situation-specific coping skills in order to enhance self-efficacy for resisting or avoiding drug use. Coping skill training is the central component of these interventions, and the acquisition of coping skills and associated self-efficacy are proposed to be the cognitive-behavioral mediators of the effect of treatment. At least two studies have evaluated their roles in the outcomes of treatment for marijuana use problems.

Stephens and colleagues (Stephens, Wertz, & Roffman, 1993, 1995) showed that self-efficacy for avoiding marijuana use in high-risk situations predicted less frequent marijuana use during the posttreatment follow-up period. Self-efficacy increased significantly from baseline to the end of treatment, and efficacy ratings at the end of treatment were generally better predictors than pretreatment ratings. Both baseline and end of treatment self-efficacy explained unique variation in outcomes after controlling for demographic, socioeconomic, psychological distress, contact with other users, and coping variables. Consistent with theory, self-efficacy was one of the strongest predictors of decreased marijuana use after treatment. Theoretical sources of self-efficacy, such as success in limiting marijuana use and the likelihood of using coping skills, were shown to predict efficacy judgments, but self-efficacy only partially mediated the effects of these variables on posttreatment outcomes (Stephens et al., 1995). Further, the RP treatment produced only marginally greater self-efficacy ratings than a group discussion comparison treatment in this study, and ratings of the likelihood of using cognitive-behavioral coping skills did not differ between conditions. Thus, although efficacy increased after treatment and predicted posttreatment outcomes, it was not clearly related to the training and acquisition of coping skills. A recent review of CBT for alcohol dependence also failed to find support for the notion that it works by increasing cognitive and behavioral coping skills (Morgenstern & Longabaugh, 2000). It remains possible that measurement of coping skill acquisition and use is inadequate, but it also may be that these treatments engender changes in marijuana or alcohol use and associated self-efficacy by increasing motivation or through other nonspecific effects rather than through the training of coping skills.

The Abstinence Violation Effect

The RP model predicts that lapses back into substance use after a period of abstinence are more likely to result in a full-blown relapse if the individual attributes the cause of the lapse to internal, stable, and global factors. The abstinence violation effect (AVE) then occurs when this attributional pattern leads to increased feelings of loss of control and guilt, which further propels the individual toward a return to regular substance use. Stephens and colleagues (Stephens, Curtin, Simpson, & Roffman, 1994) examined the attributions of 103 adult marijuana users who had completed either RP or group discussion treatment and who had achieved at least 7 days of abstinence before slipping and using marijuana at least once. Participants reported on the situation in which the slip occurred and then rated the degree to which the cause of the slip was due to something about themselves (internal), likely to be present in the future (stable), and applied to more than just their drug use (global). Participants also rated their feelings of guilt and loss of control following the slip. Participants who returned to regular marijuana use following the slip were more likely to show the proposed attributional pattern and a greater sense of loss of control than participants who returned to abstinence. Feelings of guilt did not distinguish the groups. Internal and global attributions for the cause of the first slip were also shown to predict frequency of marijuana use at future follow-up, suggesting that these attributions were more than post-hoc explanations. Interestingly, the tendency to experience the AVE did not differ between participants who had received the RP versus the group discussion treatments, despite efforts in the RP treatment to educate and prevent the pathological attributional pattern.

SUMMARY

According to the 2001 National Household Survey on Drug Abuse, more than two million individuals met diagnostic criteria for dependence on cannabis. In contrast, data from 2001 indicate that 263,718 individuals who entered drug treatment reported that cannabis was their primary drug of abuse. While it is likely that many cannabis-dependent individuals successfully resolve their dependence on their own or through interventions outside of the drug treatment system, these data suggest that cannabis dependence is an underserved phenomenon.

Promising results from trials with adults and adolescents with cannabis use disorders indicate that counseling interventions can be of positive benefit. However, the field is still at an early stage in designing and evaluating interventions for this population, and the outcomes found thus far in controlled studies are modest. Recent discoveries concerning the biological basis for cannabis dependence are likely to eventually contribute to the development and evaluation of pharmaceutical agents in the treatment of this disorder, either in terms of supporting individuals in the initial acquisition of abstinence or in maintaining behavior change in the long term.

From a harm reduction perspective, cannabis moderation deserves more study, and the testing of interventions designed to support moderation outcome goals is warranted. While clearly posing political challenges due to the illegality of cannabis, it is likely that moderation is perceived as a preferable outcome by a substantial number of individuals who seek treatment for cannabis dependence. As an example, in a currently underway controlled trial we are conducting with cannabis-dependent participants who sought treatment, 67% enrolled with the desire to achieve abstinence, while 33% wanted to achieve moderation. When reassessed at 4 months following enrollment, 27% had changed their goal from abstinence to moderation, and 7% from moderation to abstinence. Inherent in this work will be dealing with the conceptual, intervention, and measurement challenges in defining cannabis moderation and understanding factors that contribute over time to what an individual aspires to accomplish and achieves. For example, is moderation sought because abstinence has been too difficult to initiate and/or maintain, or because it is unnecessary in order to avoid adverse consequences? Is the prospect of smoking cannabis moderately and without harm more viable for individuals with selected profiles but not for others?

The relatively modest long-term outcomes reported in the trials conducted thus far also suggest that varying models of intervention time frames (e.g., duration of counseling availability, dosage-delivery intensity) ought to be developed and tested. Tested interventions in the substance abuse field have tended to involve fixed dosages delivered in a fixed time frame (e.g., 10 sessions over 10 weeks, 18 sessions over 6 months, 8 sessions plus two aftercare sessions at scheduled intervals). Because successful outcomes often follow multiple treatment exposures, chronic care intervention models that permit clients greater latitude (e.g., in taking breaks from counseling and returning for additional sessions as needed over a several-year period) need to be developed and evaluated.

Finally, there is a relative paucity of information concerning the mechanisms through which motivational enhancement therapy and cognitive-behavioral therapy interventions effect change. Greater attention is needed to assessing shifts in client readiness to change and training clinicians to be capable of sensitively refocusing their work to fit with these shifts. The "check-up" and treatment interventions discussed in this chapter offer evidence that cannabis-dependent clients at varying stages of readiness for change can be reached and enrolled. The modest outcomes, however, suggest that the intervention protocols developed thus far offer too little sensitivity to effectively meet the needs of this population.

REFERENCES

American Psychiatric Association. (1994). *Diagnostic and statistical manual of mental disorders* (4th ed.). Washington, DC: Author.

Anthony, J. C., Warner, L. A., & Kessler, R. C. (1994). Comparative epidemiology of dependence on tobacco, alcohol, controlled substances, and inhalants: Basic findings from the National Comorbidity Survey. *Experimental and Clinical Psychopharmacology, 2,* 244–268.

Babor, T. D. (in press). The classification and diagnosis of cannabis dependence. In R. A. Roffman & R. S. Stephens (Eds.), *Cannabis dependence: Its nature, consequences, and treatment.* Cambridge, UK: Cambridge University Press.

Bell, J. (Producer). (1997). *Quantum—What's Your Poison—Marijuana.* Sydney: Australian Broadcasting Corporation.

Bien, T. H., Miller, W. R., & Tonigan, S. (1993). Brief interventions for alcohol problems: A review. *Addiction, 88,* 315–336.

Budney, A. J., Higgins, S. T., Radonovich, K. J., & Novy, P. L. (2000). Adding voucher-based incentives to coping skills and motivational enhancement improves outcomes during treatment for marijuana dependence. *Journal of Consulting and Clinical Psychology, 8,* 1051–1061.

Budney, A. J., Novy, P., & Hughes, J. R. (1999). Marijuana withdrawal among adults seeking treatment for marijuana dependence. *Addiction, 94*(9), 1311–1321.

Carroll, K. M., Sinha, R., & Easton, C. (in press). Engaging young probation-referred marijuana-abusing individuals in treatment. In R. A. Roffman & R. S. Stephens (Eds.), *Cannabis dependence: Its nature, consequences, and treatment.* Cambridge, UK: Cambridge University Press.

Compton, W. M., Grant, B. F., Colliver, J. D., Glantz, M. D., & Stinson, F. S. (2004). Prevalence of marijuana use disorders in the United States: 1991–1992 and 2001–2002. *Journal of the American Medical Association, 291*(17), 2114–2121.

Copeland, J., Swift, W., & Rees, V. (2001). Clinical profile of participants in a brief intervention program for cannabis use disorder. *Journal of Substance Abuse Treatment, 20,* 45–52.

Copeland, J., Swift, W., Roffman, R., & Stephens, R. (2001). A randomized controlled trial of brief cognitive-behavioral interventions for cannabis use disorders. *Journal of Substance Abuse Treatment, 21,* 55–64.

Crowley, T. J., Macdonald, M. J., Whitmore, E. A., & Mikulich, S. K. (1998). Cannabis dependence, withdrawal, and reinforcing effects among adolescents with conduct disorder symptoms and substance use disorders. *Drug and Alcohol Dependence, 50,* 27–37.

Degenhardt, L., Hall, W., & Lynskey, M. (2001). The relationship between cannabis use, depression and anxiety among Australian adults: Findings from the national survey of mental health and well-being. *Social Psychiatry and Psychiatric Epidemiology, 36,* 219–227.

Dennis, M. L., Godley, S. H., Diamond, G., Tims, F. M., Babor, T., Donaldson, J., Liddle, H., Titus, J. C., Kaminer, Y., Webb, C., Hamilton, N., & Funk, R. (2004). The Cannabis Youth Treatment (CYT) Study: Main findings from two randomized trials. *Journal of Substance Abuse Treatment, 27,* 193–213.

Devane, W. A., Dysarz, F. A., Johnson, M. R., Melvin, L. S., & Howlett, A. C. (1988). Determination and characterization of a cannabinoid receptor in rat brain. *Molecular Pharmacology, 34,* 605–613.

Devane, W. A., Hanus, L., Breuer, A., Pertwee, R. G., Stevenson, L. A., Griffin, G., Gibson, D., Mandelbaum, A., Etinger, A., & Mechoulam, R. (1992). Isolation and structure of a brain constituent that binds to the cannabinoid receptor. *Science, 258,* 1946–1949.

Earleywine, M. (2002). *Understanding marijuana: A new look at the scientific evidence.* New York: Oxford University Press.

Gfroerer, J. C., Wu, L., & Penne, M. A. (2002). *Initiation of marijuana use: Trends, patterns, and implications.* Rockville, MD: Department of Health and Human Services, Substance Abuse and Mental Health Services Administration, Office of Applied Studies.

Grant, P. F., & Pickering, R. (1998). The relationship between cannabis use and DSM-IV cannabis use and dependence: Results from the national longitudinal alcohol epidemiology study. *Journal of Substance Abuse, 10,* 255–264.

Grenyer, B., & Solowij, N. (in press). Supportive–expressive psychotherapy for cannabis dependence. In R. A. Roffman & R. S. Stephens (Eds.), *Cannabis dependence: Its nature, consequences, and treatment.* Cambridge, UK: Cambridge University Press.

Haney, M., Ward, A. S., Comer, S. D., Foltin, R. W., & Fischman, M. W. (1999). Abstinence symptoms following smoked marijuana in humans. *Psychopharmacology, 141,* 395–404.

Hewes, R. L., & Janikowski, T. P. (1998). Readiness for change and treatment outcome among individuals with alcohol dependency. *Rehabilitation Counseling Bulletin, 42*(1), 76–93.

Jones, R. T., Benowitz, N. L., & Herning, R. I. (1981). Clinical relevance of cannabis tolerance and dependence. *Journal of Clinical Pharmacology, 21,* 1435–152S.

Lang, E., Engelander, M., & Brooke, T. (2000). Report of an integrated brief intervention with self-defined problem cannabis users. *Journal of Substance Abuse Treatment, 19,* 111–116.

Marlatt, G. A., & Gordon, J. R. (1985). *Relapse prevention: Maintenance strategies in the treatment of addictive behaviors* (1st ed.). New York: Guilford Press.

McBride, C. M., Curry, S. J., Stephens, R. S., Wells, E. A., Roffman, R. A., & Hawkins, J. D. (1994). Intrinsic and extrinsic motivation for change in cigarette smokers, marijuana smokers, and cocaine users. *Psychology of Addictive Behaviors, 8,* 243–250.

Miller, W. R., & Rollnick, S. (1991). *Motivational interviewing: Preparing people to change addictive behavior.* New York: Guilford Press.

Morakinyo, O. (1983). Aversion therapy of cannabis dependence in Nigeria. *Drug and Alcohol Dependence, 12,* 287–293.

Morgenstern, J., & Longabaugh, R. (2000). Cognitive-behavioral treatment for alcohol dependence: A review of evidence for its hypothesized mechanisms of action. *Addiction, 95,* 1474–1490.

MTP Research Group. (in press). Brief treatments for cannabis dependence: Findings from a randomized multi-site trial. *Journal of Consulting and Clinical Psychology, 72,* 455–466.

National Institute on Drug Abuse, Division of Epidemiology and Prevention Research. (1991). *National household survey on drug abuse: Main findings 1990.* Rockville, MD: Department of Health and Human Services.

Prochaska, J. O., & DiClemente, C. C. (1992). The transtheoretical approach. In J. C. Norcross & M. R. Goldfried (Eds.), *Handbook of psychotherapy integration.* New York: Basic Books.

Rinaldi-Carmona, M., Barth, F., Heaulme, M., Shire, D., Calandra, B., Congy, C., Martinez, S., Maruani, J., Neliat, G., Caput, D., Ferrara, P., Soubrie, P., Breliere, J. C., & LeFur, G. (1994). SR 141716A, a potent and selective antagonist of the brain cannabinoid receptor. *FEBS Letters, 350,* 240–244.

Roffman, R. A. (2001, January). *Motivating adolescent marijuana use cessation: Results of a pilot study.* Presentation at the 5th annual conference of the Society for Social Work and Research, Atlanta.

Smith, J. W., Schmeling, G., & Knowles, P. L. (1988). A marijuana smoking cessation clinical trial utilizing THC-free marijuana, aversion therapy, and self-management counseling. *Journal of Substance Abuse Treatment, 5,* 89–98.

Sobell, L. C., Sobell, M. B., Wagner, E. F., Agrawal, S., & Ellingstad, T. P. (in press). Guided self-change: A brief motivational intervention for cannabis users. In R. A. Roffman & R. S. Stephens (Eds.), *Cannabis dependence: Its nature, consequences, and treatment.* Cambridge, UK: Cambridge University Press.

Steinberg, K. L., Roffman, R. A., Carroll, K. M., Kabela, E., Kadden, R., Miller, M., Duresky, D., & the Marijuana Treatment Project Research Group. (2002). Tailoring cannabis dependence treatment for a diverse population. *Addiction, 97*(Suppl. 1), 135–142.

Stephens, R. S., Babor, T. F., Kadden, R., Miller, M., & the Marijuana Treatment Project Research Group. (2002). The Marijuana Treatment Project: Rationale, design, and participant characteristics. *Addiction, 97,* 109–124.

Stephens, R. S., Curtin, L., Simpson, E. E., & Roffman, R. A. (1994). Testing the abstinence violation effect construct with marijuana cessation. *Addictive Behaviors, 19,* 23–32.

Stephens, R. S., & Roffman, R. A. (2005). Assessment of cannabis use disorders. In D. Donovan & G. A. Marlatt (Eds.), *Assessment of addictive behaviors* (2nd ed.). New York: Guilford Press.

Stephens, R. S., Roffman, R. A., & Curtin, L. (2000) Comparison of extended versus brief treatments for marijuana use. *Journal of Consulting and Clinical Psychology, 68,* 898–908.

Stephens, R. S., Roffman, R. A., & Simpson, E. E. (1993). Adult marijuana users seeking treatment. *Journal of Consulting and Clinical Psychology, 61,* 1100–1104.

Stephens, R. S., Roffman, R. A., & Simpson, E. E. (1994). Treating adult marijuana dependence: A test of the relapse prevention model. *Journal of Consulting and Clinical Psychology, 62,* 92–99.

Stephens, R. S., Wertz, J. S., & Roffman, R. A. (1993). Predictors of marijuana treatment outcomes: The role of self-efficacy. *Journal of Substance Abuse, 5,* 341–353.

Stephens, R. S., Wertz, J. S., & Roffman, R. A. (1995). Self-efficacy and marijuana cessation: A construct validity analysis. *Journal of Consulting and Clinical Psychology, 63,* 1022–1031.

Substance Abuse and Mental Health Services Administration. (2003). *Results from the 2002 National Survey on Drug Use and Health: National Findings* (NHSDA Series H-22; DHHS Publication No. SMA 03–3836). Rockville, MD: Department of Health and Human Services, Substance Abuse and Mental Health Services Administration, Office of Applied Studies.

Tims, F. M., Dennis, M. L., Hamilton, D., Buchan, B. J., Diamond, G., Funk, R., & Brantley, L. B. (2002). Characteristics and problems of 600 adolescent cannabis abusers in outpatient treatment. *Addiction, 97*(1), 46–57.

Wagner, F. A., & Anthony, J. C. (2002). From first drug use to drug dependence: Developmental periods of risk for dependence upon marijuana, cocaine, and alcohol. *Neuropsychopharmacology, 26,* 479–88.

Weisbeck, G. A., Schuckit, M. A., Kalmijn, J. A., Tipp, J. E., Bucholz, K. K., & Smith, T. L. (1996). An evaluation of the history of marijuana withdrawal syndrome in a large population. *Addiction, 91,* 1469–1478.

World Health Organization (WHO). (1964). *WHO expert Committee on Addiction—Producing Drugs, 13th report, Technical report series no. 273.* Geneva: Author.

CHAPTER 8

Relapse Prevention for Abuse of Club Drugs, Hallucinogens, Inhalants, and Steroids

Jason R. Kilmer
Jessica M. Cronce
Rebekka S. Palmer

Previous chapters in this book have addressed alcohol, tobacco, cocaine, heroin, marijuana, and methamphetamine problems and the implications for treatment. Although there are several other drugs of abuse beyond those listed, this chapter focuses on substances for which trends in national data have suggested that significant treatment and relapse prevention (RP) issues in counseling, clinical, and treatment settings are emerging. These substances include club drugs (such as Ecstasy, GHB, and ketamine), hallucinogens and dissociative drugs, inhalants, and steroids.

Since 1996, the majority of high school seniors have reported illicit drug use in their lifetime, with 53.0% of students reporting such use in 2002. Illicit drug use is not unique to this age group, given that one in four eighth graders now report that they have used at least one illicit drug in their lifetime (Johnston, O'Malley, & Bachman, 2003). Increasingly, use is becoming more widespread of substances that are derivatives of other drugs or chemical creations for which no dosing information or potency is evident to the user, for which adulterants are quite likely, and from which immediate harm is possible. Despite showing an annual increase in use since 1998, with the largest increase of any drug in 2001 (Johnston et al.,

2002), data from the Monitoring the Future study (Johnston et al., 2003) indicate that Ecstasy (MDMA) use declined over 2002. While trends in past-year use of other club drugs did not change significantly from 2001 to 2002, prevalence rates among high school seniors remained higher than for heroin or PCP. The Monitoring the Future researchers also reported that use of anabolic steroids by high school seniors had increased significantly in 2001, followed by no change in 2002. Past-year use of inhalants has decreased significantly since peaking in 1999, with 12.2% of eighth graders in 1996 reporting past-year use decreasing to 7.7% in 2002. Yet there was no significant change in past-30-day use, and inhalants remain the drug of choice for substances other than alcohol, tobacco, and marijuana for eighth graders, the youngest students in the Monitoring the Future sample.

Among people 12 years of age and older, the number of new users of hallucinogens and inhalants is increasing dramatically. The National Household Survey on Drug Abuse (Substance Abuse and Mental Health Services Administration, 2001) showed that the number of new users of hallucinogens and inhalants is at its highest level since 1965. Thirty-nine percent of respondents over the age of 12 report lifetime use of at least one illicit drug.

Likely related to these substance use increases is the popularity of the "rave" or "club" scene—social events associated with "electronic" or "house" music, hundreds to thousands of people and, typically, drugs. Specifically associated with these gatherings are three club drugs that represent the focus of treatment issues in this chapter: Ecstasy (3,4-methylenedioxy-methamphetamine), ketamine, and gamma-hydroxybutyrate (GHB). The latter two have received attention as drugs used in sexual assaults (i.e., "date rape drugs") and have now joined Rohypnol (flunitrazepam) as substances that share this distinction. Ketamine and GHB are examples of drugs with legitimate medical purposes being used outside the realm of their original intent in recreational ways (Weiner, 2000).

Hallucinogens also are addressed, given the data reflecting new users, and this chapter addresses LSD. Dextromethorphan, a cough suppressant found in most over-the-counter cough syrups, is a dissociative anesthetic that, at high doses, can cause a complete sense of dissociation from one's body and can be followed by lingering perceptual problems. Clinical issues relevant to its abuse are discussed.

A peculiar classification issue for some is the inclusion of common household products in a discussion of drug use and abuse. However, when misused as inhalants, a diagnosis of abuse or dependence is possible. When one looks over the list of commonly abused inhalants, including dry-cleaning fluids, gasoline, glues, correction fluids, markers, whipping cream aerosols or dispensers, spray paints, hair sprays, deodorant sprays, and fabric protector sprays, clearly these are chemicals not meant for consumption. Nevertheless, these are substances are being used, and severe short- or long-term consequences could accompany this use.

Finally, while not a substance used socially, the increase in anabolic androgenic steroids demonstrated in the Monitoring the Future study suggests that issues related to treatment of steroid use will need closer consideration. Risky injection practices, such as needle sharing, put steroid users at risk for additional negative consequences outside the realm of the effects of the substance itself.

To understand RP and treatment issues with these substances, one must understand the effects of the use of these drugs and ways in which they may surface in clinical settings. The preceding drugs are described by reviewing what the drug is, what its street names are, the history of the drug, and the risks associated with or negative consequences following use. After this review, we discuss specific RP and treatment issues relevant to these substances.

INFORMATION ON DRUGS OF ABUSE

MDMA/Ecstasy

MDMA is a synthetic derivative of amphetamine that has both stimulant and hallucinogenic qualities (National Institute on Drug Abuse, 2001a). Commonly referred to as Ecstasy, MDMA has been distributed under several other pseudonyms, including Adam, Clarity, E, Lover's Speed, X, and XTC (Office of National Drug Control Policy, 2002a).

MDMA was initially patented by Merck, a German pharmaceutical company, in 1914 (Parrott, 2001; Shulgin, 1986). Some reports suggest that it was tested as a potential appetite suppressant (Kalant, 2001), while other sources indicate that its development was strictly experimental without planned application (McDowell, 1999). Military applications of MDMA were later explored in experimental trials conducted by the U.S. Army in the 1950s; however, the project was abandoned after disappointing results (Gahlinger, 2001; Grob & Poland, 1997). MDMA resurfaced sometime during the mid-1960s to 1970s after a biochemist, Dr. Alexander Shulgin, reproduced the drug (Parrott, 2001; Sharma, 2001). In initial experimental testing with humans, MDMA was noted for its ability to induce euphoric mental states (Shulgin & Nichols, 1978), and it was soon employed as an adjunct to psychotherapy by some members of the clinical community (Greer & Tolbert, 1986; Morgan, 1997). Although it is unclear precisely when MDMA was first used recreationally, by 1984 its large-scale production and distribution in the southern United States drew the interest of various political and law enforcement entities (McDowell, 1999; Morgan, 1997). In 1985, MDMA was classified as a Schedule I drug, making it illegal for recreational and clinical use (Lawn, 1985).

Recreational use of MDMA has been documented in a number of contexts, but it is most often associated with "raves" and dance clubs (Spiess, 2002; Schwartz & Miller, 1997). MDMA is available in tablet and powder form and is typically ingested; however, it can be snorted, smoked, inserted into the rectum, or administered intravenously (Parrott, 2001). Tablets come in a number of colors with various logos, presumably to help identify their origin (Cole, Bailey, Sumnall, Wagstaff, & King, 2002). A typical dose consists of one to two 100 milligram tablets (Drug Enforcement Administration, 2004a; Parrott & Lasky, 1998; Parrott et al., 2002); however, a percentage of more frequent users have reported using three or more tablets per occasion (Parrott et al., 2002). The exact amount of MDMA in each tablet can vary widely making its use particularly dangerous and difficult to assess. Examination of tablets purported to be MDMA has revealed that they contained one or more of a number of adulterants, including methylenedioxyamphetamine (MDA), amphetamine, ketamine, and dextromethorphan, and in some cases did not contain any MDMA at all (Cole et al., 2002; Parrott, 2004).

The positive subjective effects of MDMA, including euphoria, increased sociability and connection with others, and elevated levels of energy take effect in under an hour and can last up to six hours, usually peaking after 2 hours (Cohen, 1995; National Institute on Drug Abuse, 2001b; Tancer & Johanson, 2001). In an effort to prolong the positive effects, users of MDMA will often consume an additional dose after the first dose has peaked (National Institute on Drug Abuse, 2001a). Negative psychological effects, including depression, irritability, paranoia, and anxiety, have also been reported following ingestion of MDMA (Cohen, 1995; Williamson et al., 1997). Negative affective states are often experienced within a few days following use (Parrott & Lasky, 1998). Common physiological effects of MDMA include elevated heart rate and blood pressure, and dysregulation of body temperature (de la Torre, 2000). Often water is consumed in large quantities to help control body temperature and avoid dehydration following vigorous exercise (e.g., dancing), but this can in itself cause health complications and in some cases death by disrupting the normal balance of electrolytes in the body (Hartung, Schofield, Short, Parr, Henry, 2002; Parrott, 2001; Traub, Hoffman & Nelson, 2002). Memory impairments (Bolla, McCann, & Ricaurte, 1998), irregularities in heart rhythm, tension of the facial muscles, nausea, vomiting, disordered eating, and sleep disruptions, among a host of other health complications, have also been associated with MDMA use (Kalant, 2001; McCann, Slate, & Ricaurte, 1996; Parrott, 2001).

A recent study found that use of MDMA had a detrimental effect on immune system functioning, and that this effect was even more pronounced when alcohol was consumed concurrently (Pacifici et al., 2001).

This finding has broad implications given that alcohol is often consumed on the same occasion as MDMA (Schifano, Di Furia, Forza, Minicuci, & Bricolo, 1998). MDMA has also been implicated in adverse reactions that resulted in hospitalization and death among HIV-positive patients taking the drug in addition to their antiretroviral medication (Antoniou & Tseng, 2002; Harrington, Woodward, Hooton, & Horn, 1999).

Profound psychological and physiological effects have been reported after ingestion of MDMA on as few as one or two occasions, including catatonia (Masi, Mucci, & Floriani, 2002), psychosis (Van Kampen & Katz, 2001), panic disorder (McCann & Ricaurte, 1992), partial deafness and tinnitus (Sharma, 2001), and hepatitis (Andreu et al., 1998). Flashbacks, while more typically associated with hallucinogens such as LSD, have also been linked to isolated cases of reported MDMA use (Creighton, Black, & Hyde, 1991).

The extant scientific evidence indicates that MDMA is a neurotoxin (i.e., damages neurons in the brain), the effects of which may be present after a single use and may not be reversible. Several studies have been conducted using nonhuman primate and other animal populations to explore the nature of MDMA's effect on serotonin neurons (see Ricaurte, Yuan, & McCann, 2000, for a review). Studies with human populations have found that regular MDMA users (defined as individuals who have taken MDMA on 25 or more occasions) have significantly lower levels of 5-hydroxy-indoleacetic acid (5-HIAA) in their cerebrospinal fluid compared to controls, which may be indicative of serotonin neurotoxicity (McCann, Ridenour, Shaham, & Ricaurte, 1994) and have reduced serotonin (5-HT) transporter density compared to controls, with density being negatively correlated with the extent of previous MDMA use (McCann, Szabo, Scheffel, Dannals, & Ricaurte, 1998).

Despite the growing body of evidence showing the potential for harm associated with MDMA use, the drug continues to be used, especially by adolescents. Over 10% of high school seniors have used MDMA in their lifetime, and almost 60% of seniors say MDMA is fairly easy or very easy to get (Johnston et al., 2003). While MDMA appears to have the potential for abuse and dependence, more research needs to be conducted evaluating long-term use and outcomes of quit attempts.

Ketamine

Ketamine hydrochloride (ketamine) is a synthetic substance classified as a dissociative anesthetic (National Institute on Drug Abuse, 2001c). Ketamine has a number of legitimate medical and veterinary uses in addition to its illicit use as a consciousness-altering drug, and is known by both pharmaceutical trade names, such as Ketalar, Ketajet, Ketaset, Ketavet, and Vetelar (Gahlinger, 2001; Siegel, 1978), and street names, including Kit

Kat, Special K, Cat Valium, and Vitamin K (Office of National Drug Control Policy, 2002d).

Ketamine was originally developed as an anesthetic in the early 1960s by Calvin Stevens, a pharmacist working for Parke-Davis and Company (Gahlinger, 2001; Jansen, 2000). A chemical derivative of phencyclidine (PCP), ketamine seemingly enjoyed the same analgesic properties and ability to induce anesthesia without some of the more problematic side-effects, including depression of respiratory and cardiovascular systems (Gahlinger, 2001; Siegel, 1978). However, ketamine was soon linked to a number of undesirable effects, most notably postanesthetic hallucinations (Siegel, 1978).

Despite these effects, ketamine was and is still used within certain settings where other anesthetic agents may put the patient at increased risk. For example, ketamine was used on military personnel in Vietnam, and may continue to be a viable option in mobile field hospitals where the more rigorous monitoring necessary with other anesthetics may not be possible (Jansen, 2000; Siegel, 1978). Ketamine has been utilized and/or evaluated as a treatment for alcohol dependence (Krupitsky & Grinenko, 1997), as an alternative or adjuvant to other methods of pain management (Bell, Eccleston, & Kalso, 2003; Kariya, Shindoh, Nishi, Yukioka, & Asada, 1998; Subramaniam, Subramaniam, & Steinbrook, 2004), as a sedative or anesthetic for children during dental procedures (Saxen, Wilson, & Paravecchio, 1999), and as a pharmacotherapeutic agent for individuals with treatment-resistant disordered eating behaviors (Mills, Park, Manara, & Merriman, 1998), with mixed results.

Ketamine, in its capacity as an N-methyl-D-aspartate (NMDA) antagonist, has also been used to explore the physiological mechanisms underlying schizophrenia. Some research has shown that ketamine intensifies psychotic symptoms among individuals with schizophrenia who are currently taking haloperidol (Lahti, Koffel, LaPorte, & Tamminga, 1995). Using ketamine with schizophrenic populations, even with the goal of acquiring knowledge that will lead to refined treatments and hopefully better outcomes for these individuals, has been a matter of ethical debate (Carpenter Jr., 1999). Thus, the utility of experimentation within nonclinical populations has been explored. Krystal and colleagues (1994) demonstrated that it was possible to temporarily induce some of the cognitive and behavioral features that are characteristic of schizophrenia in mentally and socially stable volunteers with a single intravenous dose of ketamine (0.5 mg/kg). Adler and colleagues (1999) compared a group of individuals diagnosed with schizophrenia or schizoaffective disorder to a group of disorder-free individuals who were administered ketamine intravenously. They failed to find significant differences between the two groups on a measure of thought disorder, thus providing further support for the use of ketamine to study the physiological etiology of the disorder in nonclinical populations.

Publicly, ketamine has garnered far more attention for its recreational use than for its medical and research uses. Ketamine is sold in liquid, powder, tablet, and capsule form and can be injected intravenously or intramuscularly, swallowed, snorted, or smoked (Drug Enforcement Administration, 2004c). A typical dose is approximately 40 mg when taken intranasally (Diversion Control Program, 2001) and 1 to 2 mg/kg when injected (Siegel, 1978); however, individuals often take multiple doses over the course of a single drug-taking episode (Siegel, 1978). A sufficiently large dose results in a trance-like state referred to as a "k-hole." Individuals report feeling a burst of energy followed by a sense of dissociation and the inability to move (Lankenau & Clatts, 2002). Ketamine has been largely associated with rave parties and the club drug scene (Dotson & Ackerman, 1995; Riley, James, Gregory, Dingle, & Cadger, 2001). However, Lankenau and Clatts (2002) conducted a recent study of young adults (ages 18–25) with a history of ketamine use recruited from the streets of a large metropolitan city and speculated that injection of ketamine may be more closely associated with nonrave use. Although all of the participants indicated that they had attended raves, their use patterns may have been affected by a number of social and environmental factors unique to this subset of individuals, including homelessness. Thus, the sample may not have been representative of the larger ketamine-using population. This being said, future studies evaluating use among recreational users may benefit from assessing not only quantity and frequency, but also setting of use and method of induction.

As with other drugs, the onset of the effects of ketamine is dependent on the route of administration. If ketamine is introduced into the body through intravenous injection, the onset is more rapid and the effects are shorter in duration than if it is administered through intramuscular injection (Lankenau & Clatts, 2002). Effects are felt rapidly (within 2 to 20 minutes depending on route of administration; Mozayani, 2002) and can last up to an hour (Diversion Control Program, 2001). The experience is extremely subjective, influenced in large part by environmental factors, and individuals assign different values to the various effects (Krupitsky & Grinenko, 1997; Siegel, 1978). For example, knowing whether or not an individual considers the hallucinations that follow heavy use of ketamine a positive or negative effect may be especially important information when tailoring intervention and prevention efforts. Effects can include euphoria, dizziness, a feeling of floating and/or being separated from the physical body, distorted perceptions, vivid hallucinations, and confusion (Siegel, 1978). Additionally, individuals may experience amnesia, loss or impairment of motor control, slurred speech, increased heart rate, elevated blood pressure, nausea, and anxiety (Kuhn, Swartzwelder, & Wilson, 2003; Siegel, 1978; van Berckel, Oranje, van Ree, Verbaten, & Kahn, 1998). Although relatively infrequent, large doses can lead to respiratory depression, coma, and death (Kuhn et al., 2003; Lalonde & Wallage, 2004). Ketamine has also been associated with sexual assault. Because it is essentially taste-less and colorless in its liquid form, it could be added to a beverage with-out the recipient's knowledge (Drug Enforcement Administration, 2001; Smith, Larive, & Romanelli, 2002).

Very little information exists in the current literature on the long-term health consequences of either occasional recreational use or of prolonged, heavy use. Some reports suggest that ketamine may have lasting effects on cognitive functioning (Curran & Morgan, 2000; Morgan, Monahan, & Curran, 2004) although the fact that participants were not ketamine naive at the time baseline measurements were taken hinders the ability to draw strong conclusions. Over time, users may develop tolerance, which may lead to more risky use (Jansen & Darrcot-Cankovic, 2001; Lankenau & Clatts, 2002; Moore & Bostwick, 1999). Individuals may also become de-pendent; however, withdrawal symptoms are not typically present (Jansen & Darracot-Cankovic, 2001; Moore & Bostwick, 1999; Siegel, 1978).

GHB

GHB is naturally produced within the human body (Nelson, Kaufman, Kline, & Sokoloff, 1981) and existing evidence suggests it acts as a neuromodulator or neurotransmitter (Cash, 1994; Maitre, 1997; Vayer, Mandel, & Maitre, 1987). GHB is also a manufactured drug that acts as a central nervous system depressant. GHB has been distributed under several names including Easy Lay, Georgia Home Boy, Grievous Bodily Harm, Liquid Ecstasy, Salty Water, and Scoop (Office of National Drug Control Policy, 2002b). GHB is available as a liquid, powder, or tablet (Nicholson & Balster, 2001; Center for Disease Control, 1990).

GHB was initially synthesized in 1960 by Dr. Henri Laborit as a gamma-aminobutric acid (GABA) analog that could be tested as an anesthetic (O'Connell, Kaye, & Plosay, 2000; Tunnicliff, 1997). Unlike ex-ogenously synthesized GABA, GHB was able to cross the blood–brain bar-rier (Laborit, 1964; Tunnicliff, 1997). Early tests indicated that the drug precipitated seizure activity and was not effective in blocking pain; thus, its use in this capacity has been limited (Dyer, 1991; Gahlinger, 2001). A num-ber of other therapeutic uses for GHB have been explored (Levy et al., 1983; Sherman, Saibil, & Janossy, 1994), including as a treatment for alcohol dependence (Gallimberti, Ferri, Ferrara, Fadda, & Gessa, 1992), alcohol withdrawal (Nimmerrichter, Walter, Gutierrez-Lobos, & Lesch, 2002), and opioid withdrawal (Gallimberti et al., 1993).

GHB has also been evaluated as a potential treatment for symptoms associated with the neurological sleep disorder narcolepsy. Individuals with narcolepsy most often experience excessive daytime sleepiness, which may or may not be characterized by unexpected, involuntary sleep episodes or "sleep attacks" (Aldrich, 1998). Sudden loss of muscle tone and motor control precipitated by a strong emotional response (i.e., cataplexy) and temporary paralysis and/or hallucinations that occur during the transition between sleeping and waking states are also experienced by some individuals with narcolepsy (Aldrich, 1998; Overeem, Mignot, van Dijk, & Lammers, 2001). GHB has been found to significantly decrease the percentage of time spent in stage 1 (i.e., light sleep) and the number of awakenings after sleep onset, as well as significantly increase the amount of stage 3 sleep and delta sleep during stages 3 and 4 (i.e., deep sleep) in individuals with narcolepsy (Scrima, Hartman, Johnson, Thomas, & Hiller, 1990). GHB has also been found to help reduce episodes of cataplexy (Scrima, Hartman, Johnson, & Hiller, 1989). Currently, Xyrem, manufactured by Orphan Medical, Inc., is the only GHB medication approved by the U.S. Food and Drug Administration (FDA) for the treatment of narcolepsy with cataplexy (Fuller & Hornfeldt, 2003; National Institute of Neurological Disorders and Stroke, 2003).

Prior to restrictions being placed on the over-the-counter sale of products containing GHB by the FDA in 1990, the drug was available commercially as an organic diet supplement and sleep aid (Chin, Kreutzer, & Dyer, 1992). It was largely advertised to body builders because of its documented ability to induce release of growth hormone (Centers for Disease Control, 1991; Takahara et al., 1977). GHB has come to be more prominently associated with rave parties and used for its reported ability to induce euphoria (Weir, 2000). A wide range of negative physical symptoms have been connected with GHB use, including dizziness, nausea, vomiting, drowsiness, vertigo, loss of consciousness, amnesia, slowed respiration and pulse, seizure-like activity, coma, and death (Centers for Disease Control, 1991; Chin et al., 1992; Dyer, 1991; Nordenberg, 2000). Several factors may heighten the risk associated with GHB consumption, including questionable purity and concentration (i.e., a single dose may contain from 500 mg to 5 g of GHB but may also contain adulterants) (Freese, Miotto, & Reback, 2002), disparate dose regulation (i.e., individual doses are sold by the capful or teaspoon) (Chin et al., 1992), and potentiation (i.e., amplification of the drug's effect) by other drugs including alcohol (McCabe, Layne, Sayler, Slusher, & Bessman, 1971; Schwartz, Milteer, & LeBeau, 2000). A 10 mg/kg dose induces amnesia and loss of muscle tone, a 20–30 mg/kg dose precipitates drowsiness and sleep, and doses upward of 50 mg/kg can lead to seizure-like activity, difficulty breathing, depressed heart rate, and coma (Center for Disease Control, 1991). Effects are felt within 15–30 minutes of ingestion, and can last anywhere from 3 to 6 hours (Lloyd, 2002).

Given the physiological impact, which can hinder a recipient's ability to fight back, it not surprising that GHB, much like flunitrazepam (i.e., Rohypnol or "roofies"), has gained notoriety as a drug used to facilitate sexual assault. The fact that GHB is colorless and odorless with only a salty taste makes it difficult to detect if mixed with a drink (Schwartz et al., 2000). In its liquid form, GHB looks exactly like water and is often kept in water bottles (Nordenberg, 2000). Despite its focus in public safety campaigns, studies have only identified GHB in a relatively small percentage of reported sexual assault cases perpetrated in the United States. This could be due, however, to failure to directly test for the presence of the drug, as well as its relatively quick elimination from the body.

One study (ElSohly & Salamone, 1999) analyzed 1,179 urine samples collected by various public health and law enforcement agencies within 72 hours of the alleged assault. Approximately 60% of the samples tested positive for one or more substances. Of these 711 cases, only 48 (6.8%) tested positive for GHB, while alcohol was found in 451 (63.4%) of the samples, and cannabinoids were found in 218 (30.7%) cases. In many of the drug-positive samples, multiple substances were detected. Within the 48 samples that tested positive for GHB, 16 also tested positive for alcohol, 6 for amphetamines, 1 for barbiturates, 10 for benzodiazepines, 4 for cocaine, 10 for cannabinoids, and 2 for opiates.

Another study (Slaughter, 2000) evaluated urine specimens collected from 2,003 victims of sexual assault. GHB was identified in only 3% of those samples that screened positive for a single substance ($n = 793$), and 4% of samples positive for more that one drug ($n = 426$), whereas alcohol was present in 69% of single-drug samples and 24% of multidrug samples. GHB is rapidly metabolized and evacuated, making immediate testing necessary if the drug is to be detected (Schwartz et al., 2000; Slaughter, 2000). If GHB is suspected, it should be reported to the individual collecting the sample, given that GHB is not included in routine toxicology screens (Elsohly & Salamone, 1999).

Chronic use of GHB may lead to tolerance and/or withdrawal symptoms when use is discontinued. Individuals have reported taking higher, more frequent doses of the drug in order to maintain relatively normal sleep patterns and to avoid tremors and feelings of anxiety (Dyer, Roth, & Hyma, 2001). Reports indicate that some individuals for whom GHB tolerance has developed ingest multiple doses every 30 minutes to 3 hours, resulting in increasingly higher daily doses (Dyer et al., 2001; McDaniel & Miotto, 2001). When use is terminated, symptoms of withdrawal, including nausea, vomiting, sweating, elevated heart rate, anxiety, insomnia, paranoia, agitation, hallucinations, and tremors, are experienced within a matter of hours (Chin, 2001; Dyer et al., 2001; McDaniel & Miotto, 2001), but usually resolve within 2 weeks following presentation for treatment (McDaniel & Miotto, 2001).

Club Drug Initiative

In response to nationally reported trends of increased use of club drugs by adolescents and young adults, in December 1999 the National Institute on Drug Abuse (NIDA), partnered with the American Academy of Child and Adolescent Psychiatry, the Community Anti-Drug Coalitions of America, Join Together, and National Families in Action, announced that they would be implementing a nationwide prevention initiative (National Institute on Drug Abuse, 1999a; Zickler, 2000). The focus of this initiative was the dissemination of general information and empirical findings regarding use and abuse of, and negative consequences associated with, club drugs. As a first step, 250,000 copies of a Community Drug Alert Bulletin (www.nida.nih.gov/ClubAlert/ClubDrugAlert.html), detailing information about MDMA/Ecstasy, GHB, Rohypnol, ketamine, methamphetamine and LSD, and 330,000 postcards showing the effects of MDMA on human brain function were distributed (National Institute on Drug Abuse, 1999a; Zickler, 2000). The initiative also established a website, www.clubdrugs.org, in order to provide the most currently available scientific evidence concerning the harm associated with club drugs to a broader base of treatment providers, researchers, and current or potential drug users. In addition to these direct prevention measures, NIDA announced that it would be increasing the amount of money allocated for club drug research from $38.5 million dollars to $54 million dollars (National Institute on Drug Abuse, 1999a; Zickler, 2000).

Hallucinogens

LSD (lysergic acid diethylamide) is the drug typically considered the most representative among the class of hallucinogenic drugs. These are drugs that cause alterations in an individual's thoughts, moods, and perceptions of reality. Street names for LSD include, among several others, acid, blotter, microdot, trip, and yellow sunshine (Kuhn et al., 2003).

The literature consistently reports Dr. Albert Hofmann's discovery and accidental consumption of LSD in 1943. When LSD was initially made available to physicians and the scientific community, it was believed to have two potential purposes: a method of studying psychoses and an adjunct to analytical psychotherapy (Bowers, 1987; Mangini, 1998). It was also thought of as method of reaching psychotherapeutically resistant patients (Abraham, Aldridge, & Gogia, 1996). Originating in the 1950s and continuing though the mid-1970s a number of studies resulted from what was thought to be potentially useful applications of LSD (Abraham et al., 1996; Mangini, 1998).

LSD was utilized widely as a tool for therapeutic purposes until 1965, when the Drug Abuse Control amendments to the Harrison Narcotics Act were passed (Abraham et al., 1996). Although extensive research and testing were conducted on LSD during this period, data were not supportive of its continued use as an addition to psychotherapy. Research was also conducted on the use of LSD to treat other disorders, most notably alcoholism. However, data suggested that LSD did no better than traditional treatments for alcoholism (Abraham et al., 1996).

Ingestion of LSD has been shown to have psychological, physiological, and behavioral effects. The effects an individual may experience while under the influence of LSD are highly unpredictable and may be impacted by a number of different contextual variables, such as the person's surroundings, personality, mood, and expectations of what the experience will be like (Diaz, 1997). LSD taken orally is quickly absorbed through the stomach and intestines, resulting in dispersion to body tissues and crossing the blood–brain barrier (Diaz, 1997; Ungerleider & Pechnick, 1999). Typically, the initial effects of LSD may be felt approximately 30–90 minutes after ingestion (National Institute on Drug Abuse, 2001c; Ungerleider & Pechnick, 1999). Physiological effects of use may result in increased body temperature, heart rate, and blood pressure, as well as sweating, dilated pupils, dry mouth, nausea and tremors (Abraham et al., 1996; National Institute on Drug Abuse, 2001c; Ungerleider & Pechnick, 1999). Psychological or behavioral effects of LSD use may include intense mood swings or experiencing several different emotions at one time, ranging from fear or anxiety to happiness (National Institute on Drug Abuse, 2001c; Ungerleider & Pechnick, 1999). LSD use can cause acute dysphoric reactions or acute adverse reactions. Also known as "bad trips," the user may experience severe, very frightening thoughts and feelings, including fears of death, insanity, or losing control (National Institute on Drug Abuse, 2001c). These adverse reactions often cause severe anxiety and panic resultant from hypervigilance, overreading of the environment, and bizarre thoughts, all while under the influence of the hallucinogen (Ungerleider & Pechnick, 1999).

The senses are also highly impacted by LSD, such that sounds, smells, and colors are highly intensified. While under the drug's influence, some individuals may experience "synesthesia," a crossing of senses such that users may "hear" images and "see" sounds (Abraham et al., 1996). Additionally, one's sense of time can be affected, such that a user may feel that minutes are more like hours (Ungerleider & Pechnick, 1999). Considered one of the strongest hallucinogens, LSD can bring about hallucinations or behavioral effects at low doses such as 20 micrograms, with synesthesia occurring when doses exceed 30 micrograms (Giannini, 1994); however, street doses have been reported ranging from 70 to 300 micrograms (Ungerleider & Pechnick, 1999).

Total duration of the drug's action can range between 6 and 12 hours (Abraham et al., 1996; Diaz, 1997; Ungerleider & Pechnick, 1999). Typically the drug's effects wear off before individuals seek medical treatment for an acute adverse reaction. Treatment of these reactions generally consists of preventing the user from harming him- or herself or others (Ungerleider & Pechnick, 1999), talking to the user in a reassuring manner in a quiet environment, and reminding the user that the drug produced his or her current thoughts. It is also helpful to keep the individual's eyes open by having him or her sit up or walk around, because closing the eyes can intensify the experience. Unfortunately, acute adverse reactions often do not end until the drug is eliminated from the body. Acute anxiety reactions have also been treated medically with a benzodiazepine (Abraham et al., 1996).

Individuals who use LSD can quickly develop a tolerance for the drug's effects. The tolerance for LSD is short-lived, but also produces a cross-tolerance for other hallucinogens, such as psilocybin and mescaline. There is little evidence for any physical withdrawal symptoms even when chronic use has ended (Diaz, 1997). Flashbacks are a well-known aversive reaction to hallucinogens, and, diagnostically, their experience is part of hallucinogen persisting perception disorder (HPPD) described in the *Diagnostic and Statistical Manual of Mental Disorders*, fourth edition, text revision (DSM-IV-TR; American Psychiatric Association, 2000). The behavioral effects may consist of "brief visual, temporal, or emotional recurrence, complete with perceptive (time) and reality distortion, that may appear days or months after the last drug exposure" (Ungerleider & Pechnick, 1999, p. 201).

Flashbacks can appear unexpectedly and, although the initial experience with the hallucinogen may have been positive, the occurrence of a flashback can be anxiety-provoking due to spontaneous and unexpected nature (Ungerleider & Pechnick, 1999). The use of other psychoactive drugs can exacerbate HPPD (Smith & Seymour, 1994). Psychotherapy can be helpful for individuals with HPPD to assist them in adjusting to chronic visual disturbances, and a range of medications may be prescribed to prevent recurrence of flashbacks. Ungerleider and Pechnick (1999) report that the mechanism causing flashbacks is still unknown; however, they typically reduce their intensity, duration, and frequency whether treated with anxiolytics and/or reassurance or left untreated. In addition, smoking marijuana can trigger a flashback in a heavy LSD user (Kuhn et al., 2003).

Bowers (1987) suggested that individuals with a predisposition for schizophrenia may experience a number of adverse reactions to the use of potent hallucinogens. Pechnick and Ungerleider (1997) support this idea, suggesting that hallucinogen use could lead to psychosis that would otherwise have remained latent, could cause psychosis to develop more rapidly, or could precipitate the relapse of a psychotic disorder within an individual previously diagnosed with the disorder.

Dextromethorphan

Dextromethorphan is frequently used and quite effective as a cough suppressant available in a number of medications that can be purchased over the counter (Bem & Peck, 1992). Street names for dextromethorphan may include DXM and Robo (described as "roboshots" when consumed in liquid form) (National Institute on Drug Abuse, 2001c). Use of dextromethorphan has been increasingly popular among adolescents and young adults. Often because this drug is available over-the-counter in "extrastrength" cough syrup, it is an easily accessible intoxicant. The amount of dextromethrophan found within a cough syrup or cold tablet can vary. Hilmas (2001) reports that the majority of cold medications, either in the form of cough syrup or pills, contain dextromethrophan in an approximate dose of 10–15 mg, although over-the-counter medications can be found that contain as much as 30 mg per dose. When used properly, suggested doses of cough medicine can range from $\frac{1}{6}$ to $\frac{1}{3}$ oz, which may include a dose of 15–30 mg of dextromethrophan (National Institute on Drug Abuse, 2001c). Much larger amounts of cough syrup can result in intoxication, such as doses greater than 4 oz, which may induce PCP- or ketamine-like experiences of dissociation (Darboue, 1996; National Institute on Drug Abuse, 2001c). The effect of the drug typically lasts 6 hours and can vary by the amount or form taken (National Institute on Drug Abuse, 2001c). NIDA reports that users of dextromethorphan experience "dose-dependent 'plateaus' ranging from a mild stimulant effect with distorted visual perceptions at low (approximately 2 ounce) doses, to a sense of complete dissociation from one's body at doses of 10 ounces or more" (National Institute on Drug Abuse, 2001c, p. 7). Other effects such as hallucinations, rapid heart rate, lethargy, confusion, and seizures may also occur at high doses (Hilmas, 2001).

Unfortunately, dextromethorphan is perceived by some to be safe because it is an over-the-counter medication and is manufactured by drug companies. Nevertheless, serious side effects, including death, have occurred. Dextromethorphan is absorbed through the gastrointestinal tract and absorption can be impacted by the ingestion of a sustained release form of dextromethorphan (Hilmas, 2001). Medications containing dextromethorphan frequently contain other active ingredients, such as chlorpheniramine, diphenhydramine, and acetaminophen, that when taken at higher than recommended doses can have a number of potentially serious side effects such as altering nervous system function, increased risk of cardiac side effects, or liver damage (Hilmas, 2001). Banerji and Anderson (2001) reported that dextromethorphan is also obtainable as the hydrobromide salt. This results in more risk factors, as some forms of over-the-counter medications may contain dextromethorphan hydrobromide and abuse of this medication can cause bromide poisoning (Banerji & Anderson, 2001; Wolfe & Caravati, 1995). Impairment of central nervous system functioning can result in changes in behavior, irritation, apathy, headache, and hallucinations, any of which can be potential symptoms of bromide poisoning (Wolfe & Caravati, 1995).

Inhalants

The other substances discussed in this chapter are individual drugs with specific properties. The term "inhalants" is applied to a growing number of chemicals that are misused for their psychoactive properties and describes the primary route of administration of these substances—inhalation through the nose and/or mouth; however, not all drugs that can be inhaled (e.g., marijuana, ketamine) are considered inhalants (Beauvais & Oetting, 1987; Edwards & Oetting, 1995). Some of the chemical compounds used as inhalants include acetone, benzene, hexane, xylene, trichloroethylene (Cohen, 1984), amyl nitrite, butane, isobutyl nitrite, methylene chloride, nitrous oxide, propane, and toluene (National Inhalant Prevention Coalition, 2004b). They are present in numerous items that can be found in the home, such as gasoline, lighter fluid, felt-tip markers, glue, correction fluid, paint thinners, spray paints, nail polish removers, cleaning products, air fresheners, cooking sprays, and whipped cream dispensers. These products are easily obtainable by the general public from legitimate retailers such as grocery stores, hardware and home improvement warehouses, and office supply stores.

Despite the recent attention they have garnered because of the prevalence of their use among adolescents in the United States, inhalants are not new drugs of abuse. Use of carbon dioxide to induce altered mental states was recorded in ancient Greece, and misuse of other inhalants (e.g., various anesthetics) have been documented throughout history (Cohen, 1977). Large-scale inhalant use first emerged in the United States sometime during the 1950s or 1960s (Bass, 1970; Cohen, 1977, 1984). Because they have legitimate uses, there are very few restrictions on the sale and distribution of products that can be used as inhalants. However, given their potential for abuse and harmful consequences, some states have enacted laws restricting their sale to and/or use by individuals under the age of 18 (Lloyd, 2003; National Inhalant Prevention Coalition, 2004d), a group which comprises the largest percentage of inhalant users (Johnston, O'Malley, Bachman, & Schulenberg, 2003).

Inhalants are known by a number of different names, some of which refer to all inhalants, such as air blast, huff, medusa, oz, and spray, and others that refer to a specific substance, such as amys (amyl nitrite), rush or white out (isobutyl nitrite), poppers (amyl or isobutyl nitrite), laughing gas or whippets (nitrous oxide), and tolly or Texas shoe shine (toluene) (Office of National Drug Control Policy, 2002c). Inhalants can be *sniffed* or *snorted* directly from their original container or, in the case of aerosols, directly dispensed into the mouth. Individuals may also engage in *huffing* or *bagging*. Huffing involves saturating a rag with the inhalant and then placing the rag directly over the nose and mouth, whereas bagging involves inhaling the substance from a plastic bag. Because the effects of most inhalants peak rapidly and dissipate within a few minutes (Cohen, 1984), individuals may engage in more covert means of using these substances in the presence of other people (Drug Enforcement Administration, 2004b; Keriotis & Upadhyaya, 2000).

Most inhalants (i.e., volatile solvents and anesthetic gases) have a depressant effect on the central nervous system, and induce feelings of euphoria and intoxication (Kurtzman, Otsuka, & Wahl, 2001). While under the influence of these inhalants, individuals may appear inebriated, exhibiting impaired motor control, disinhibition, slurred speech, and belligerent behavior, and may also experience hallucinations and delusions (American Psychiatric Association, 2000; Dinwiddie, 1994; Kurtzman, Otsuka, & Wahl, 2001). Other negative effects of inhalant use include coughing, wheezing, dizziness, stupor, skin irritation around the nose and mouth ("sniffer's rash"), headache, tremor, muscle weakness, abdominal pain, nausea, and vomiting (American Psychiatric Association, 2000; Dinwiddie, 1994; Lloyd, 2003). Individuals who engage in repeated use over a discrete period of time to prolong the intoxicating effect may put themselves at risk for experiencing some of the more severe negative consequences associated with use including loss of consciousness and irregular heart rhythms leading to heart failure and death (Bass, 1970; King, Smialek, & Troutman, 1985; National Institute on Drug Abuse, 2004a).

"Sudden sniffing death" (SSD) can occur in novice as well as chronic users. Numerous chemicals have been associated with SSD, including butane, propane (Steffee, Davis, & Nichol, 1996), 1,1,1-trichloroethane; trichloroethylene (King et al., 1985), toluene, and benzene (Bass, 1970). Death may also be caused by asphyxiation or suffocation, and may be a particular risk when bagging; because many of these chemicals are flammable, users may also sustain burns or other injuries if these substances ignite (Center for Substance Abuse Treatment, 2003; Kurtzman et al., 2001).

Nitrites are unique among other inhalants in that their use results in vasodilation, smooth muscle relaxation, elevated heart rate, and other signs of stimulation (e.g., feelings of warmth and exhilaration) (National Institute on Drug Abuse, 2004b; Balster, 1998). Nitrites also induce euphoria, but are most often used for their purported ability to enhance sexual pleasure and performance, and specifically among men who have sex with men (MSM) (Brouette & Anton, 2001). Nitrite use was associated with increases in risky sexual behavior in a large sample of MSM, placing users at heightened risk for contracting sexually transmitted diseases (Ostrow et al., 1990). Short-term physical consequences can include headache, nausea, vomiting, loss of control over bodily functions, weakness, chills (Brouette & Anton, 2001), decreased blood pressure, and increased heart rate (Hadjimiltiades, Panidis, McAllister, Ross, & Mintz, 1991).

The consequences of long-term use have been evaluated for a number of specific chemicals typically abused as inhalants. Research and case reports have linked many of them to serious and often irreversible damage to the brain, heart, lungs, liver, kidneys, and hematological system (Kurtzman et al., 2001; Meadows & Verghese, 1996; Sharp & Rosenberg, 1997). Nitrite use has been specifically linked to impaired immune system functioning and may be a risk factor for contracting HIV and/or developing a specific type of cancer called Kaposi's sarcoma (Brouette & Anton, 2001; Soderberg, 1998). The health consequences associated with a particular chemical may not represent the total risk to the individual, since products used as inhalants often contain multiple chemicals, many of which may not be listed on packaging or labels (Sharp & Rosenberg, 1997). Some individuals may also combine different inhalants to produce the desired positive effects, and often use other drugs in addition to inhalants, making it even more difficult to determine which substances are responsible for the resulting health consequences (Dinwiddie, 1994).

Use of inhalants by adolescents is troubling for reasons beyond the known physical consequences. Inhalant use in adolescence may increase the risk for use of other substances in young adulthood. Bennett, Walters, Miller, and Woodall (2000) found that college students who reported using inhalants prior to the age of 18 were approximately 16 times more likely to report use of drugs including inhalants, MDMA, steroids, crack or powder cocaine, amphetamines, sedatives, hallucinogens, and opiates during the past month and nearly 14 times more likely to report use of any of these substances in the past year relative to students who had not initiated use of inhalants or marijuana before age 18. Use among adolescents also tends to occur in peer groups (American Psychiatric Association, 2000; Edwards & Oetting, 1995), which may promote more widespread use among adolescents of approximately the same age (Edwards & Oetting, 1995) and may make cessation of use more difficult because of normative peer pressure.

Various reports have noted tolerance to inhalants among heavy users (American Psychiatric Association, 2000; Kono et al., 2001). Individuals may also develop dependence (American Psychiatric Association, 2000) and experience symptoms typically associated with withdrawal, such as craving, anxiety, irritability, restlessness, difficulty concentrating or paying attention, and sleep disturbances (Keriotis & Upadhyaya, 2000; Kono et al., 2001). Additionally, individuals may experience increased heart rate, headache, hallucinations, excessive perspiration, shivering, tremors, nausea, diarrhea, and fluctuations in appetite after discontinuation of inhalant use (Keriotis & Upadhyaya, 2000; Kono et al., 2001; National Inhalant Prevention Coalition, 2004a).

Anabolic–Androgenic Steroids

Anabolic–androgenic steroids are the commonly used terms for the synthetic derivatives of the male hormone testosterone. These drugs can be taken orally or injected and act to increase muscle growth. Often when steroids are taken, they are used in doses far above what is considered medically appropriate, ranging from as much as 2 to 26 times an appropriate dose (Brower, Blow, Young, & Hill, 1991). Anabolic–androgenic steroids are used medically to treat conditions such as delayed puberty, wasting of the body from HIV or other diseases, and types of impotence (National Institute on Drug Abuse, 2000). Street names for anabolic–androgenic steroids may include "juice" and "roids" (Galloway, 1997). Many different types of steroids have been developed over the years and require a prescription for use, although anabolic–androgenic steroids are frequently smuggled from other countries (National Institute on Drug Abuse, 2000).

Professional and Olympic-level competitors have been tested for years to prevent the use of performance-enhancing drugs. However, the use of these drugs has become increasingly popular among adolescents, high school athletes, and college athletes. The Monitoring the Future study reporting data from 2002 demonstrated that approximately 2.5% of eighth graders, 3.5% of tenth graders, and 4.0% of twelfth graders have misused anabolic–androgenic steroids at least once in their life (Johnston et al., 2003). Prevalence of steroid use is higher among males than females, although young women are the group experiencing the most rapid increase of steroid abuse (National Institute on Drug Abuse, 2000). Galloway (1997) reports that estimates for lifetime use in the United States ranges from 1.8 to 11% in males and from 0.2 to 3.2% in females, with athletes reporting the highest prevalence of use. Steroid abuse in the adult population is much more difficult to report due to a lack of studies.

Steroids are frequently used in a cyclic pattern which can be characterized as the use of one or multiple steroids for a set length of time, then a period of abstinence, followed by a re-initiation of use. The cycles can range from 4 to 18 or more weeks and periods of abstinence can extend from 1 month to 1 year (Brower, Blow, Young, & Hill, 1991; Frankle, 1984; Galloway, 1997). Another type of cycle, called a "pyramid," involves building up to a maximum dose, then slowly reducing use over time (Frankle, 1984; Galloway, 1997). It is considered "stacking" when multiple steroids are used at one time, which can entail the use of both oral and injectable steroids in a period of use (Brower, Blow, et al., 1991; Frankle, 1984; Galloway, 1997).

Much is known about the adverse effects of anabolic–androgenic steroids on males and females. Among the most commonly reported side effects are acne and oily hair and skin. In males, side effects may consist of testicular atrophy, impotence, decreased testosterone production, male-pattern baldness, and breast development (gynecomastia) (Galloway, 1997). Among women, hormonal changes due to steroid use can cause the voice to become lower, growth of body hair, a loss of scalp hair, enlarged clitoris, and reductions in body fat and breast size (Galloway, 1997; Pärssinen & Seppälä, 2002). The literature reports a number of cardiovascular risks, which may include changes in cholesterol (increases in low-density lipoprotein and decreases in high-density lipoprotein), an increased risk of blood clots, and diseases such as strokes and heart attacks (Galloway, 1997; Pärssinen & Seppälä, 2002). Other negative health consequences reported by Pärssinen and Seppälä (2002) are increased risk of cancer (liver, kidney, and prostate), early closure of bone growth plates (Hallagan, Hallagan, & Snyder, 1989), and higher risk of tendon tears. In addition, a number of complications can arise from injection drug or steroid use because of needle-sharing practices, such as hepatitis B, HIV infection, and infections to the skin (National Institute on Drug Abuse, 2000).

Behaviorally, Galloway (1997) reports that steroid use has been shown to increase aggressive behavior, sometimes called "roid rage." Other problems reported by steroid users include increased irritability; euphoria; mood swings; cognitive impairment such as distractibility, forgetfulness, and confusion; anxiety; paranoia; and depression (Brower, Catlin, Blow, Eliopulos, & Beresford, 1991; Galloway, 1997; Pärssinen & Seppälä, 2002). Another significant problem often cited in the literature is steroid dependence. In a study by Brower, Blow, et al. (1991) among 49 anabolic–androgenic steroid users, 94% reported at least one symptom of dependence, with 57% meeting the DSM-III-R (American Psychiatric Association, 1987) diagnostic criteria for dependence. The most frequently reported symptoms of dependence in the previous study included withdrawal symptoms, spending a large amount of time in substance-related activities, and taking more of the substance than intended (Brower, Blow, et al., 1991). Withdrawal symptoms are behavioral in nature and may present in the form of restlessness, rapid changes in mood, fatigue, loss of appetite, reduced sex drive, and the desire to resume steroid use (Brower, Blow, et al., 1991).

Research suggests that steroid users are much more likely to also abuse other substances and be at risk for significant negative consequences. Meilman, Crace, Presley, and Lyerla (1995) found that among collegiate steroid users, average weekly alcohol consumption was 26.0 drinks per week, compared to 8.3 drinks per week for nonusers. Users also demonstrated heavier consumption patterns of other drugs than nonusers, and a greater percentage of users experienced negative consequences related to their substance use. Due to the increased risk to collegiate athletes, Meilman and colleagues (1995) suggest a possible method of identifying college athletes who may be using steroids. Typically, university athletic departments have a sports medicine trainer on staff. Trainers could be made aware of potential symptoms of steroid use. Common signs trainers could watch for are increased irritability; large or unusual gains in muscle mass, strength, and endurance; any cardiovascular or liver abnormalities; or signs of water retention (Meilman et al., 1995). Additionally, physicians and team doctors should be aware of common laboratory abnormalities.

TREATMENT ISSUES AND RELAPSE PREVENTION

There are no efficacy studies evaluating RP strategies specifically for the drugs described in this chapter, and a review of psychology and medical databases resulted in only two case studies in which RP was mentioned. One of these is a Spanish-language article, in which the English-language abstract details the case of a man whose use of Ecstasy led to opiate addiction that was treated through individual therapy, family therapy, and social-interpersonal therapy using, among other approaches, RP (Sanchez Hervas & Tomas Gradoli, 1998). The other is a study of a male dependent on GHB, and mentions only that "the patient was engaged in relapse prevention" and was referred to additional counseling (Price, 2000).

While not a focal point of the articles and therefore not identified through literature reviews, some articles discussing treatment issues do mention RP in their treatment suggestions. Brower (1992) names RP an important strategy for rehabilitation from steroid use. He explains that dependent steroid users may experience strong internal urges and external pressures to resume use, and sees RP techniques for developing coping strategies as an important component of counseling. Corcoran and Longo (1992) similarly state that "relapse prevention techniques used in the substance abuse field are helpful" in discussing costs and benefits or myths and realities associated with steroid abuse (p. 233). Further, Jansen and Darracot-Cankovic (2001), after reporting that most individuals who use large quantities of ketamine eventually stop doing so without formal treatment, suggest that RP with the ketamine user primarily involves identifying the "danger signs" that could lead to a relapse. They suggest that there are two periods in a ketamine user's recovery during which risk for relapse is increased. Within 6–12 weeks in recovery, an individual may have trouble deriving pleasure from traditional activities and see a return to ketamine use as a solution. Additionally, at 6 months in recovery, life may seem "flat" to the user, and ketamine may be seen as the solution to change that. The authors conclude that the client should work to generate alternative responses to those that would previously have led to substance use.

Few if any treatments exist solely for inhalant abuse; however, clinicians and inhalant researchers have proposed a number of key elements necessary to any inhalant treatment or RP program (National Inhalant Prevention Coalition, 2004c). Among these guidelines are that (1) treatment programs must take into consideration the level of cognitive impairment of individuals seeking treatment; (2) follow-up sessions may be necessary to address ongoing issues with familial and peer relations that may precipitate relapse; and (3) once in the body, inhalants are taken up into fat stores and can be present in the body for an extended period after cessation of use, thus a longer period may be necessary to completely detoxify.

In the absence of a body of literature evaluating the application of RP to these substances, a look to efficacy studies of other treatment approaches is indicated. Similarly, very little information exists other than documenting issues in the treatment of HPPD (i.e., not LSD dependence itself) (Aldurra & Crayton, 2001; Giannini, 1994; Lerner, Finkel, Oyffe, Merenzon, & Sigal, 1998; Lerner, Oyffe, Isaacs, & Sigal, 1997; Lerner, Skladman, Kodesh, Sigal, & Shufman, 2001; Morehead, 1997) and describing treatment of GHB dependence with medications (Addolorato, Caputo, Capristo, & Gasbarrini, 2001; McDaniel & Miotto, 2001). Duggal, Sinha, and Nizamie (2000) state that there is no standard acceptable treatment for inhalant use. To look, then, at approaches to treating dependence and abuse of these substances, one can look at general treatment issues deemed effective with drugs to examine the applicability of RP to these issues.

The National Institute on Drug Abuse (1999b) has outlined principles of effective drug abuse treatment, and has identified RP as an example of an effective treatment approach. We will consider ways in which RP can or cannot be applied to meet NIDA's principles with the drugs discussed in this chapter, in addition to acknowledging relevant treatment issues for these substances where they do exist in the literature. In all, 13 principles are proposed.

1. *No single treatment is appropriate for all individuals.* While preventing a relapse is a goal for all going through drug abuse treatment, the strategies utilized with each client will differ based on the individual. This involves appropriate and detailed needs assessment and treatment planning, and also involves strategizing with the client to identify and develop coping skills for the high-risk situations he or she sees as most threatening. Additionally, RP involves working with a client to determine the treatment or outcome goal. This may involve eliminating use, reducing use, or working to avoid the combination of several substances (i.e., eliminating use of multiple substances at once). Regardless, as the goal differs, as high-risk situations each person faces differ, and as the strategies needed to address high-risk situations differ, treatment will differ as well.

2. *Treatment needs to be readily available.* Several studies have demonstrated that most relapses occur within the first 90 days after changing behavior. So, with RP itself, there clearly is a window of opportunity. This window may be particularly small for certain substance users, as McDaniel and Miotto (2001) report that relapse to GHB occurred soon after the treatment of withdrawal. The key is to ensure that those who want treatment are getting it. For inhalant abusers, many find themselves turned away from drug treatment facilities because of a perception that they are resistant to treatment (Sharp & Rosenberg, 1997). This is unfortunate and is somewhat ironic given that the rejection of a seemingly motivated individual may be based on the perception that this population is "resistant" to treatment. As a field, we must meet our clients and patients where they are in terms of their readiness to make changes, and do what we can to admit into treatment anyone asking for this very opportunity. Given the risks for relapse with a number of substances, timely offering of RP strategies in treatment or counseling should be made.

3. *Effective treatment attends to multiple needs of the individual, not just his or her drug use.* Substance use does not occur in a vacuum, and, therefore, should be put into a larger context for the individual. Identifying other sources of stress for a client can allow one to anticipate possible threats, challenges, or barriers to maintaining abstinence or reducing use. Self-esteem issues may drive a person's steroid use, so building self-esteem through exercises while in counseling will likely be of importance to this type of client. A person's Ecstasy or methamphetamine use may have originated because of the perception that there is no other way to have fun, so lowering the threshold on access to alternative activities (or even identifying other activities) may be necessary.

In some instances it will be necessary to illustrate for the client the ways in which substance use may be impacting other problems in his or her life, particularly if the individual is passionate about addressing a particular problem in therapy and is reluctant to make changes in substance use. In motivation enhancement approaches to counseling (e.g., motivational interviewing; Miller & Rollnick, 2002), clients may receive feedback about their use in a way that seeks to develop discrepancies between how a person sees him- or herself and what might be going on for the individual (or, between where a person is and where he or she wants to be). A client who reports occasional Ecstasy use and seeks treatment for problems with job functioning that he or she sees as related to memory problems may initially attribute the problems to feeling overwhelmed, busy, and somewhat depressed. This person may not see Ecstasy use, and the possible memory problems that can accompany this, as the source of his or her problems. Feedback on effects of substance use can serve to get a person thinking differently about the impact of his or her use as the clinician works to elicit personally relevant reasons for changing.

Various measures can allow the practitioner to assess and identify other life problems for an individual, as well as to hear the client's report of the perceived involvement of substance use in his or her experience of that problem (e.g., Miller & Marlatt's "Other Life Problems" section of the Brief Drinker Profile, 1987). Once completed, this sets the stage for understanding the context of one's use, and perhaps heightens one's motivation to change by allowing the person to see his or her use differently.

Once other treatment needs of the client are identified, these too can become a focus of therapy, particularly if their continued existence serves as a high-risk situation for an individual. As an example, steroid users find that decreased sexual function can occur following cessation of use. Addressing this, therefore, will be of utmost importance if problems with sexual functioning lead to resuming use. In a case study of a man with impotence, no spontaneous erections, and diminished libido after stopping anabolic steroid use, Bickelman, Ferries, and Eaton (1995) report that relapse to steroid use occurred to achieve a level of sexual performance greater than that of medications used to support changes in potency of his libido. Sexual functioning may, therefore, need to be evaluated during treatment with steroid users, given the relapse risk because of problems in this domain. Brower, Blow, et al. (1991) examined correlates of anabolic–androgenic steroid dependence and found that the best predictors of dependence were dosage used and dissatisfaction with body size. They suggest that both prevention and treatment programs may need to target body image to maximize effectiveness. Similarly, Galloway (1997) and Brower (1992) suggest that consultation with a fitness expert and generating a diet and exercise plan can be components of treatment with steroid users.

Brower (1992) reviews his past work and notes that treatment issues with steroid users can be different from those who use other drugs. First, the immediate gratification inherent to the use of many drugs is not present—it can often take days to weeks to develop the somatic and psychoactive effects of steroids. Second, there may be a greater commitment to fitness, success, victory, and goal-directed behavior among steroid users than among other illicit drug users. Finally, preoccupation with physical attributes like body size may distinguish those inclined to use steroids.

Our clients can tell us a great deal about what is most important to them and what can be most helpful for them in counseling and treatment. When these goals are attainable, these can and should be addressed. Because of RP's emphasis on identifying high-risk situations, coping skills training, and working toward a balanced lifestyle, concerns about other life problems can be targeted during treatment with users of the substances addressed in this chapter.

4. *An individual's treatment and services plan must be assessed continually and modified as necessary to ensure that the plan meets the person's changing needs.* RP strategies often include monitoring and record-

ing cravings, thoughts, and outcomes. While many clients are able to identify their most significant high-risk situations, others may not. Consequently, their treatment efforts, to some degree, may be a "work in progress" as they learn about threats to goals, unanticipated high-risk situations, and patterns related to urges and cravings. Monitoring on its own can be a valuable intervention. Monitoring exercises may uncover date- or time-specific cues associated with use (e.g., payday, end of the working day, weekends, etc.) which could be risky situations for a client. When the client becomes aware of these issues, appropriate coping strategies can be explored. This is another instance of a routine RP component that can be used with people having problems with club drugs, inhalants, hallucinogens, or steroids.

5. *Remaining in treatment for an adequate period of time is critical for treatment effectiveness.* The National Institute on Drug Abuse (1999b) reports that the threshold for significant improvement occurs at about 3 months. Perhaps not surprisingly, this is the same 90-day window in which two-thirds of relapses occur. People are not necessarily "home free" once 3 months have been exceeded, but the emphasis on providing ongoing counseling during this 3-month period can be made to the client given this window of risk.

6. *Counseling (individual and/or group) and other behavioral therapies are critical components of effective treatment for addiction.* If a person is able to execute a coping response in the face of a high-risk situation, the probability of relapse decreases. Consequently, appropriate coping skills training efforts are indicated as part of RP. These may take the form of coping with social pressures to use, dealing with cravings and urges, coping with cognitive distortions, relaxation strategies, or other behavioral approaches. Corcoran and Longo (1992) suggest that group treatment for steroid users can be useful after an initial period of individual treatment, and that strategies for restructuring cognitive distortions can also be of value.

7. *Medications are an important element of treatment for many patients, especially when combined with counseling and other behavioral therapies.* While a variety of medications are available for maintaining abstinence from alcohol (e.g., Antabuse, naltrexone), opiates (e.g., methadone, LAAM, buprenorphine, naltrexone), and cocaine (e.g., bromocriptine, amantadine), there are no specific medications indicated for maintenance of abstinence from the substances discussed in this chapter. Diazepam (i.e., Valium) may be utilized to suppress GHB-related withdrawal symptoms (Addolorato et al., 2001), and McDaniel and Miotto (2001) describe use of, among others, clonazepam, gabapentin, baclofen, trazodone, lorazepam, valproic acid, chlordiazepoxide, and bromocriptine in their case study descriptions of GHB withdrawal. Sharp and Rosenberg (1997) report that pharmacotherapy is not usually useful for people in treatment for

problems with inhalant abuse. Once detoxified, use of antidepressants, anxiolytics, or neuroleptics could be utilized, following a full medical consultation and evaluation, as an adjunct to counseling, depending on the symptoms or problems that initially contributed to or have resulted from a person's use (e.g., depression from Ecstasy use, hallucinations from LSD or mushroom use, etc.). There are, nevertheless, instances in which these treatment options may be contraindicated. For example, risperidone for the treatment of HPPD can actually exacerbate these symptoms (Abraham & Mamen,1996; Morehead, 1997; Solhkhah, Finkel, & Hird, 2000).

8. *Addicted or drug-abusing individuals with coexisting mental disorders should have both disorders treated in an integrated way.* True. Additionally, addicted or drug-abusing individuals with other coexisting addiction problems should have use of both or more substances treated in an integrated way. The client who declares that he or she has stopped drinking alcohol entirely may have accomplished this feat by now using GHB daily or smoking marijuana. Sharp and Rosenberg (1997) suggest that alcohol is a common secondary drug of abuse with abusers of inhalants, so sensitivity and attention to issues around alcohol use for these individuals is needed.

Corcoran and Longo (1992) note that other substances may be abused by steroid users in early stages of treatment to alleviate symptoms of depression. In response, then, to this treatment component, issues around depression should be addressed, with strategies for coping with depression being a focus both to help the client deal with depression and to reduce the risk of relapse.

9. *Medical detoxification is only the first stage of addiction treatment and by itself does little to change long-term drug use.* As mentioned previously in this chapter, several studies discuss issues involved in the medical treatment of withdrawal or acute substance-induced psychosis (e.g., Abraham & Mamen, 1996; Li et al., 1998; McDaniel & Miotto, 2001; Miller, Gay, Ferris, & Anderson, 1992; Morehead, 1997) including use of medications to address emerging drug-related symptoms, withdrawal itself, and possible medical contraindications. Li and colleagues (1998) suggest that research trials have demonstrated reversal of GHB effects using neostigmine and physostigmine, and both, along with atropine, have shown promise in situations where bradycardia (an abnormally slow heart rate) or coma due to GHB use is worsening. McDaniel and Miotto (2001) describe five case studies involving medically supervised withdrawal from GHB or GBL, a GHB analog, noting that withdrawal symptoms lasted from 3 to 13 days. Relevant to this treatment recommendation from NIDA is that four of the five individuals relapsed after discharge, including one resumption of use in the hospital parking lot. It is clear from these and other examples that additional counseling is necessary beyond discharge from detoxification. Attempting to prevent an initial lapse or reducing the

severity of a lapse can be an important part of these treatment and counseling efforts.

10. *Treatment does not need to be voluntary to be effective.* There are no published studies on mandated treatment for the substances discussed in this chapter. Theoretically, however, Prochaska and DiClemente's (1986) transtheoretical model makes clear that not everyone will be at the same level of readiness to change, and it would seem that most mandated or involuntary clients may be "precontemplative" (not yet thinking about their use as problematic) or "contemplative" (thinking about but not yet initiating change). An approach like motivational interviewing (discussed in treatment point 3 in this list) is indicated for people who have not yet begun to see, nor even think about, their substance use as problematic. Nevertheless, evaluation of the effectiveness of mandated or involuntary-selected treatment with persons using the substances discussed in this chapter is needed.

11. *Possible drug use during treatment must be monitored continuously.* Again, Sharp and Rosenberg (1997) report that alcohol is a common secondary drug of abuse by users of inhalants, and suggest that a program targeting alcohol use may be needed as well. Corcoran and Longo (1992) warn treatment providers to be aware of the tendency for steroid users to abuse other substances to alleviate depression when use of steroids stops, and also advise the provider to be aware of and informed about alternative substances that may be substituted for anabolic–androgenic steroids. Galloway (1997) notes that toxicology screens can be a positive component of treatment for those making changes in steroid use. Urine toxicology screens could be used as a complement to counseling utilizing RP strategies, but is by no means an RP approach itself. Since exclusive reliance on urinalysis will miss alcohol use that occurred outside of treatment (granted, a breathalyzer will detect if a client is actively intoxicated), the treatment provider using RP could request that a client monitor cravings for use of a substance. Alternatively, a provider could make assessments of other reported use throughout treatment or counseling.

12. *Treatment programs should provide assessment for HIV/AIDS, hepatitis B and C, tuberculosis, and other infectious diseases, and counseling to help patients modify or change behaviors that place themselves or others at risk of infection.* While RP itself would not provide the testing for various infectious diseases, the emphasis on work toward a balanced lifestyle could include reducing other risky behaviors and increasing health-promoting behaviors. If a physical examination has not occurred by the time one is considering RP options, a referral can be made.

13. *Recovery from drug addiction can be a long-term process and frequently requires multiple episodes of treatment.* Contributing to a long-term process can be a pace dictated by the cognitive functioning of the client. Sharp and Rosenberg (1997) note that treatment becomes slower and,

in time, more difficult when brain damage due to inhalant use is an issue for a client. Memory problems in Ecstasy abusers can potentially contribute to slowing treatment as well. Given the lack of information about treatment with these substances, the case for multiple episodes of treatment can, nevertheless, be made.

SPECIFIC RELAPSE PREVENTION ISSUES AND APPLICATIONS

Looking at the 13 principles established by NIDA, RP is certainly an appropriate approach for working with people trying to make changes in their use of steroids, inhalants, club drugs, or hallucinogens. Specific strategies, along with existing research implications, have been detailed here, and continue to be explored in the remainder of the chapter.

As discussed earlier in this book, strategies aiming to prevent or reduce relapse can include improving skills for coping with high-risk situations, environmental coping strategies, and behavior-change strategies. An important step in working with clients who are using any of the substances discussed in this chapter involves identifying potential high-risk situations so that appropriate cognitive and behavioral strategies can be selected. These high-risk situations can include wanting to enhance positive emotional states or cope with negative emotional states (e.g., wanting to "party," feeling down and wanting to feel better, self-esteem and self-confidence issues contributing to use), interpersonal variables (e.g., pressure to use), environmental variables (e.g., exposure to cues associated with use in the past, such as places, paraphernalia, or music), spiritual variables (e.g., trying to find a sense of inner meaning, particularly with use of hallucinogens or Ecstasy), and, of course, any combination of the preceding factors. Research reported in the first edition of this book demonstrated that the three primary high-risk situations associated with relapse are coping with negative emotional states, coping with interpersonal conflict, and social pressure. The most common high-risk situations among users of the substances discussed in this chapter may not necessarily be among these three, so identifying cues associated with substance use relevant to an individual client is of obvious importance early in the treatment process. Once identified, cognitive and behavioral strategies for coping with these situations can be discussed in therapy. These are discussed in detail by Marlatt and Witkiewicz (Chapter 1 of this volume).

If specific environmental cues or situations are identified by the client as high-risk, stimulus-control techniques that aim to minimize exposure to these cues can be utilized. For example, going to a different gym if one's steroid use has been associated with a particular locker room may be indicated. Altering routines, avoiding places or people, and getting rid of paraphernalia can also be important. For inhalant abusers, eliminating (if possible) the substance of choice by finding alternative sources of the product without an abuse potential (e.g., purchasing whipped cream in a tub in place of a can or canister) can reduce immediate risks due to exposure in the environment. In time, exposure with response prevention could be used if indicated and appropriate.

Working with the client to generate alternative activities to substance use can also be of great benefit in therapy. If a significant contributor to substance use is the perception that there is "nothing else to do," or if there are a number of positive outcome expectancies associated with the use of a substance, cessation of that use will likely result in a risk for relapse if these issues are not addressed.

Use of Multiple Substances

Clients may report using multiple substances, potentially simultaneously. For example, Meilman et al. (1995) showed that a significantly higher percentage of steroid users than nonusers also reported use of tobacco, marijuana, cocaine, amphetamines, sedatives, hallucinogens, opiates, inhalants, and club drugs. Such polysubstance use carries with it a range of dangerous negative consequences, and the dangers of drug interactions should be discussed with the individual.

With two drugs that have a depressant effect on the central nervous system (CNS), for example, alcohol and GHB, the risk of a potentiation interaction arises. The depressant effects are much more pronounced for these two drugs than the cumulative effect of each drug individually (as we often say, "one plus one is greater than two"). A similar potentiation interaction is possible with two drugs with stimulant effects on the CNS (e.g., methamphetamine and Ecstasy).

With drugs having an opposite impact on the CNS (i.e., a depressant and a stimulant), an antagonistic drug interaction becomes possible. This can be dangerous in multiple ways. When taking drugs in this way, the body gets put in a physiological "tug of war," with one drug telling the body to speed up, and with the other drug telling the body to slow down. This alone can result in lethal consequences. The cues associated with use of the stimulant alone or the depressant alone are not obvious to the user because of the other drug's impact to the CNS such that, in time, an individual might consume much more of either drug than was ever intended. Finally, an antagonistic drug interaction can have lethal consequences if, despite steps taken to control and hold constant the rate of consumption and absorption of the two substances, the drugs leave the body at differential rates. A person can be left with a debilitating and potentially lethal dose of one of the two drugs if the other leaves the system more rapidly than the other does.

Making other changes in one's substance use can also be important. Use of a particular substance could be a behavior or cue associated with use of another substance (e.g., people frequently note that they seem to smoke more when they drink alcohol). Consequently, if a person tries to eliminate or reduce use of one drug, use of a substance with strong associations could lead to urges and cravings to use the "target" drug. This could mean stopping use of a related substance for a period of time, and/or altering situations in which the substance is used.

If a barrier to staying in treatment is the concern that "they'll try and change everything about me," it will be important to go at a pace that feels manageable to the client. Suggestions about behavior change that include time-specific goals (e.g., "for a while," "for the time being," "for 30 days," etc.) and that reframe a behavior change as trying to heighten one's chances for success could be made.

CONCLUSIONS

It is an understatement to say that there is little that has been empirically demonstrated in evaluating the impact of RP strategies with the class of club drugs, hallucinogens, inhalants, and anabolic–androgenic steroids. Future studies could evaluate feasibility and efficacy trials of RP with any one of these substances, and could examine predictors of treatment success within users of these substances.

If the future follows past trends, use of new substances or of old substances in new ways will continue as chemical alterations are explored, as drugs are combined, and as substances are used outside of the realm or dose of what they were intended for. Following closely behind will be attempts to understand both the substances and the consequences associated with their use. Yet further behind that will be efforts to address problems associated with this use through intervention and prevention efforts. For those who have developed abuse or dependence problems from their substance use, efforts to change this use can be supported by RP. Absence of specific research applications of this approach to users of these substances does not necessarily mean the research has simply not been conducted. Rather, a limitation to conducting research in this area may involve treatment utilization and appropriate assessment and screening of these substances. Disseminating information both about treatment successes and failures will allow us, as a field, to meet the changing needs of the populations we serve.

REFERENCES

Abraham, H. D., Aldridge, A. M., & Gogia, P. (1996). The psychopharmacology of hallucinogens. *Neuropsychopharmacology, 14*(4), 285–298.

Abraham, H. D., & Mamen, A. (1996). LSD-like panic from risperidone in post-LSD visual disorder. *Journal of Clinical Psychopharmacology, 16*(3), 238–241.

Addolorato, G., Caputo, F., Capristo, E., & Gasbarrini, G. (2001). Diazepam in the treatment of GHB dependence. *British Journal of Psychiatry, 178,* 183.

Adler, C. M., Malhotra, A. K., Elman, I., Goldberg, T., Egan, M., Pickar, D., & Breier, A. (1999). Comparison of ketamine-induced thought disorder in healthy volunteers and thought disorder in schizophrenia. *American Journal of Psychiatry, 156,* 1646–1649.

Aldrich, M. S. (1998). Diagnostic aspects of narcolepsy. *Neurology, 50*(Suppl. 1), S2–S7.

Aldurra, G., & Crayton, J. W. (2001). Improvement of hallucinogen persisting perception disorder by treatment with a combination of fluoxetine and olanzapine: Case report. *Journal of Clinical Psychopharmacology, 21*(3), 343–344.

American Psychiatric Association. (1986). *Diagnostic and statistical manual of the mental disorders* (3rd ed., rev.). Washington, DC: Author.

American Psychiatric Association. (2000). *Diagnostic and statistical manual of mental disorders* (4th ed., text revision). Washington, DC: Author.

Andreu, V., Mas, A., Bruguera, M., Salmeron, J. M., Moreno, V., Nogue, S., & Rodes, J. (1998). Ecstasy: A common cause of severe acute hepatotoxicity. *Journal of Hepatology, 29,* 394–397.

Antoniou, T., & Tseng A. L. (2002). Interactions between recreational drugs and antiretroviral agents. *Annals of Pharmacotherapy, 36,* 1598–1613.

Balster, R. L. (1998). Neural basis of inhalant abuse. *Drug and Alcohol Dependence, S1,* 207–214.

Banerji, S., & Anderson, I. B. (2001). Abuse of Coricidin HBP Cough & Cold tablets; episodes recorded by a poison control center. *American Journal of Health System Pharmacy, 58,* 1811–1814.

Bass, M. (1970). Sudden sniffing death. *Journal of the American Medical Association, 212,* 2075–2079.

Beauvais, F., & Oetting, E. R. (1987). Toward a clear definition of inhalant abuse. *International Journal of the Addictions, 22,* 779–784.

Bell, R. F., Eccleston, C., & Kalso, E. (2003). Ketamine as adjuvant to opioids for cancer pain: A qualitative systematic review. *Journal of Pain and Symptom Management, 26,* 867–875.

Bem, J. L., & Peck, R. (1992). Dextromethorphan: An overview of safety issues. *Drug Experience, 7*(3), 190–199.

Bennett, M. E., Walters, S. T., Miller, J. H., & Woodall, W. G. (2000). Relationship of early inhalant use to substance use in college students. *Journal of Substance Abuse, 12,* 227–240.

Bickelman, C., Ferries, L., & Eaton, R. P. (1995). Impotence related to anabolic steroid use in a body builder response to clomiphene citrate. *Western Journal of Medicine, 162*(2), 158–160.

Bolla, K. I., McCann, U. D., & Ricaurte, G. A. (1998). Memory impairment in abstinent MDMA ("Ecstasy") users. *Neurology, 51,* 1532–1537.

Bowers, M. B. (1987). The role of drugs in the production of schizophreniform psychoses and related disorders. In H. U. Meltzer (Ed.), *Psychopharmacology: The third generation of progress* (pp. 819–823). New York: Raven Press.

Brouette, T., & Anton, R. (2001). Clinical review of inhalants. *American Journal on Addictions, 10,* 79–94.

Brower, K. J. (1992). Clinical assessment and treatment of anabolic steroid users. *Psychiatric Annals, 22*(1), 35–40.

Brower, K. J., Blow, F. C., Young, J. P., & Hill, E. M. (1991). Symptoms and correlates of anabolic–androgenic steroid dependence. *British Journal of Addiction, 86*(6), 759–768.

Brower, K. J., Catlin, D. H., Blow, F. C., Eliopulos, G. A., & Beresford, T. P. (1991). Clinical assessment and urine testing for anabolic–androgenic steroid abuse and dependence, *17*(2), 161–171.

Carpenter, W. T., Jr. (1999). The schizophrenia ketamine challenge study debate. *Biological Psychiatry, 46*, 1081–1091.

Cash, C. D. (1994). Gammahydroxybutyrate: An overview of the pros and cons for it being a neurotransmitter and/or a useful therapeutic agent. *Neuroscience and Biobehavioral Reviews, 18*, 291–304.

Centers for Disease Control. (1991). Multistate outbreak of poisoning associated with illicit use of gamma hydroxy butyrate. *Journal of the American Medical Association, 265*, 447–448.

Center for Substance Abuse Prevention. (2000). Club drugs: GHB, an anabolic steroid. *Prevention Alert, 3*(27).

Center for Substance Abuse Treatment. (2003). Inhalants. *Substance Abuse Treatment Advisory, 3*(1).

Chin, R. L. (2001). A case of severe withdrawal from gamma-hydroxybutyrate. *Annals of Emergency Medicine, 37*, 551–552.

Chin, M. Y., Kreutzer, R. A., & Dyer, J. E. (1992). Acute poisoning from gamma-hydroxybutyrate in California. *Western Journal of Medicine, 156*, 380–384.

Cohen, R. S. (1995). Subjective reports on the effects of the MDMA ("Ecstasy") experience in humans. *Progress in Neuro-Psychopharmacology in Biological Psychiatry, 19*, 1137–1145.

Cohen, S. (1977). Inhalant abuse: An overview of the problem. In C. W. Sharp & M. L. Brehm (Eds.), *Review of inhalants: Euphoria to dysfunction* (NIDA Research Monograph 15; pp. 2–11). Rockville, MD: National Institute on Drug Abuse.

Cohen, S. (1984). The hallucinogens and the inhalants. *Psychiatric Clinics of North America, 7*, 681–688.

Cole, J. C., Bailey, M., Sumnall, H. R., Wagstaff, G. F., & King, L. A. (2002). The content of Ecstasy tablets: Implications for the study of their long-term effects. *Addiction, 97*, 1531–1536.

Corcoran, J. P., & Longo, E. D. (1992). Psychological treatment of anabolic–androgenic steroid-dependent individuals. *Journal of Substance Abuse Treatment, 9*(3), 229–235.

Creighton, F. J., Black, D. L., & Hyde, C. E. (1991). "Ecstasy" psychosis and flashbacks. *British Journal of Psychiatry, 159*, 713–715.

Curran, H. V., & Morgan, C. (2000). Cognitive, dissociative and psychotogenic effects of ketamine in recreational users on the night of drug use and 3 days later. *Addiction, 95*, 575–590.

Darboue, M. N. (1996). Abuse of dextromethorphan-based cough syrup as a substitute for licit and illicit drugs: A theoretical framework. *Adolescence, 31*(121), 239–245.

Diaz, J. (1997). *How drugs influence behavior: Neuro-behavioral approach.* Upper Saddle River, NJ: Prentice-Hall.

Dinwiddie, S. H. (1994). Abuse of inhalants: A review. *Addiction, 89*, 925–939.

Diversion Control Program. (2001). *Drugs and chemicals of concern: Ketamine.* Re-

trieved March 31, 2004, from www.deadiversion.usdoj.gov/drugs_concern/
    ketamine/summary.htm.
Dotson, J. W., & Ackerman, D. L. (1995). Ketamine abuse. *Journal of Drug Issues*,
    25, 751–757.
Drug Enforcement Administration. (2001). *Drug intelligence brief: club drugs. An
    update.* Retrieved March 31, 2004, from www.usdoj.gov/dea/pubs/intel/01026/
    index.html.
Drug Enforcement Administration. (2004a). *MDMA (Ecstasy).* Retrieved March 29,
    2004, from www.dea.gov/concern/mdma/mdma_factsheet.html.
Drug Enforcement Administration. (2004b). *Inhalants.* Retrieved March 25, 2004,
    from www.usdoj.gov/dea/concern/inhalants.html.
Drug Enforcement Administration. (2004c). *Ketamine.* Retrieved March 29, 2004,
    from www.usdoj.gov/dea/concern/ketamine_factsheet.html.
Duggal, H. S., Sinha, B. N. P., & Nizamie, S. H. (2000). Gasoline inhalation depend-
    ence and bipolar disorder. *Australian and New Zealand Journal of Psychiatry*,
    34(3), 531–532.
Dyer, J. E. (1991). Gamma-hydroxybutyrate: A health-food product producing coma
    and seizurelike activity. *American Journal of Emergency Medicine*, *9*, 321–324.
Dyer, J. E., Roth, B., & Hyma, B. A. (2001). Gamma-hydroxybutyrate withdrawal
    syndrome. *Annals of Emergency Medicine*, *37*, 147–153.
Edwards, R. W., & Oetting, E. R. (1995). Inhalant use in the United States. In N.
    Kozel, Z. Sloboda, & M. De La Rosa (Eds.), *Epidemiology of inhalant abuse:
    An international perspective* (NIDA Research Monograph 148; pp. 8–28).
    Rockville, MD: National Institute on Drug Abuse.
ElSohly, M. A., & Salamone, S. J. (1999). Prevalence of drugs used in cases of alleged
    sexual assault. *Journal of Analytical Toxicology*, *23*, 141–146.
Frankle, M. (1984). Use of androgenic anabolic steroids by athletes. *Journal of the
    American Medical Association*, *252*(4), 482.
Freese, T. E., Miotto, K., & Reback, C. J. (2002). The effects and consequences of se-
    lected club drugs. *Journal of Substance Abuse Treatment*, *23*, 151–156.
Fuller, D. E., & Hornfeldt, C. S. (2003). From club drug to orphan drug: Sodium
    oxybate (xyrem) for the treatment of cataplexy. *Pharmacotherapy*, *23*, 1205–
    1209.
Gahlinger, P. M. (2001). *Illegal drugs: A complete guide to their history, chemistry,
    use and abuse.* Salt Lake City, UT: Sagebrush Press.
Gallimberti, L., Cibin, M., Pagnin, P., Sabbion, R., Pani, P. P., Pirastu, R., Ferrara, S.
    D., & Gessa, G. L. (1993). Gamma-hydroxybutyric acid for treatment of opiate
    withdrawal syndrome. *Neuropsychopharmacology*, *9*, 77–81.
Gallimberti, L., Ferri, M., Ferrara, S. D., Fadda, F., & Gessa, G. L. (1992). Gamma-
    hydroxybutyric acid in the treatment of alcohol dependence: A double-blind
    study. *Alcoholism: Clinical and Experimental Research*, *16*, 673–676.
Galloway, G. P. (1997). Anabolic–androgenic steroids. In J. H. Lowinson, P. Ruiz, R.
    B. Millman, & J. G. Langrod (Eds.), *Substance abuse: A comprehensive text-
    book* (3rd ed., pp. 308–318). Baltimore, MD: Williams & Wilkins.
Gerra, G., Zaimovic, A., Giucastro, G., Maestri, D., Monica, C., Sartori, R.,
    Caccavari, R., & Delsignore, R. (1998). Serotonergic function after (+/–) 3,4-
    methylene-dioxymethamphetamine ("Ecstasy") in humans. *International Clini-
    cal Psychopharmacology*, *13*, 1–9.

Giannini, A. J. (1994). Inward the mind's I: Description, diagnosis, and treatment of acute and delayed LSD hallucinations. *Psychiatric Annals, 24*(3), 134–136.

Greer, G., & Tolbert, R. (1986). Subjective reports of the effects of MDMA in a clinical setting. *Journal of Psychoactive Drugs, 18*, 319–327.

Grob, C. S., & Poland, R. E. (1997). MDMA. In J. H. Lowinson, P. Ruiz, R. B. Millman, & J. G. Langrod (Eds.), *Substance abuse: A comprehensive textbook* (3rd ed., pp. 269–275). Baltimore: Williams & Wilkins.

Hadjimiltiades, S., Panidis, I. P., McAllister, M., Ross, J., & Mintz, G. S. (1991). Dynamic changes in left ventricular outflow tract flow velocities after amyl nitrite inhalation in hypertrophic cardiomyopathy. *American Heart Journal, 121*, 1143–1148.

Hallagan, J. B., Hallagan, L. F., & Snyder, M. B. (1989). Anabolic–androgenic steroid use by athletes. *New England Journal of Medicine, 321*, 1042–1045.

Harrington, R. D., Woodward, J. A., Hooton, T. M., & Horn, J. R. (1999). Life-threatening interactions between HIV-1 protease inhibitors and the illicit drugs MDMA and ?-hydroxybutyrate. *Archives of Internal Medicine, 159*, 2221–2224.

Hartung, T. K., Schofield, E., Short, A. I., Parr, M. J. A., & Henry, J. A. (2002). Hyponatraemic states following 3,4-methylenedioxymethamphetamine (MDMA, "Ecstasy") ingestion. *Quarterly Journal of Medicine, 95*, 431–437.

Hilmas, E. (2001). Adolescent dextromethorphan abuse. *Toxalert Maryland Poison Center, 18*(1), 1–3.

Jansen, K. L. R. (2000). A review of the nonmedical use of ketamine: Use, users and consequences. *Journal of Psychoactive Drugs, 32*, 419–433.

Jansen, K. L. R., & Darracot-Cankovic, R. (2001). The nonmedical use of ketamine, part two: A review of problem use and dependence. *Journal of Psychoactive Drugs, 33*, 151–158.

Johnston, L. D., O'Malley, P. M., & Bachman, J. G. (2002). *Monitoring the Future national survey results on adolescent drug use: Overview of key findings, 2001* (NIH Publication No. 02-5105, pp. 1–56). Bethesda, MD: National Institute on Drug Abuse.

Johnston, L. D., O'Malley, P. M., & Bachman, J. G. (2003). *Monitoring the Future national survey results on adolescent drug use: Overview of key findings, 2002* (NIH Publication No. 03-5374, pp. 1–56). Bethesda, MD: National Institute on Drug Abuse.

Johnston, L. D., O'Malley, P. M., Bachman, J. G., & Schulenberg, J. E. (2003). *Monitoring the Future national survey results on drug use, 1975–2003: Volume I, secondary school students* (NIH Publication No. 04-5507). Bethesda, MD: National Institute on Drug Abuse.

Kalant, H. (2001). The pharmacology and toxicology of "Ecstasy" (MDMA) and related drugs. *Canadian Medical Association Journal, 165*, 917–928.

Kariya, N., Shindoh, M., Nishi, S., Yukioka, H., & Asada, A. (1998). Oral clonidine for sedation and analgesia in a burn patient. *Journal of Clinical Anesthesia, 10*, 514–517.

Keriotis, A. A., & Upadhyaya, H. P. (2000). Inhalant dependence and withdrawal symptoms. *Journal of the American Academy of Child and Adolescent Psychiatry, 39*, 679–680.

King, G. S., Smialek, J. E., & Troutman, W. G. (1985). Sudden death in adolescents resulting from the inhalation of typewriter correction fluid. *Journal of the American Medical Association, 253*, 1604–1606.

Kono, J., Miyata, H., Ushijima, S., Yanagita, T., Miyasato, K., Ikawa, G., & Hukui, K. (2001). Nicotine, alcohol, methamphetamine, and inhalant dependence: A comparison of clinical features with the use of a new clinical evaluation form. *Alcohol, 24*, 99–106.

Krupitsky, E. M., & Grinenko, A. Y. (1997). Ketamine psychedelic therapy (KPT): A review of the results of ten years of research. *Journal of Psychoactive Drugs, 29*, 165–183.

Krystal, J. H., Karper, L. P., Seibyl, J. P., Freeman, G. K., Delaney, R., Bremner, J. D., Heninger, G. R., Bowers, M. B., & Charney, D. S. (1994). Subanesthetic effects of the noncompetitive NMDA antagonist, ketamine, in humans. Psychotomimetic, perceptual, cognitive, and neuroendocrine responses. *Archives of General Psychiatry, 51*, 199–214.

Kuhn, C., Swartzwelder, S., & Wilson, W. (2003). *Buzzed: The straight facts about the most used and abused drugs from alcohol to Ecstasy, Second edition.* New York: Norton.

Kurtzman, T. L., Otsuka, K. N., & Wahl, R. A. (2001). Inhalant abuse by adolescents. *Journal of Adolescent Health, 28*, 170–180.

Laborit, H. (1964). Sodium 4-hydroxybutyrate. *International Journal of Neuropharmacology, 3*, 433–452.

Lahti, A. C., Koffel, B., LaPorte, D., & Tamminga, C. A. (1995). Subanesthetic doses of ketamine stimulate psychosis in schizophrenia. *Neuropsychopharmacology, 13*, 9–19.

Lalonde, B. R., & Wallage, H. R. (2004). Postmortem blood ketamine distribution in two fatalities. *Journal of Analytical Toxicology, 28*, 71–74.

Lankenau, S. E., & Clatts, M. C. (2002). Ketamine injection among high risk youth: Preliminary findings from New York City. *Journal of Drug Issues, 32*, 893–905.

Lawn, J. C. (1985). Schedules of controlled substances; temporary placement of 3,4-methylenedioxymethamphetamine (MDMA) into Schedule I. *Federal Register, 50*, 23118–23120.

Lerner, A. G., Finkel, B., Oyffe, I., Merenzon, I., & Sigal, M. (1998). Clonidine treatment for hallucinogen persisting perception disorder. *American Journal of Psychiatry, 155*(10), 1460.

Lerner, A. G., Oyffe, I., Isaacs, G., & Sigal, M. (1997). Naltrexone treatment of hallucinogen persisting perception disorder. *American Journal of Psychiatry, 154*(3), 437.

Lerner, A. G., Skladman, I., Kodesh, A., Sigal, M., & Shufman, E. (2001). LSD-induced hallucinogen persisting perception disorder treated with clonazepam: Two case reports. *Israel Journal of Psychiatry and Related Sciences, 38*(2), 133–136.

Levy, M. I., Davis, B. M., Mohs, R. C., Trigos, G. C., Mathe, A. A., & Davis, K. L. (1983). Gamma-hydroxybutyrate in the treatment of schizophrenia. *Psychiatry Research, 9*, 1–8.

Li, J., Stokes, S. A., & Woeckener, A. (1998). A tale of novel intoxication: A review of the effects of ?-Hydroxybutyric acid with recommendations for management. *Annals of Emergency Medicine, 31*(6), 729–736.

Lloyd, J. (2002). *Gammahydroxybutyrate (GHB)*. Retrieved April 4, 2004, from www.whitehousedrugpolicy.gov/publications/factsht/gamma/index.html.

Lloyd, J. (2003). *Inhalants*. Retrieved March 31, 2004, from www.whitehousedrugpolicy. gov/publications/factsht/inhalants/inhalants.pdf.

Maitre, M. (1997). The gamma-hydroxybutyrate signally system in brain: Organization and functional implications. *Progress in Neurobiology, 51,* 337–361.

Mangini, M. (1998). Treatment of alcoholism using psychedelic drugs: A review of the program of research. *Journal of Psychoactive Drugs, 30*(4), 381–418.

Masi, G., Mucci, M., & Floriani, C. (2002). Acute catatonia after a single dose of Ecstasy. *Journal of the American Academy of Child and Adolescent Psychiatry, 41,* 892.

McCabe, E. R., Layne, E. C., Sayler, D. F., Slusher, N., & Bessman, S. P. (1971). Synergy of ethanol and a natural soporific—gamma hydroxybutyrate. *Science, 171,* 404–406.

McCann, U. D., & Ricaurte, G. A. (1992). MDMA ("Ecstasy") and panic disorder: Induction by a single dose. *Biological Psychiatry, 32,* 950–953.

McCann, U. D., Ridenour, A., Shaham, Y., & Ricaurte, G. A. (1994). Serotonin neurotoxicity after (+/_)3,4-methylenedioxymethamphetamine (MDMA; "Ecstasy"): A controlled study in humans. *Neuropsychopharmacology, 10,* 129–138.

McCann, U. D., Slate, S. O., & Ricaurte, G. A. (1996). Adverse reactions with 3,4-methylenedioxymethamphetamine (MDMA; "Ecstasy"). *Drug Safety, 15,* 107–115.

McCann, U. D., Szabo, Z., Scheffel, U., Dannals, R. F., & Ricaurte, G. A. (1998). Positron emission tomographic evidence of toxic effect of MDMA ("Ecstasy") on brain serotonin neurons in human beings. *Lancet, 352,* 1433–1437.

McDaniel, C. H., & Miotto, K. A. (2001). Gamma hydroxybutyrate (GHB) and gamma butyrolactone (GBL) withdrawal: Five case studies. *Journal of Psychoactive Drugs, 33*(2), 143–149.

McDowell, D. M. (1999). MDMA, Ketamine, GHB, and the "club drug" scene. In M. Galanter & H. D. Kleber (Eds.), *The American Psychiatric Press textbook of substance abuse treatment* (2nd ed., pp. 295–305). Washington, DC: American Psychiatric Press.

McQueen, A. L., & Baroletti, S. A. (2002). Adjuvant ketamine analgesia for the management of cancer pain. *Annals of Pharmacotherapy, 36,* 1614–1619.

Meadows, R., & Verghese, A. (1996). Medical complications of glue sniffing. *Southern Medical Journal, 89,* 455–462.

Meilman, P. W., Crace, R. K., Presley, C. A., & Lyerla, R. (1995). Beyond performance enhancement: Polypharmacy among collegiate users of steroids. *Journal of American College Health, 44*(3), 98–104.

Miller, P. L., Gay, G. R., Ferris, K. C., & Anderson, S. (1992). Treatment of acute, adverse psychedelic reactions: "I've tripped and I can't get down." *Journal of Psychoactive Drugs, 24,* 277–279.

Miller, W. R., & Marlatt, G. A. (1987). *Brief Drinker Profile*. Odessa, FL: Psychological Assessment Resources.

Miller, W. R., & Rollnick, S. (2002). *Motivational interviewing: Preparing people for change* (2nd ed.). New York: Guilford Press.

Mills, I. H., Park, G. R., Manara, A. R., & Merriman, R. J. (1998) Treatment of compulsive behaviour in eating disorders with intermittent ketamine infusions. *Quarterly Journal of Medicine, 91,* 493–503.

Moore, N. N., & Bostwick, J. M. (1999). Ketamine dependence in anesthesia providers. *Psychosomatics, 40,* 356–359.

Morehead, D. B. (1997). Exacerbation of hallucinogen-persisting perception disorder with risperidone. *Journal of Clinical Psychopharmacology, 17*(4), 327–328.

Morgan, J. P. (1997). Designer drugs. In J. H. Lowinson, P. Ruiz, R. B. Millman, & J. G. Langrod (Eds.), *Substance abuse: A comprehensive textbook* (3rd ed., pp. 264–275). Baltimore, MD: Williams & Wilkins.

Mozayani, A., (2002). Ketamine—Effects on human performance and behavior. *Forensic Science Review, 14,* 123–131.

National Inhalant Prevention Coalition. (2004a). *About inhalants.* Retrieved March 31, 2004, from www.inhalants.org/about.htm.

National Inhalant Prevention Coalition. (2004b). *Chemical found in inhalants.* Retrieved March 30, 2004, from www.inhalants.org/chemical.htm.

National Inhalant Prevention Coalition. (2004c). *Inhalant treatment guidelines.* Retrieved March 31, 2004, from www.inhalants.org/guidelines.htm.

National Inhalant Prevention Coalition. (2004d). *State inhalant legislation.* Retrieved March 30, 2004, from www.inhalants.org/laws.htm.

National Institute of Neurological Disorders and Stroke. (2003). *Narcolepsy fact sheet.* Retrieved April 5, 2004, from www.ninds.nih.gov/health_and_medical/pubs/narcolepsy.htm.

National Institute on Drug Abuse. (1999a). *Club drugs take center stage in new national education and prevention initiative by NIDA and national partners. Initiative includes research funding and community outreach.* Retrieved March 31, 2004, from www.nida.nih.gov/MedAdv/99/NR-122.html.

National Institute on Drug Abuse. (1999b). *Principles of drug addiction treatment: A research based guide* (NIH Publication No. 99–4180).

National Institute on Drug Abuse. (2000). About anabolic steroids. *NIDA Notes, 16*(3).

National Institute on Drug Abuse. (2001a). *Ecstasy: What we know and don't know about MDMA. A scientific review.* Retrieved March 29, 2004, from www.drugabuse. gov/Meetings/MDMA/MDMAExSummary.html.

National Institute on Drug Abuse. (2001b). MDMA/Ecstasy—A drug with complex consequences. *NIDA Notes, 16*(5).

National Institute on Drug Abuse. (2001c). *Research report series—Hallucinogens and dissociative drugs.* Retrieved April 4, 2004, from www.drugabuse.gov/ResearchReports/Hallucinogens/.

National Institute on Drug Abuse. (2004a). *NIDA Info Facts—Inhalants.* Retrieved April 4, 2004, from www.drugabuse.gov/Infofax/inhalants.html.

National Institute on Drug Abuse. (2004b). *Research report series—Inhalant abuse.* Retrieved April 4, 2004, from www.drugabuse.gov/ResearchReports/Inhalants.

National Institute on Drug Abuse. (2004c). *Research report series – MDMA abuse (Ecstasy).* Retrieved March 31, 2004, from www.drugabuse.gov/ResearchReports/MDMA/.

Nelson, T., Kaufman, E., Kline, J., & Sokoloff, L. (1981). The extraneural distribution of gamma-hydroxybutyrate. *Journal of Neurochemistry, 37,* 1345–1348.

Nicholson, K. L., & Balster, R. L. (2001). GHB: A new and novel drug of abuse. *Drug and Alcohol Dependence, 63,* 1–22.

Nimmerrichter, A. A., Walter, H., Gutierrez-Lobos, K. E., & Lesch, O. M. (2002). Double-blind controlled trial of gamma-hydroxybutyrate and clomethiazole in the treatment of alcohol withdrawal. *Alcohol and Alcoholism, 37,* 67–73.

Nordenberg, T. (2000). The death of the party: All the rave, GHB's hazards go unheeded. *FDA Consumer Magazine, 34*(2), 14–16, 18–19.

O'Connell, T., Kaye, L., & Plosay, J. J., III. (2000). Gamma-hydroxybutyrate (GHB): A newer drug of abuse. *American Family Physician, 62,* 2478–2482.

Office of National Drug Control Policy. (2002a). *Street terms: Drugs and the drug trade. Drug type: Ecstasy (methylenedioxymethamphetamine; MDMA).* Retrieved April 3, 2004, from www.whitehousedrugpolicy.gov/streetterms/ByType.asp?intTypeID=7.

Office of National Drug Control Policy. (2002b). *Street terms: Drugs and the drug trade. Drug type: GHB (gamma hydroxybutyrate).* Retrieved April 5, 2004, from www.whitehousedrugpolicy.gov/streetterms/ByType.asp?intTypeID=48.

Office of National Drug Control Policy. (2002c). *Street terms: Drugs and the drug trade. Drug type: Inhalants.* Retrieved March 31, 2004, from www.whitehousedrugpolicy.gov/streetterms/ByType.asp?intTypeID=34.

Office of National Drug Control Policy. (2002d). *Street terms: Drugs and the drug trade. Drug type: Ketamine.* Retrieved April 3, 2004, from www.whitehousedrugpolicy.gov/streetterms/ByType.asp?intTypeID=32.

Ostrow, D. G., Van Raden, M. J., Fox, R., Kingsley, L. A., Dudley, J., & Kaslow, R. A. (1990). *Recreational drug use and sexual behavior change in a cohort of homosexual men.* The Multicenter AIDS Cohort Study (MACS). *AIDS, 4,* 759–765.

Overeem, S., Mignot, E., van Dijk, J. G., & Lammers, G. J. (2001). Narcolepsy: Clinical features, new pathophysiologic insights, and future perspectives. *Journal of Clinical Neurophysiology, 18,* 78–105.

Pacifici, R., Zuccaro, P., Lopez, C. H., Pichini, S., Di Carlo, S., Farre, M., Roset, P. N., Ortuno, J., Segura, J., & De La Torre, R. (2001). Acute effects of 3,4-methylenedioxymethamphetamine alone and in combination with ethanol on the immune system in humans. *Journal of Pharmacology and Experimental Therapeutics, 296,* 207–215.

Parrott, A. C. (2001). Human psychopharmacology of Ecstasy (MDMA): A review of 15 years of empirical research. *Human Psychopharmacology, 16,* 557–577.

Parrott, A. C. (2004). Is Ecstasy MDMA? A review of the proportion of Ecstasy tablets containing MDMA, their dosage levels, and the changing perceptions of purity. *Psychopharmacology, 173,* 234–241.

Parrott, A. C., Buchanan, T., Scholey, A. B., Heffernan, T., Ling, J., & Rodgers, J. (2002). Ecstasy/MDMA attributed problems reported by novice, moderate and heavy recreational users. *Human Psychopharmacology, 17,* 309–312.

Parrott, A. C., & Lasky J. (1998). Ecstasy (MDMA) effect upon mood and cognition: Before, during and after a Saturday night dance. *Psychopharmacology, 139,* 261–268.

Pärssinen, M., & Seppälä, T. (2002). Steroid use and long-term health risks in former athletes. *Sports Medicine, 32*(2), 83–94.

Pechnick, R. N., & Ungerleider, J. T. (1997). Hallucinogens. In J. H. Lowinson, P.

Ruiz, R. B. Millman, & J. G. Langrod (Eds.), *Substance abuse: A comprehensive textbook* (3rd ed., pp. 230–238). Baltimore, MD: Williams & Wilkins.

Price, G. (2000). In-patient detoxification after GHB dependence. *British Journal of Psychiatry, 177,* 181.

Prochaska, J. O., & DiClemente, C. C. (1986). Toward a comprehensive model of change. In W. R. Miller & N. Heather (Eds.), *Treating addictive behaviors: Processes of Change* (pp. 3–27). New York: Plenum Press.

Ricaurte, G. A., Yuan, J., & McCann, U. D. (2000). (+/-)3,4-methylenedioxymethamphetamine ('Ecstasy')-induced serotonin neurotoxicity: Studies in animals. *Neuropsychology, 42,* 5–10.

Riley, S. C. E., James, C., Gregory, D., Dingle, H., & Cadger, M. (2001). Patterns of recreational drug use at dance events in Edinburgh, Scotland. *Addiction, 96,* 1035–1047.

Roth, R. H., & Giarman, N. J. (1970). Natural occurrence of gamma-hydroxybutyrate in mammalian brain. *Biochemical Pharmacology, 19,* 1087–1093.

Sanchez Hervas, E., & Tomas Gradoli, V. (1998). Use of MDMA (Ecstasy): Analysis of a multiple drug-addiction case. *Analisis y Modificacion de Conducta, 24*(98), 907–922.

Saxen, M. A., Wilson, S., & Paravecchio, R. (1999). Anesthesia for pediatric dentistry. *Dental Clinics of North America, 43,* 231–245.

Schifano, F., Di Furia, L., Forza, G., Minicuci, N., & Bricolo, R. (1998). MDMA ('Ecstasy') consumption in the context of polydrug abuse: A report on 150 patients. *Drug and Alcohol Dependence, 52,* 85–90.

Schwartz, R. H., & Miller, N. S. (1997). MDMA (Ecstasy) and the rave: A review. *Pediatrics, 100,* 705–708.

Schwartz, R. H., Milteer, R., & LeBeau, M. A. (2000). Drug-facilitated sexual assault ("date rape"). *Southern Medical Journal, 94,* 655–656.

Scrima, L., Hartman, P. G., Johnson, F. H., Jr., & Hiller, F. C. (1989). Efficacy of gamma-hydroxybutyrate versus placebo in treating narcolepsy-cataplexy: Double-blind subjective measures. *Biological Psychiatry, 26,* 331–343.

Scrima, L., Hartman, P. G., Johnson, F. H., Jr., Thomas, E. E., & Hiller, F. C. (1990). The effects of gamma-hydroxybutyrate on the sleep of narcolepsy patients: A double-blind study. *Sleep, 13,* 479–490.

Sharma, A. (2001). A case of sensorineural deafness following ingestion of Ecstasy. *Journal of Laryngology and Otology, 115,* 911–915.

Sharp, C. W., & Rosenberg, N. L. (1997). Inhalants. In J. H. Lowinson, P. Ruiz, R. B. Millman, & J. G. Langrod (Eds.), *Substance abuse: A comprehensive textbook* (3rd ed., pp. 246–264). Baltimore, MD : Williams & Wilkins.

Sherman, I. A., Saibil, F. G., & Janossy, T. I. (1994). Gamma-hydroxybutyrate mediated protection of liver function after long-term hypothermic storage. *Transplantation, 57,* 8–11.

Shulgin, A. T. (1986). The background and chemistry of MDMA. *Journal of Psychoactive Drugs, 18,* 291–304.

Shulgin, A. T., & Nichols, D. E. (1978). Characterization of three new psychotomimetics. In R. C. Stillman & R. E. Willette (Eds.), *The pharmacology of hallucinogens.* New York: Pergamon.

Siegel, R. K. (1978). Phencyclidine and ketamine intoxication: A study of four populations of recreational users. In R. C. Peterson & R. C. Stillman (Eds.),

Phencyclidine (PCP) abuse: An appraisal (National Institute on Drug Abuse Research Monograph 21, pp. 119–147). Rockville, MD: National Institute on Drug Abuse, Division of Research.

Slaughter, L. (2000). Involvement of drugs in sexual assault. *Journal of Reproductive Medicine, 45*, 425–430.

Smith, D. E., & Seymour, R. B. (1994). LSD: History and toxicity. *Psychiatric Annals, 24*(3), 145–147.

Smith, K. M., Larive, L. L., & Romanelli, F. (2002). Club drugs: Methylenedioxymethamphetamine, flunitrazepam, ketamine hydrochloride, and gamma-hydroxybutyrate. *American Journal of Health-System Pharmacists, 59*, 1067–1076.

Soderberg, L. S. F. (1998). Immunomodulation by nitrite inhalants may predispose abusers to AIDS and Kaposi's sarcoma. *Journal of Neuroimmunology, 83*, 157–161.

Solhkhah, R., Finkel, J., & Hird, S. (2000). Possible resperidone-induced visual hallucinations. *Journal of the American Academy of Child and Adolescent Psychiatry, 39*(9), 1074–1075.

Spiess, M. (2002). *MDMA (Ecstasy)*. Retrieved June 18, 2002, from www.whitehousedrugpolicy.gov.publications/factsht/mdma/index.html.

Steffee, C. H., Davis, G. J., & Nichol, K. K. (1996). A whiff of death: Fatal volatile solvent inhalation abuse. *Southern Medical Journal, 89*, 879–884.

Subramaniam, K., Subramaniam, B., & Steinbrook, R. A. (2004). Ketamine as adjuvant analgesic to opioids: A quantitative and qualitative systematic review. *Anesthesia and Analgesia, 99*, 482–495.

Substance Abuse and Mental Health Services Administration. (2001). *Summary of findings from the 2000 National Household Survey on Drug Abuse*. NHSDA Series H-13, DHHS Publication No. (SMA) 01-3549. Rockville, MD: Office of Applied Studies.

Takahara, J., Yunoki, S., Yakushiji, W., Yamauchi, J., Yamane, Y., & Ofuji, T. (1977). Stimulatory effects of gamma-hydroxybutyric acid on growth hormone and prolactin release in humans. *Journal of Clinical Endocrinology and Metabolism, 44*, 1014–1017.

Tancer, M. E., & Johanson, C. E. (2001). The subjective effects of MDMA and mCPP in moderate MDMA users. *Drug and Alcohol Dependence, 65*, 97–101.

Traub, S. J., Hoffman, R. S., & Nelson, L. S. (2002). The "Ecstasy" hangover: Hyponatremia due to 3,4-methylenedioxymethamphetamine. *Journal of Urban Health, 79*, 549–555.

Tunnicliff, G. (1997). Sites of action of gamma-hydroxybutyrate (GHB)—A neuroactive drug with abuse potential. *Clinical Toxicology, 35*, 581–590.

Ungerleider, J. T., & Pechnick, R. N. (1999). Hallucinogens. In M. Galanter & H. D. Kleber (Eds.), *The American Psychiatric Press textbook of substance abuse treatment* (2nd ed., pp. 195–203). Washington, DC: American Psychiatric Press.

van Berckel, B. N. M., Oranje, B., van Ree, J. M., Verbaten, M. N., & Kahn, R. S. (1998). The effects of low dose ketamine on sensory gating, neuroendocrine secretion and behavior in healthy human subjects. *Psychopharmacology, 137*, 271–281.

Van Kampen, J., & Katz, M. (2001). Persistent psychosis after a single ingestion of "Ecstasy." *Psychosomatics, 42,* 525–527.

Vayer, P., Mandel, P., & Maitre, M. (1987). Gamma-hydroxybutyrate, a possible neurotransmitter. *Life Sciences, 41,* 1547–1557.

Weiner, A. L. (2000). Emerging drugs of abuse in Connecticut. *Connecticut Medicine, 64,* 19–23.

Weir, E. (2000). Raves: A review of the culture, the drugs and the prevention of harm. *Canadian Medical Association Journal, 162,* 1843–1848.

Williamson, S., Gossop, M., Powis, B., Griffiths, P., Fountain, J., & Strang, J. (1997). Adverse effects of stimulant drugs in a community sample of drug users. *Drug and Alcohol Dependence, 44,* 87–94.

Wolfe, T. R., & Caravati, E. M. (1995). Massive dextromethorphan ingestion and abuse. *American Journal of Emergency Medicine, 13*(2), 174–176.

Zickler, P. (2000). NIDA launches initiative to combat club drugs. *NIDA Notes, 14*(6).

CHAPTER 9

Relapse Prevention for Eating Disorders and Obesity

R. Lorraine Collins

H. B. is a 24-year-old unmarried female from a European American background. She has a high school diploma and currently works full-time in a clerical position. She described her bulimia as having started during her teens. She was highly preoccupied with her weight and caloric intake, and reports spending 81–90% of her day thinking about these issues. Her preoccupation was such that she described her thoughts, images, or impulses related to food as interfering in her social and work life. She described both of her parents as overweight, but not obese. H. B. grew up in a family that emphasized achievement, perfection, and physical appearance. She endorsed a number of cognitions that are typical of bulimics, including a high level of preoccupation with shape, weight, and physical appearance. She had an exaggerated fear of being fat and a strong desire to lose weight. In a typical month, H. B. engaged in binge eating about half of the days and engaged in secret eating about 75% of the days. She dieted by setting rules about eating and avoiding specific foods. She used purging (two to four times each week) and daily ingestion of two over-the-counter diet pills to control her weight so that it was within the normal range for her height. Her score on the Beck Depression Inventory was 53, indicating a high level of clinical depression.

H. B. has an eating disorder: bulimia nervosa with co-occurring depression. H. B.'s gender reflects the fact that, with the exception of obesity, the preponderance of individuals who experience eating disorders are female. For example, 90% of the cases of anorexia nervosa and bulimia nervosa involve females (American Psychiatric Association, 2000). Eating disorders are indicative of an individual's maladaptive relationship with food, and the treatment of eating disorders is challenging. It raises some unique issues that are not seen when treating addictions to substances such as tobacco and alcohol, where abstinence often serves as a viable treatment goal. To successfully treat eating disorders, individuals must learn to regulate their food intake. Unfortunately for many, regulation of intake is a difficult undertaking and they either underregulate and eat too much, as in binge-eating and obesity, or overregulate and eat too little, as in anorexia nervosa. What might the relapse prevention (RP) model (Marlatt & Gordon, 1980, 1985) offer to researchers and clinicians seeking to treat eating disorders? In this chapter, the RP model is presented as a useful framework for integrating a variety of approaches and maintenance strategies that are effective in the treatment of various eating disorders. More specifically, the chapter focuses on psychological treatments for bulimia nervosa, binge-eating disorder, and obesity, each of which is treated using interventions that can be integrated within the RP framework. Given the rarity of anorexia nervosa, the fact that it is the only eating disorder that does not involve the underregulation of food intake, and the unique elements of its treatment (e.g., inpatient hospitalization), anorexia nervosa will only be discussed to make specific points.

This chapter begins with a description of the RP model and related conceptualizations of the processes involved in changing behavior and maintaining behavior change. I then describe standard multicomponent treatments that integrate cognitive and behavioral interventions for eating disorders and highlight successful empirically supported interventions that share commonalities with, or are derived from, components of the RP model. Such interventions are drawn from cognitive-behavioral therapy, interpersonal psychotherapy, motivational interviewing, and other treatment approaches that overlap with the principles of the RP model. All of these approaches acknowledge that initial treatment success often is followed by the immense challenges of long-term maintenance. This acknowledgment is supported by empirical data indicating that most treatments for eating disorders are not effective in the long term. For example, Garner and Wooley (1991) cited the lack of long-term efficacy of a range of commonly used behavioral and dietary treatments for obesity. Relapse rates for the treatment of bulimia nervosa, binge-eating, and anorexia nervosa are similarly high.

As previously mentioned, one major difference between eating disorders and other substance use disorders is the fact that the goal of treatment has to be the regulation of food intake rather than abstinence. The components of the RP model are easily applicable to the processes involved in regulating behavior and maintaining behavior change (Marlatt & Gordon,

1980, 1985). When applied to treating eating disorders, they can be summarized as follows. The woman who is trying to overcome an eating disorder experiences a high-risk situation (e.g., stress) for which she has no coping response. The lack of a coping response leads to decreased self-efficacy (i.e., low confidence about handling the situation) and positive beliefs that eating will help her to handle the situation and/or to feel better. This leads to initial maladaptive eating (a lapse). The lapse is experienced as a failure to which she responds with the abstinence violation effect (AVE). The AVE involves self-blame for the lapse and a negative affective reaction. To cope with the AVE, including to feel better and repair her negative mood, the woman engages in further maladaptive eating, thereby moving to a full blown relapse.

Although the RP model is the focus in this chapter, researchers have proposed other models to explain the processes involved in the regulation of behavior and/or the failure to maintain behavior change. Two models that are compatible with RP are the *self-control strength model* (Muraven & Baumeister, 2000; Muraven, Tice, & Baumeister, 1998), which is based on research on self-regulation (Baumeister, Heatherton, & Tice, 1998), and the *false-hope syndrome model* (Polivy & Herman, 2002), which seeks to account for repeated attempts to change behavior in light of the high rates of relapse and failure.

Baumeister and colleagues (1998) focus on self-regulation as the key to changing behavior and maintaining the change over time. They describe the failure to self-regulate as involving factors such as having conflicting goals, failing to monitor oneself, and failing to manage attention and negative affect. Consistent with the AVE described in the RP model, they describe the paradox of holding *zero tolerance beliefs*. Such beliefs initially aid efforts to self-regulate because they provide a strict rule by which to govern behavior. However, over time they can undermine or weaken self-regulation because, when the inevitable lapse occurs, the individual has no alternative response to the lapse and reverts to engaging in the behavior she sought to change. In the case of a bulimic who has a zero tolerance belief that no purging is acceptable, once the first purge occurs and she has no way to handle it, she then finds it difficult to refrain from purging. Based on research on self-regulation, Muraven and Baumeister (2000; Muraven et al., 1998) have proposed a *self-control strength model* in which self-control is conceptualized as a finite resource. When individuals exert self-control in one situation, it undermines their capacity to exert self-control in a subsequent situation. Thus, a female whose supply of self-control strength is depleted by coping with a stressful day at work will have less self-control strength available to regulate her binge-eating at dinner that night and so will engage in excessive binge-eating. This may be particularly the case because women who binge-eat appraise stressors as more stressful than their non-eating-disordered peer controls (Hansel & Wittrock, 1997).

Polivy and Herman (2002) have proposed a *false-hope syndrome model* to explain the processes that may account for the high rates of relapse and continued attempts to change behavior. In their model, an individual trying to change a behavior optimistically expects and experiences initial success. Over time, as she finds it difficult to maintain the effort to change, failures occur. Once failures or relapses accumulate, she experiences negative affect. However, to the extent that she makes attributions to explain away the failures, it becomes possible to begin the cycle of change all over again.

Findings concerning the high rates of relapse in response to various treatments as well as the explanatory models that have been proposed highlight the need to focus on strategies that enhance the maintenance of behavior change and treatment gains. As will become apparent, the components of the RP model have relevance both to initial interventions for eating disorders and the maintenance of the positive effects of treatment over time. However, the model's strengths lie in providing a conceptual framework for understanding the issues faced during the maintenance phase and developing useful strategies for enhancing long-term maintenance.

ASSESSMENT OF EATING DISORDERS AS A PRELUDE TO TREATMENT

Eating disorders are multiply determined and therefore can truly be characterized as biopsychosocial disorders. Biological factors, including genetic influences, play a role in some of these disorders. For example, the melanocortin 4 receptor gene is related to some forms of obesity, and a mutation of that gene was found among a small percentage of obese binge-eaters, suggesting a genetic cause for their eating disorder (Branson et al., 2003). Even so, current research suggests that social and psychological factors predominate in the etiology of eating disorders. One only has to consider the fact that during the past century the prevalence of obesity in the U.S. population has increased to 54.9% of persons 20 years or older (National Heart, Lung, and Blood Institute, 1998), even though the genetic make-up of the U.S. population generally has not changed. Psychological factors that are related to eating disorders may include using food as a way to cope with stress and other negative affective states. Social factors that are related to eating disorders include internalizing sociocultural pressure to be thin, or modeling maladaptive patterns of excessive eating. The wide availability of a variety of foods and the sensory aspects (including taste) of these foods also contribute to increased intake (Raynor & Epstein, 2001). In addition, behavioral changes in day-to-day activities such as driving rather than walking or taking the elevator rather than the stairs lessen caloric expenditures and thereby contribute to increased rates of obesity. Given the central role of psychological, social, and behavioral factors in the etiology of many eating disorders, such factors must be considered as central to treatment. Individualized assessment to pinpoint the specific etiological and maintenance factors that need to be addressed in treatment can then lead to selection of the specific interventions that can be used to address these biopsychosocial factors.

In formal taxonomies such as the fourth edition of the *Diagnostic and Statistical Manual of Mental Disorders* (DSM-IV; American Psychiatric Association, 2000), the diagnostic criteria for eating disorders change over time and as a function of research and clinical experience. Diagnostic criteria often are controversial and may not provide appropriate guidance for intervention (Herzog & Delinsky, 2001). Although treatment of eating disorders often begins with examination of the DSM criteria, within the cognitive-behavioral framework provided by the RP model, assessment includes the wide range of behavioral and psychosocial factors that are related to current eating behavior (see Collins & Ricciardelli, 2005). In some cases, eating disorders co-occur with other addictions (e.g., bulimia with substance abuse) or with other mental health problems (e.g., binge-eating disorder with depression). Dependent on the aspect of the eating behavior that is being assessed, there are a variety of strategies and psychometrically sound measures that can be used to assess the presenting symptoms (see Collins & Ricciardelli, 2005). Following a thorough assessment of etiological and maintenance factors, the clinician develops a plan for intervening to change the eating disorder.

APPLICATION OF THE RELAPSE PREVENTION MODEL TO THE TREATMENT OF EATING DISORDERS

To lessen the probability of a full-blown relapse, Marlatt and Gordon (1980, 1985) outlined cognitive and behavioral interventions to address each of the components of their RP model. Many of these RP-based interventions have been incorporated into cognitive-behavioral treatments for the different eating disorders. The efficacy of such interventions vary, possibly in part due to the selective inclusion of different components of the model. Perri and colleagues directly compared RP with other strategies designed to enhance maintenance of weight loss (Perri, Shapiro, Ludwig, Twentyman, & McAdoo, 1984). They compared 12-month maintenance of weight loss related to three different treatments (behavioral, nonbehavioral, behavioral + RP) and two maintenance conditions (mail or telephone therapist contact vs. no therapist contact). At posttreatment, all three treatments produced similarly good weight loss. However, at the 12-month follow-up, only those participants who had received behavior therapy + RP treatment combined with posttreatment therapist contact maintained their weight loss. The efficacy of this combined approach was related to having provided training in the use of coping strategies and to greater use of behavioral procedures. In contrast, the failure of those who received behavior therapy + RP with no posttreatment contact was attributed to limited time for teaching RP, which meant that participants could not master the various techniques and failed to appropriately implement the other maintenance procedures. The efficacy of a behavior therapy treatment followed by RP + therapist contact during maintenance has been replicated (cf. Baum, Clark, & Sandler, 1991).

It has been suggested that one possible limitation of comprehensive approaches such as RP is the level of demand that it places on the individuals who are in treatment. Perri et al. (2001) compared relapse prevention therapy (RPT) to problem-solving therapy (PST) for long-term maintenance of weight loss for obese women who had completed a standard behavioral weight management program. Participants in an extended maintenance (i.e., 1 year) component received either 24 biweekly sessions of RPT based on Marlatt and Gordon's (1985) model or 24 biweekly sessions of PST. RPT consisted of biweekly psychoeducational sessions that focused on topics such as identifying high-risk situations, coping with high-risk situations, and balancing one's lifestyle. Participants in PST reported on specific difficulties encountered since the previous session. The group then engaged in a five-stage problem solving model that included activities such as defining problems and goals, decision making, and evaluating the efficacy of their plan. Results indicated that although RPT and PST were not significantly different over time, weight loss for those in RPT was not significantly better than the behavior therapy (BT) waiting-list control condition. PST was significantly different from BT. In trying to explain the failure to replicate previous successes of RPT for obesity, Perri et al. (2001) noted the differences between the two extended-care conditions. Namely, RPT participants had to learn a wide range of skills and thus may not have had sufficient opportunity to develop mastery of each of the specific skills. In contrast, the PST condition consisted of multiple opportunities to apply the same model to solving different problems. This insight provides a useful critique of multicomponent interventions such as RP and suggests the need to more carefully consider the therapeutic context in which RP is presented, such as the individual's level of motivation to change. It also enhances the case for focusing on RP, either in the context of a structured intervention (cf. Annis, Schober, & Kelly, 1996) or by selecting one or more specific components of the RP model that have relevance to the specific issues faced by a particular individual.

STAGES OF CHANGE AND MOTIVATIONAL INTERVIEWING

The individual's motivation to change her eating disorder is an important issue that has to be considered in treatment planning (Rossi, Rossi, Velicer,

& Prochaska, 1995; Treasure & Schmidt, 2001). Regardless of the treatment approach, research based on the transtheoretical model of stages of change (Prochaska, DiClemente, & Norcross, 1992) suggests that understanding the individual's orientation toward change will enhance treatment matching, thereby influencing the course and outcome of treatment. Particularly in the case of eating disorders, where an individual may feel ambivalent about treatment, identification of the individual's stage of readiness may help the clinician to engage her in treatment. The transtheoretical model describes five stages of readiness: (1) *precontemplation*, not prepared to change; (2) *contemplation*, seriously thinking about engaging in the change process; (3) *preparation*, intending to take action to change; (4) *action*, actively engaged in changing behaviors and/or cognitions; and (5) *maintenance*, working to maintain positive outcomes and prevent relapse.

Standard measures of the stages and processes of the transtheoretical model have been applied to eating disorders. For example, the 32-item *Stages of Change Questionnaire* (SCQ; McConnaughy, Prochaska, & Velicer, 1983) and the *Processes of Change Questionnaire* (PCQ; Ward, Troop, Todd, & Treasure, 1996) have been modified for use in the treatment of bulimia nervosa (Stanton, Rebert, & Zinn, 1986; Treasure et al., 1999). New measures have been developed to assess the application of the transtheoretical model to anorexia nervosa (Jordan, Redding, Troop, Treasure, & Serpell, 2003). The applicability of the transtheoretical model has been enhanced by the development of a psychometrically sound semistructured *Readiness and Motivation Interview* (RMI) that focuses on the symptoms of eating disorders (Geller, Cockell, & Drab, 2001; Geller & Drab, 1999). The RMI incorporates the diagnostic items of the *Eating Disorder Examination* (EDE; Cooper & Fairburn, 1987) so that both diagnostic (frequency and severity of symptom from the EDE) and readiness/motivation items can be jointly assessed. In an initial assessment of the RMI with a clinical sample, readiness to change differed across symptom domains (Geller et al., 2001). For example, clients were more ready to change bingeing, but less ready to change caloric restriction or exercise. In addition, clients in the action stage reported fewer symptoms and lower levels of psychiatric problems. These differences may help to explain the inconsistencies previously found in studies of the role of stages of change in the outcome of treatment for eating disorders.

Applications of the transtheoretical model to treating eating disorders have shown some clinical utility (Blake, Turnbull, & Treasure, 1997), although findings have not been consistent. In some cases, stages of change have been linked to treatment outcome (e.g., Treasure et al., 1999), particularly the outcome for interpersonal therapy (Wolk & Devlin, 2001). In other cases, it has not predicted outcome, particularly for cognitive-behavioral therapy (Wolk & Devlin, 2001). Geller and colleagues found that understanding readiness across symptom domains is likely to be important for enhancing the clinician's ability to respond to clients so as to engage and retain them in treatment. For example, the clinician can begin to actively work on symptoms that the client is ready to change while helping her to move along the earlier stages (precontemplation, contemplation, preparation) toward taking action on other symptoms (Geller et al., 2001).

The clinical intervention most directly associated with the transtheoretical model is motivational interviewing (MI; DiClemente & Velasquez, 2002). In MI, the clinician's goals are to create in the client an awareness of the need for change, to increase the client's motivation to make a change, and to discuss plans for change (Miller & Rollnick, 1991, 2002). MI techniques include (1) eliciting self-motivational statements, (2) listening with empathy, (3) asking open-ended questions about the client's feelings, ideas, concerns, and plans, (4) affirming the client in a way that acknowledges her serious consideration of and steps toward change, (5) deflecting resistance by reflecting the client's feelings or by shifting focus away from a problematic issue, rather than arguing with or confronting the client, (6) reframing problematic thoughts or perceptions so that the client sees a given issue from a more productive point of view, and (7) reflecting and summarizing concerns raised by the client during the decision-making process (Miller & Rollnick, 1991, 2002). In some adaptations of MI, the clinician provides objective personalized feedback and related factual information and uses an empathic style to move the client toward seeing behavior change as necessary (e.g., Miller et al., 1993). Once the client decides to change, she is provided with a menu of treatment strategies from which interventions are selected and implemented.

DiLillo, Siegfried, and West (2003) have described methods for integrating MI into an individualized, comprehensive weight-loss program. Their recommendations reflect the MI techniques that already have been listed. For example, DiLillo et al. provide detailed descriptions of methods for eliciting self-motivational statements (i.e., statements in favor of losing weight) from a client and methods for providing personalized feedback about objective data (e.g., information about cholesterol and/or blood pressure) to reinforce the decision to lose weight. Although their recommendations for clinical integration are useful, they are based only on the promise of using MI to treat eating disorders; there is a paucity of research on the topic.

In a recent meta-analysis of research that included adaptations of MI, Burke, Arkowitz, and Menchola (2003) identified only five studies that focused on eating behaviors. Four of the studies focused on diet and exercise and one focused on eating disorders. Comparisons of the efficacy of MI with other interventions and control conditions yielded medium effect-sizes for changes in the target behaviors (e.g., blood pressure, physical activity score). However, the MI-based interventions achieved their effects in much less time than standard interventions, an important consideration in these days of concern about the cost-effectiveness of treatment. Burke et al. concluded that the effects of MI for diet and exercise were equivalent to other active treatments and superior to control conditions. In addition, the results were sustained at follow-up, showed evidence of clinical impact, and showed evidence of affecting life areas beyond the target symptoms. Although links have been made between the transtheoretical model and MI, Burke et al. also concluded that MI interventions did not appear to increase readiness to change, relative to other interventions. The questions raised by this review as well as the overall lack of research on the application of MI and its adaptations to treating eating disorders clearly indicate the need for more research on this topic.

The RP approach can be combined with the transtheoretical model to produce an effective intervention for maladaptive behaviors, including eating disorders. An example of such a successful combination is *structured relapse prevention* (SRP) counseling for addictions (Annis et al., 1996). Their five-stage approach links each of the five stages of change with RP assessment and treatment in the following pairings: precontemplation + assessment; contemplation + motivational interviewing; preparation + the development of individual treatment plans; action + initial treatment; and maintenance + longer-term treatment. Results for the use of SRP to treat clients with alcohol and drug abuse problems indicate findings that are consistent with the RP model. As summarized by Annis et al. (1996), SRP clients reduced their substance use, showed good use of coping strategies for handling high-risk situations, and showed high self-efficacy as a function of effective treatment. Those who used a greater number and variety of coping strategies were at reduced risk for experiencing a relapse. Although Annis et al.'s SRP approach has not been applied to the treatment of eating disorders, its applicability is clear and its potential for success may match that found for the treatment of other addictions.

COGNITIVE-BEHAVIORAL TREATMENT FOR EATING DISORDERS

There are many consistencies across differing approaches for treating different eating disorders, suggesting that there are stable elements across different versions of multicomponent cognitive-behavioral treatment (CBT) and other psychological treatments for eating disorders. Many of these elements overlap with aspects of the RP model, and some approaches even incorporate the RP model into treatment, particularly in the maintenance phases of their programs. In numerous qualitative reviews and meta-analyses of the literature on treating eating disorders, CBT has been identified as the treatment of choice (e.g., Lewandowski, Gebing, Anthony, & O'Brien, 1997; Wilson & Fairburn, 2002). In comparison to other commonly used treatments including medication and interpersonal therapy, CBT is the most effective treatment for bulimia nervosa that currently is available, even through long-term (up to 1 year) follow-ups (e.g., Anderson & Maloney, 2001; Lewandowski et al., 1997). CBT for bulimia nervosa is effective in applied contexts that do not include the controls found in research settings (Tuschen-Caffier, Pook, & Frank, 2001) and a version of CBT was effective for treating binge-eating (Telch, Agras, Rossiter, Wilfley, & Kenardy, 1990). Often CBT is used to treat obesity (Cooper & Fairburn, 2001). As such, CBT serves as the gold-standard and an excellent point of departure for considering RP-based intervention strategies for treating eating disorders.

Fairburn, Marcus, and Wilson (1993) presented a comprehensive and commonly used approach to CBT for bulimia nervosa. Their semistructured, 20-session program is divided into three stages. Stage 1 consists of eight sessions that are designed to provide a rationale for CBT and to establish a stable pattern of regular eating. During this phase the client learns to self-monitor eating, identify and use pleasurable alternative behaviors, and engage in weekly weigh-ins. They also receive educational information about the adverse effects of dieting, purging, and laxative use as ways of controlling weight. Stage 2 consists of eight sessions that focus on reducing dieting and other controls (e.g., banned foods) on eating. Clients are taught the steps to effective problem solving, and cognitive restructuring is used to address concerns about the body, weight, and shape. Stage 3 consists of three sessions that focus on preparation for maintaining treatment gains. Sessions focus on encouragement to practice the cognitive and behavioral techniques learned in the previous sessions and development of a written maintenance plan. This stage includes highlighting the distinction between a *lapse* (a situational change that can be self-corrected) and a *relapse* (a longer-term deterioration that requires help from a clinician). The maintenance plan can include reminders of the interventions that the individual has found to be most helpful. One useful aspect of the approach outlined by Fairburn et al. (1993) is that with a few modifications, it can be applied to the treatment of other eating disorders, such as binge-eating among the obese as well as anorexia nervosa.

Similar programs that involve approximately 20 sessions/weeks of treatment that are organized into three or four stages/phases have been described by Spangler (1999) and Wonderlich, Mitchell, Peterson, and Crow (2001). In all of these multicomponent treatments, the final stage/phase focuses on maintaining treatment gains and preventing relapse. Thus, Spangler described a treatment program that consisted of three phases that occur over 20 weeks. The phases involve (1) establishing a regular pattern of eating, (2) identifying and changing beliefs about body shape and weight, and (3) preventing relapse. Phase 1 includes interventions such as self monitoring of food intake, eating at regular mealtimes, weighing only once per week and learning accurate information to correct maladaptive beliefs related to food and bulimic behaviors. There also is a focus on developing positive alternatives to bulimic behaviors. Once a regular pattern of eating is established, treatment moves to the second phase. Phase 2 interventions include increasing the number and types of foods that are eaten, identifying and changing beliefs that promote body dissatisfaction and developing positive alternatives to thoughts and behaviors that maintain bulimic behaviors. There also is a focus on developing problem-solving and coping skills. Phase 3 focuses on preparation to maintain the changes that were made in the previous two phases. A *relapse plan* for handling the possible return of bulimia is developed. Components of the plan include identifying "recurrences" and relapse, using interventions to lessen recurrences and relapse, and continuing to use effective cognitive-behavioral strategies to maintain treatment gains.

Wonderlich et al.'s (2001) program is based on an integrative cognitive therapy approach that is said to go beyond standard CBT in its inclusion of issues such as enhancing motivation for treatment, focusing on self-oriented cognition, interpersonal relationships, emotions, and cultural factors. *Phase I* consists of three sessions that incorporate ideas from MI (Miller & Rollnick, 1991), develop the client's understanding about the discrepancy between her actual and ideal body shape and weight, and discuss the role of cultural factors (idealization of thinness) in her eating disorder. Self-monitoring of eating serves as an important behavioral task. *Phase II* consists of five sessions that focus on normalizing eating (e.g., planning and consuming of nutritious meals) and developing eating-specific coping skills. These coping skills include learning to identify, express, and handle negative emotional states using techniques such as relaxation training. *Phase III* consists of 10 sessions that focus on interpersonal and intrapersonal factors. This includes an analysis of interpersonal situations to identify the ways in which the client uses specific interaction patterns to manage negative affect. The analysis of intrapersonal, mainly cognitive, processes focuses on changing the discrepancy between the actual and the ideal self. The two sessions of *Phase IV* are based in part on the RP model. They focus on preventing relapses and lifestyle management as well as education about the nature of relapse (e.g., the distinction between a lapse and a relapse). Clients identify different types of high-risk situations and develop strategies for coping with them. Following a review of treatment success the client develops a maintenance plan that includes strategies for continued improvement in the context of a healthy lifestyle.

Using an approach that shares commonalities with aspects of the RP approach, Page, Sutherby, and Treasure (2002) describe the use of "relapse management cards" in the maintenance phase of inpatient treatment of anorexia nervosa. The use of the cards is predicated on the notion that anorexia nervosa is a chronic illness within which relapse is common. Just prior to discharge, the cards are prepared in collaboration with the anorexia nervosa client, family members, and a representative of the treatment team. The items on the relapse management cards are individualized and are based on a semistructured menu that includes the following items: "Treatment on discharge; Plans to decrease likelihood of relapse; Signs of relapse; Interventions which have been helpful in the past when relapsing: Interventions which have been unhelpful in the past when relapsing; Plans in the event of a relapse; Specific refusals in the event of a relapse; Reasons to be re-admitted to hospital" (p. 284). Although the relapse management cards address issues that are much broader than those addressed by the RP model, the focus on maintaining treatment gains, identifying the precursors of relapse, and reducing the likelihood of relapse share much in common with Marlatt and Gordon's (1980, 1985) approach. Data from a sample of 41 patients indicated that some items on the cards were more readily endorsed than others. For example, 77.5% of the patients identified changes in food habits and social withdrawal as signs of a relapse. Only 42.5% of the patients wanted their families to be involved in the event of a relapse. To date there are no data on whether the use of these relapse management cards will reduce relapse rates among anorexics; however, the cards are seen as an effective way of involving clients in their care following discharge, thereby opening up communication and empowering the client to focus on maintaining treatment gains.

APPLICATION OF RELAPSE PREVENTION: SPECIFIC INTERVENTIONS FOR TREATING EATING DISORDERS AND MAINTAINING POSITIVE OUTCOMES

Identification of High-Risk Eating Situations: The Role of Negative Affect

The RP model describes high-risk situations as those that challenge the individual's ability to cope. When faced with such situations, individuals tend to use the maladaptive strategies with which they are familiar and comfortable, including excessive eating. The failure to cope with high-risk situations leads to lapses and/or relapses, which can occur during the course of treatment or after treatment, during the maintenance phase. Thus, identifying high-risk situations and developing coping strategies that preclude maladaptive eating are highly relevant to the RP approach to treating eating disorders. Cummings, Gordon, and Marlatt (1980) categorized high-risk situations for relapse following treatment for various addictions (smoking, alcohol abuse, overeating) and identified consistencies across substances. For overeaters, relapses occurred in situations that involved both intrapersonal (46%) and interpersonal (52%) determinants. The most important intrapersonal determinants (33%) involved negative emotional states (e.g., depression, anxiety). Urges and temptations (10%) played a smaller role. Unique to overeaters was the fact that the most important interpersonal determinants (28%) involved positive emotional states (e.g., happy). However, overeaters were similar to other substance abusers in reporting relapses in which interpersonal conflict (14%) and social pressure (10%) played a role. Similarly, Grilo, Shiffman, and Wing (1989) identified high-risk situations for overeating by analyzing the posttreatment reports of obese participants in a behavioral weight-loss program. Overeating relapses were most likely during social (with family, friends) mealtimes as well as in situations involving negative affect (anger, anxiety, depression) and low arousal (alone, bored). The presence of food or affective cues was common. In these and other studies, negative affect appears to be a particularly potent high-risk situation that either precipitates or maintains maladaptive eating.

The pervasiveness of negative affect as a precursor to maladaptive eating is acknowledged in the models such as Heatherton and Baumeister's (1991) escape model of binge-eating, which posits that binge-eating occurs as an attempt to escape from aversive self-awareness, accompanied by negative affect. Other researchers have acknowledged the importance of negative affect by developing measures that assess it as specifically related to eating. For example, the *Emotional Eating Scale* (Arnow, Kenardy, & Agras, 1995) includes subscales that measure anger/frustration, depression, and anxiety as precursors to eating. All three subscales were associated with binge-eating, such that the authors proposed that negative-affect eating may precipitate binge episodes. Negative affect prior to maladaptive eating also has been identified in a self-monitoring study of bulimics, who tended to report more negative mood prior to a binge episode (Davis, Freeman, & Garner, 1988) and in a laboratory study of obese women with binge-eating disorder (Agras & Telch, 1998).

Wegner et al. (2002) examined the covariation of mood and binge-eating among a sample of 27 female college students who reported subclinical levels of binge-eating behavior. The women used handheld computers to self-monitor moods, eating, and related phenomena multiple times per day in their natural environments for 2 weeks. Their results indicated that moods were more negative on binge as compared to nonbinge days, with mood just after a binge being much worse than mood just prior to a binge. Interestingly, transient negative mood did not seem to precipitate a binge, as proposed in some theories of eating disorders. In addition, food did not provide relief from negative mood, as described by models, including RP, that conceptualize eating as a coping strategy. The fact that this study included ecologically valid, ongoing assessment of mood in the natural environment is a major methodological plus, particularly when compared to the many studies that are based on retrospective reports that are subject to forgetting, the aggregation of affect over time, and other biases. However, the sample did not meet diagnostic criteria for eating disorders, and so the results may not generalize to the processes that occur in clinical populations

Coping with High-Risk Eating Situations

In their study of relapse precipitants, Grilo et al. (1989) were able to identify the situational determinants of actual episodes of overeating as well as
the type of coping used to address the situation. In most cases, participants
used behavioral and/or cognitive coping and were able to overcome the
lapse/relapse. Combining behavioral and cognitive coping produced better
outcomes than using either one alone. All situations in which the dieters
used no coping response ended in a lapse/relapse in which overeating occurred. Paxton and Diggens (1997) examined the role of avoidance coping
in binge-eating. Generally, avoidance coping is conceptualized as being
maladaptive. Thus, within the RP framework, use of avoidance coping
would likely lead to failure to cope with high-risk situations, thereby precipitating maladaptive eating. The results of Paxton and Diggens study
suggested that use of avoidance coping was confounded with depression,
and therefore it was negative affect rather than use of maladaptive coping
that precipitated binge-eating.

One strategy for assessing the individual's ability to cope with high-
risk situations before they occur in the field is to expose them to potential
high-risk scenarios/situations, for which they have to provide a coping response other than substance use (cf. Chaney, O'Leary, & Marlatt, 1978).
High-risk situations can be generic or can be developed based on the triggers faced by specific individuals. In Chaney et al.'s study, alcoholics were
presented with audiotaped versions of high-risk scenarios. The latency
with which the participants generated a coping response was measured as
an indication of their potential to experience a lapse/relapse. The idea being that longer latencies indicate a lack of a coping response, which in turn
means that the individual will use her typical maladaptive coping response
of using substances. Along with the latency of the response, the nature and
efficacy of the coping response also can be measured. In this way, gaining
an understanding of the individual's ability to cope with high-risk situations can set the stage for the subsequent component of the RP model,
which is providing training in coping strategies.

Drapkin, Wing, and Shiffman (1995) used an approach similar to
Chaney et al.'s (1978) to examine the responses of persons who were faced
with situations that presented high risks for eating. At the start of a weight-
control program, clients listened to descriptions of four hypothetical high-
risk scenarios in which dieters might choose to go off their diets. The four
clinically relevant scenarios depicted (1) a family celebration involving favorite foods; (2) an argument that ends with escape to a kitchen filled with
favorite foods; (3) visiting the kitchen during a commercial break in a television show; and (4) taking a break from pressure at work and being faced
with delicious snacks brought in by a coworker. For each situation, participants were asked to describe what they would think or do to avoid overeating. In addition, they rated their temptation to eat and their self-efficacy

regarding not overeating. Latency to respond, type of coping (behavioral vs. cognitive), and consistency of coping (over 6 months) also were examined. The results indicated that the number of situations in which participants generated a coping response was related to long-term (6-month) weight loss. Actual lapses during the program were similar to the type of scenarios (negative vs. positive affect) that the participants judged to be their most difficult. This latter finding was said to reflect the participants' accurate knowledge of themselves and their ability to predict their own behavior. Implications for treatment included the suggestion that identifying difficult scenarios could indicate areas for which specific coping skills could be taught. Also of note, most coping responses involved behavioral coping, suggesting that training in this form of coping might be very effective, particularly in treatment using the group format that was used by Drapkin et al. (1995).

Hansel and Wittrock (1997) assessed women's coping in laboratory tasks as well as their use of self-monitoring in the natural environment. The laboratory tasks varied in the level of stress. They consisted of a videotaped interpersonal situation involving two women in conversation and an academic stressor that involved solving anagrams. Results indicated that women with binge-eating disorder reported more stress than the nonbinge-eating controls, particularly related to the high-stress condition. Although the binge-eaters reported more positive coping, they also reported more catastrophizing both in the laboratory tasks and in the natural environment. It was concluded that although binge and nonbinge eaters did not differ in the number of stressors they reported, bingers reported each event as more stressful and used more positive and negative coping strategies. The efficacy of a particular coping strategy is more important than the number of coping strategies used. Hansel and Wittrock's finding may indicate that binge-eaters and others with eating disorders are using many coping strategies because they either are not selecting efficacious strategies or their implementation of a particular strategy is poor. In either case, the RP model suggests that the acquisition and use of effective coping is an important strategy for maintaining treatment gains.

Enhancement of Coping Responses: Alternatives to Maladaptive Eating

In some etiological models of eating disorders, food serves as a readily available source of psychological comfort that helps the individual to cope with internal or external sources of stress and negative affect (cf. Heatherton & Baumeister, 1991). The use of eating and other maladaptive ways of coping is common among individuals with eating disorders. Troop, Holbrey, Trowler, and Treasure (1994) compared problem areas and use of coping strategies among women with anorexia nervosa, those with bulimia nervosa, and a control group of women with no eating disorders. Compared to the controls, women with eating disorders tended to describe more psychological problems. They also used more avoidance coping, more wishful thinking, and less social support and less problem-focused coping than the controls. Reliance on nonproblem-focused coping strategies is less adaptive and has been linked to the development of disorders such as depression, which might further contribute to problems with eating. The authors concluded that teaching coping strategies would be a useful component of treatment for eating disorders (Troop et al., 1994). Given the variety of high-risk situations, these techniques take many forms.

Providing Alternatives to Maladaptive Eating

It is important that individuals with eating disorders develop positive alternatives to maladaptive eating. These alternatives can counter high-risk situations that include boredom/lack of activities, and they can foster the development of skills for coping with a variety of situations. These positive alternatives include exercise, meditation, and other forms of relaxation as a component of developing a healthy lifestyle. Initially such activities may seem difficult, but over time regular practice of exercise or meditation can transform them into *positive addictions*, habits that "feel unpleasant in the short run . . . but are associated with positive consequences in the long run" (Marlatt, 1985, p. 299).

Exercise serves as a useful positive alternative to eating, which may be particularly useful during the maintenance phase of treatment for eating disorders such as obesity (Garner & Wooley, 1991; Jakicic, Wing, & Winters-Hart, 2002; Wadden, Vogt, Foster, & Anderson, 1998), binge-eating (Pendleton, Goodrick, Poston, Reeves, & Foreyt, 2002), and bulimia nervosa (Sundgot-Borgen, Rosenvingne, Bahr, & Schneider, 2002). Exercise confers benefits related to burning calories, thereby enhancing maintenance of reduction in weight among the obese. For example, Jakicic et al. (2002) examined the role of physical activity in a behavioral weight-loss program. Over an 18-month period, they found that increased physical activity was associated with decreases in body weight and body-mass index (BMI) as well as increases in eating behaviors that promote weight loss. They concluded that interventions that combine both behavior change and increased activity are necessary for improving long-term weight loss. In the treatment of binge-eating, adding exercise and a maintenance program to CBT led to significant reductions in binge-eating frequency, body weight, and BMI (Pendleton et al., 2002). In the treatment of bulimia nervosa, exercise reduced the frequency of bingeing and purging and was useful for addressing the pursuit of thinness and body dissatisfaction (Levine, Marcus, & Moulton, 1996; Sundot-Borgen et al., 2002).

The regulation of negative affect may play a role in the etiology and/or maintenance of eating disorders (Penas-Lliedo, Vaz Leal, & Waller, 2002). Exercise promotes positive affect, thereby countering the negative affective states that can increase risk for relapse following treatment (Nieman, Custer, Butterworth, Utter, & Henson, 2000; Stice, 1999). Moderate exercise training has led to decreases in anxiety (Cramer, Nieman, & Lee, 1991) and depression (Hayward, Sullivan, & Libonati, 2000) as well as improvements in general well-being (Cramer et al., 1991; Nieman et al., 2000) among obese women. These findings suggest that exercise confers many psychological benefits that promote maintenance of treatment gains.

Although exercise provides many benefits, it can be a double-edged sword because excessive or obligatory exercise can play an etiological role in eating disorders, particularly anorexia nervosa (Ackard, Brehm, & Steffen, 2002; Davis et al., 1997; Penas-Lliedo et al., 2002). In such cases, during treatment and maintenance, the focus must be on lessening rather than increasing the level and frequency of exercise. For example, results of a pilot study on using a graded exercise program to treat anorexia nervosa showed that it increased compliance with treatment and did not interfere with short-term gains in body fat or BMI (Thien, Thomas, Markin, & Birmingham, 2000). Thus, even in situations where excessive exercise may be problematic, a well-structured exercise program can confer benefits related to maintaining treatment gains.

Meditation and other forms of relaxation can serve as strategies for coping with stress and for regulating negative affective states. Marlatt (1985) has noted that the regular practice of relaxation can lead to a subjective feeling similar to being *high* on psychoactive drugs. This altered state of consciousness can be a goal in and of itself or can serve as a useful strategy for coping with cognitive (e.g., urges, cravings) and affective states that inevitably serve as risks during the maintenance phase. Similarly, the practice of meditation also can serve as a positive alternative that is effective in enhancing the maintenance of treatment for behavioral problems, including eating disorders (Marlatt & Kristeller, 1999). Mindfulness training, which incorporates meditation, relaxation, and attentional control is growing in popularity as a stand-alone treatment and as a component of cognitive-behavioral interventions for various stress-related medical conditions, anxiety, and depression (Baer, 2003; Teasdale et al., 2000). In a unique study, Kristeller and Hallett (1999) examined the efficacy of a meditation-based intervention for binge-eating disorder. Their results indicated significant reductions in measures of binge-eating, depression, and anxiety. The more time spent on meditation, the greater the decrease in scores on their measure of binge-eating. Although this exploratory study showed the promise of using meditation to treat eating disorders, its methodology was limited by the lack of a control group and long-term follow-up. Research is needed to examine the therapeutic efficacy of meditation alone and as an ingredient in multicomponent interventions for eating disorders. Researchers also need to examine the range of strategies that serve as positive alternatives for coping with high-risk eating situations and for regulating affect during longer-term maintenance.

Building Self-Efficacy

Self-efficacy involves an individual's confidence in her ability to effectively handle a stressful situation (Bandura, 1977). High self-efficacy is linked to effective coping, including the handling of high-risk situations that can undermine treatment gains. RP theory suggests that when faced with situations with which they cannot cope, persons with eating disorders may experience decreases in self-efficacy that will undermine their ability to regulate their food intake. Consistent with these notions, research suggests that changes in self-efficacy are associated with treatment-related changes in eating-related behavior. To assess self-efficacy concerning eating behaviors, researchers have developed psychometrically sound scales. Clark, Abrams, Niaura, Eaton, and Rossi (1991) developed the *Weight Efficacy Life-Style Questionnaire* (WEL), a 20-item measure that contains five subscales that assess self-efficacy for resisting food: (1) when experiencing negative emotions, (2) when it is readily available, (3) in response to social pressure, (4) when experiencing physical discomfort, and (5) when participating in positive activities. Each of these areas corresponds to high-risk situations identified by Marlatt and Gordon (1980, 1985). In studies to validate the WEL, Clark et al. found that obese participants lost weight and showed improvements in self-efficacy following a 19-week CBT weight-loss program that included training in RP versus a self-help program. Specifically, there were changes in the scores for the two WEL subscales that assessed resisting eating as a function of negative emotions and during positive activities. A second study included a 26-week weight-reduction program that involved CBT (including RP) plus a very low-calorie diet. At posttreatment, participants had lost weight and showed significant improvements in WEL scores in the areas of negative emotions, availability, and social pressure. These findings suggest that success in weight loss is associated with improvements in self-efficacy. Drapkin et al. (1995) assessed self-efficacy related to four hypothetical situations that posed increased risk for overeating. Results indicated that participants' ratings of confidence for not overeating were not related to losing weight. This contrasts to the relationship typically found between weight loss and self-efficacy as assessed using questionnaire measures such as the WEL. Inconsistencies between studies are likely the result of methodological differences that influence the nature of the relationships found between self-efficacy and treatment outcome for eating disorders. More research, including consideration of methodological issues, is needed to increase our understanding of this topic.

Countering Maladaptive Positive Beliefs That Maintain Eating Disorders

Beliefs about the positive effects of ingesting a substance (i.e., positive expectancies) exist for a variety of addictive substances, including alcohol (Goldman, Del Boca, & Darkes, 1999), tobacco (Copeland, Brandon, & Quinn, 1995), cocaine, and marijuana (Aarons, Brown, Stice, & Coe, 2001; Jaffe & Kilbey, 1994; Schafer & Brown, 1991). The content of these learned beliefs tend to be specific to the pharmacological and/or psychological features of the particular substance as well as the individual's learning history for the particular substance. Learning can occur directly via actual experience with the substance or indirectly through portrayals and messages from the broader culture, media, and other sources of modeling. In many cases, the positive beliefs that promote substance use are immediate, whereas the negative effects of substance use are distal and longer term. Regardless of the source, expectancies motivate behavior. Particularly after a period of abstinence or moderated use, the RP model suggests that when faced with a high-risk situation, no coping response, and low self-efficacy, these positive beliefs or expectancies can contribute to relapse because they reinforce the decision to reinstate or continue substance use.

As described in Collins and Ricciardelli (2005), during the past decade psychometrically sound measures have been developed to assess outcome expectancies for eating-related phenomena. They include the *Weight Loss Expectancy Scale* (WLES; Allen, Thombs, Mahoney, & Daniel, 1993), which consists of five factors: social confidence, social approval, self-worth, positive performance, and negative consequences. The *Eating Expectancy Inventory* (EEI; Hohlstein, Smith, & Atlas, 1998) consists of five factors/subscales that cover positive beliefs related to "eating helps manage negative affect," "eating is pleasurable and useful as a reward," "eating leads to feeling out of control," "eating enhances cognitive competence," "eating alleviates boredom." The *Thinness and Restricting Expectancy Inventory* (TREI; Hohlstein et al., 1998) consists of single factor that assesses the expectation that thinness and restricting food intake lead to overgeneralized self-improvement. The scales of both the EEI and the TREI measures were found to distinguish among women with symptoms for bulimia nervosa, anorexia nervosa, a psychiatric control, and a normal control group.

The items of the various measures of outcome expectancies came from sources that range from the self-reports of persons (typically women) with eating disorders to information from models of the etiology and correlates of eating disorders. As with expectancies for other substances, knowledge of specific positive beliefs provides a starting point for interventions. For example, the belief that eating helps to manage negative affect or boredom can be addressed by providing training in noneating-related strategies for coping with these negative affective states. The expectation that weight loss provides social confidence could be addressed with interventions to boost self-acceptance as well as with assertiveness training, and so on. Some of these interventions already exist in CBT and RP-based treatments, but assessment of specific expectancies can guide the targeting of interventions to specific individuals and/or specific eating disorders. By intervening to counter positive outcome expectancies, particularly those beliefs that are maladaptive, clinicians can help to change the individual's learned reinforcement contingencies and challenge the influence of the cognitions that maintain eating disorders.

Interpretation and Encapsulation of a Lapse

Although abstinence from eating any food is not an option for treatment of eating disorders, it is possible to set goals related to lessening or stopping certain behaviors. For example, the self-help program Overeaters Anonymous recommends abstinence from certain foods, and a clinician might recommend that a bulimic client abstain from purging. When the individual inevitably deviates from the abstinence goal, her reaction to that deviation will either allow her to interpret the deviation as a lapse (a situational occurrence over which she has control) versus a relapse (a global failure that is indicative of her lack of ability to change her eating habits). Viewing the deviation as situational leads to efforts to understand the causes of the lapse and based on that understanding to redouble efforts to maintain the positive behavior change. Viewing the deviation as a relapse leads to a return to her maladaptive eating behavior and maintenance of her eating disorder. Thus, programs that forbid the eating of particular foods may prime the occurrence of relapses, as proposed in the AVE.

The Abstinence Violation Effect

A reduction in dietary restraint has been cited as an important mediator of posttreatment improvement in CBT for bulimia nervosa (Wilson, Fairburn, Agras, Walsh, & Kraemer, 2002). Herman and Mack (1975) introduced the construct of dietary restraint as a way to account for differences in eating behavior of dieters and the obese as compared to persons of normal weight. Restrained individuals are concerned about their weight and try to regulate their food intake, but are highly responsive to external cues for eating. Later elaboration of the eating restraint model introduced the idea of upper and lower *boundaries* within which eating is regulated (Herman & Polivy, 1984). Restrained eaters successfully regulate their food intake (i.e., diet) until their restraint is broken by disinhibitors that range from the consumption of forbidden foods to the experience of negative affect. Once their restraint is broken they tend to engage in counterregulatory eating. That is, they binge or overeat until dietary regulation can be reestablished (Polivy & Herman, 1985). In survey, laboratory, and clinical studies, persons with eating disorders such as bulimia nervosa and binge-eating have been shown to be high in dietary restraint, as measured by self-report scales (Davis et al., 1988; Johnson, Corrigan, Crusco, & Schlundt, 1986).

There is much overlap between the conceptualization of dietary restraint and the AVE described in the RP model. Marlatt and Gordon (1980, 1985) describe the AVE as involving two stages: a cognitive attribution for the lapse or other violation of self-selected abstinence followed by an affective reaction to the attribution. Individuals who make internal causal attributions for the lapse and see it as a general failure to regulate their intake ("I lack willpower and so I'll never be able to do this") experience negative affective states. To feel better and to cope with the negative mood, they engage in further maladaptive eating, thereby moving to a full-blown relapse.

Aspects of the AVE have been substantiated in studies of persons with eating disorders that include obesity (Mooney, Burling, Hartman, & Brenner-Liss, 1992; Ogden & Wardle, 1990) and binge-eating (Grilo & Shiffman, 1994) as well as in theoretical notions about the role of attributions in bulimia nervosa (Ward, Hudson, & Bulik, 1993). Ogden and Wardle (1990) assessed the role of attributional style in the dieting success of moderately overweight women. As predicted by the AVE, those who reported higher levels of internal attributions for negative events also reported more lapses and relapses during their diet. Similar findings were reported by Mooney et al. (1992), who examined the AVE among a sample of morbidly obese clients in a very low-calorie (500 calories/day) diet and behavioral education program. Compared to those who made situational attributions, clients who reported greater internal attributions for their first lapse during the diet lost less weight. Among program dropouts, those who experienced a more intense AVE dropped out of the program earlier than those who experienced a less intense AVE. Grilo and Shiffman (1994) conducted a longitudinal study of AVE reactions following food binges in which they administered a binge-eating measure of attributional style to community women. Their results were consistent with the AVE, in that participants saw the causes of their binges as being internal, global, and uncontrollable, and they experienced negative affect and decreased self-efficacy. There was a positive association between the strength of the AVE and the speed with which a subsequent binge occurred. Of interest, the researchers found variation in the attributional and cognitive reactions to binges *within* individuals, thus highlighting the need for individualized approaches to treatment planning.

CONCLUSIONS

This overview of the application of the RP model to eating disorders makes the case that it clearly applies to conceptualizing the issues that are likely to be faced in planning and intervening to change maladaptive eating and maintain treatment gains. The RP model is compatible with other cognitive and behavioral approaches currently being used to treat eating disorders. It complements other models of the processes involved in initiating treatment (e.g., the transtheoretical model) and/or maintaining positive treatment outcomes. Dependent on the specific case, the components of the RP model can be applied in whole or in part. In fact, much of the research in support of the RP conceptualization of treating eating disorders has focused on specific components such as the role of positive expectancies or the abstinence violation effect. There are a few studies that have applied the entire RP model to conceptualizing treatment. While they have shown that RP has promise, there also is the suggestion that researchers and clinicians have to consider the complexity of integrating the various intervention strategies suggested by the model with the time needed for the client to fully assimilate all the treatment components. To more fully understand and evaluate the contributions of RP to treating eating disorders, we need more research and clinical applications of the RP model.

REFERENCES

Aarons, G. A., Brown, S. A., Stice, E., & Coe, M. T. (2001). Psychometric evaluation of the Marijuana and Stimulant Effect Expectancy Questionnaires for adolescents. *Addictive Behaviors, 26,* 219–236.

Ackard, D. M., Brehm, B. J., & Steffen, J. J. (2002). Exercise and eating disorders in college-aged women: Profiling excessive exercisers. *Journal of Treatment and Prevention, 10,* 31–47.

Agras, W. S., & Telch, C. F. (1998). The effects of caloric deprivation and negative affect on binge eating in obese binge-eating disordered women. *Behavior Therapy, 29,* 491–503.

Allen, K. M., Thombs, D. L., Mahoney, C. A., & Daniel, E. L. (1993). Relationships between expectancies and adolescent dieting behaviours. *Journal of School Health, 63,* 176–181.

American Psychiatric Association. (2000). *Diagnostic and statistical manual of mental disorders* (4th ed., text rev.). Washington, DC: Author.

Anderson, D. A., & Maloney, K. C. (2001). The efficacy of cognitive-behavioral therapy on the core symptoms of bulimia nervosa. *Clinical Psychology Review, 21,* 971–988.

Annis, H. M., Schober, R., & Kelly, E. (1996). Matching addiction outpatient counseling to client readiness for change: The role of structured relapse prevention counseling. *Experimental and Clinical Psychopharmacology, 4,* 37–45.

Arnow, B., Kenardy, J., & Agras, W. S. (1995). The Emotional Eating Scale: The development of a measure to assess coping with negative affect by eating. *International Journal of Eating Disorders, 18*, 79–90.

Baer, R. A. (2003). Mindfulness training as a clinical intervention: A conceptual and empirical review. *Clinical Psychology: Science and Practice, 10*, 125–143.

Bandura, A. (1977). Self-efficacy: Toward a unifying theory of behavior change. *Psychological Review, 84*, 191–215.

Baum, J. G., Clark, H. B., & Sandler, J. (1991). Preventing relapse in obesity through posttreatment maintenance systems: Comparing the relative efficacy of two levels of therapist support. *Journal of Behavioral Medicine, 14*, 287–302.

Baumeister, R. F., Heatherton, D. F., & Tice, D. M. (1998). *Losing control: How and why people fail at self-regulation.* San Diego, CA: Academic Press.

Blake, W., Turnbull, S., & Treasure, J. (1997). Stages and processes of change in eating disorders: Implications for therapy. *Clinical Psychology and Psychotherapy, 4*, 186–191.

Branson, R., Potoczna, N., Kral, J. G., Lentes, K-U., Hoehe, M. R., & Horber, F. F. (2003). Binge eating as a major phenotype of melanocortin 4 receptor gene mutations. *New England Journal of Medicine, 348*, 1096–1103.

Burke, B. L., Arkowitz, H., & Menchola, M. (2003). The efficacy of motivational interviewing: A meta-analysis of controlled clinical trials. *Journal of Consulting and Clinical Psychology, 71*, 843–861.

Chaney, E. F., O'Leary, M. R., & Marlatt, G. A. (1978). Skill training with alcoholics. *Journal of Consulting and Clinical Psychology, 46*, 1092–1104.

Clark, M. M., Abrams, D. B., Niaura, R. S., Eaton, C. A., & Rossi, J. S. (1991). Self-efficacy in weight management. *Journal of Consulting and Clinical Psychology, 59*, 739–744.

Collins, R. L., & Ricciardelli, L. A. (2005). Assessment of eating disorders. In D. M. Donovan & G. A. Marlatt (Eds.), *Assessment of addictive behaviors* (2nd ed.). New York: Guilford Press.

Cooper, Z., & Fairburn, C. G. (1987). The Eating Disorder Examination: A semistructured interview for the assessment of the specific psychopathology of eating disorders. *International Journal of Eating Disorders, 6*, 1–8.

Cooper, Z., & Fairburn, C. G. (2001). A new cognitive behavioral approach to the treatment of obesity. *Behaviour Research and Therapy, 39*, 499–511.

Copeland, A. L., Brandon, T. H., & Quinn, E. P. (1995). The Smoking Consequences Questionnaire—Adult: Measurement of smoking outcome expectancies of experienced smokers. *Psychological Assessment, 7*, 484–494.

Cramer, S. R., Nieman, D. C., & Lee, J. W. (1991). The effects of moderate exercise training on psychological well-being and mood state in women. *Journal of Psychosomatic Research, 35*, 437–449.

Cummings, C., Gordon, J. R., & Marlatt, G. A. (1980). Relapse: Prevention and prediction. In W. R. Miller (Ed.), *The addictive behaviors* (pp. 291–321). Oxford, UK: Pergamon Press.

Davis, C. S., Katzman, D. K., Kaptein, S., Kirsh, C., Brewer, H., Kalmbach, K., et al. (1997). The prevalence of high-level exercise in the eating disorders: Etiological implications. *Comprehensive Psychiatry, 38*, 321–326.

Davis, R., Freeman, R. J., & Garner, D. M. (1988). A naturalistic investigation of eating behavior in bulimia nervosa. *Journal of Consulting and Clinical Psychology*, 56, 273–279.

DiClemente, C. C., & Velasquez, M. M. (2002). Motivational interviewing and the stages of change. In W. R. Miller & S. Rollinck (Eds.), *Motivational interviewing: Preparing people for change* (2nd ed., pp. 201–216). New York: Guilford Press.

DiLillo, V., Siegfried, N. J., & West, D. S. (2003). Incorporating motivational interviewing into behavioral obesity treatment. *Cognitive and Behavioral Practice*, 10, 120–130.

Drapkin, R. G., Wing, R. R., & Shiffman, S. (1995). Responses to hypothetical high risk situations: Do they predict weight loss in a behavioral treatment program or the context of dietary lapses? *Health Psychology*, 14, 417–434.

Fairburn, C. G., Marcus, M. D., & Wilson, G. T. (1993). Cognitive-behavioral therapy for binge eating and bulimia nervosa: A comprehensive treatment manual. In C. G. Fairburn & G. T. Wilson (Eds.), *Binge eating: Nature, assessment, and treatment* (pp. 361–404). New York: Guilford Press.

Garner, D. M., & Wooley, S. C. (1991). Confronting the failure of behavioral and dietary treatments for obesity. *Clinical Psychology Review*, 11, 729–780.

Geller, J., Cockell, S. J., & Drab, D. L. (2001). Assessing readiness for change in the eating disorders: The psychometric properties of the readiness and motivation interview. *Psychological Assessment*, 13, 189–198.

Geller, J., & Drab, D. L. (1999). The Readiness and Motivation Interview: A symptom-specific measure of readiness for change in the eating disorders. *European Eating Disorders Review*, 7, 259–278.

Goldman, M. S., Del Boca, F. K., & Darkes, J. (1999). Alcohol expectancy theory. The application of cognitive neuroscience. In K. E. Leonard & H. T. Blane (Eds.), *Psychological theories of drinking and alcoholism* (pp. 203–246). New York: Guilford Press.

Grilo, C. M., & Shiffman, S. (1994). Longitudinal investigation of the abstinence violation effect in binge eaters. *Journal of Consulting and Clinical Psychology*, 62, 611–619.

Grilo, C. M., Shiffman, S., & Wing, R. R. (1989). Relapse crises and coping among dieters. *Journal of Consulting and Clinical Psychology*, 57, 488–495.

Hansel, S. L., & Wittrock, D. A. (1997). Appraisal and coping strategies in stressful situations: A comparison of individuals who binge eat and controls. *International Journal of Eating Disorders*, 21, 89–93.

Hayward, L. M., Sullivan, A. C., & Libonati, J. R. (2000). Group exercise reduces depression in obese women without weight loss. *Perceptual and Motor Skills*, 90, 204–208.

Heatherton, T. F., & Baumeister, R. F. (1991). Binge eating as escape from self-awareness. *Psychological Bulletin*, 110, 86–108.

Herman, C., & Mack, D. (1975). Restrained and unrestrained eating. *Journal of Personality*, 43, 647–660.

Herman, C. P., & Polivy, J. (1984). A boundary model for the regulation of eating. In A. J. Stunkard & E. Stellar (Eds.), *Eating and its disorders* (pp. 141–156). New York: Raven Press.

Herzog, D. B., & Delinsky, S. S. (2001). Classification of eating disorders. In R. H. Striegel-Moore & L. Smolak (Eds.), *Eating disorders: Innovative directions in research and practice* (pp. 31–50). Washington, DC: American Psychological Association.

Hohlstein, L. A., Smith, G. T., & Atlas, J. G. (1998). An application of expectancy theory to eating disorders: Development and validation of measures of eating and dieting expectancies. *Psychological Assessment, 10,* 49–58.

Jaffe, A. J., & Kilbey, M. M. (1994). The Cocaine Expectancy Questionnaire (CEQ): Construction and predictive utility. *Psychological Assessment, 6,* 18–26.

Jakicic, J. M., Wing, R. R., & Winters-Hart, C. (2002). Relationship of physical activity to eating behaviors and weight loss in women. *Medicine and Science in Sports and Exercise, 34,* 1653–1659.

Johnson, W. G., Corrigan, S. A., Crusco, A. H., & Schlundt, D. G. (1986). Restraint among bulimic women. *Addictive Behaviors, 11,* 351–354.

Jordan, P. J., Redding, C. A., Troop, N. A., Treasure, J., & Serpell, L. (2003). Developing a stage of change measure for assessing recovery from anorexia nervosa. *Eating Behaviors, 3,* 365–385.

Kristeller, J. L., & Hallett, C. B. (1999). An exploratory study of a meditation-based intervention for binge eating disorder. *Journal of Health Psychology, 4,* 357–363.

Levine, M. D., Marcus, M. D., & Moulton, P. (1996). Exercise in the treatment of binge eating disorder. *International Journal of Eating Disorders, 19,* 171–177.

Lewandowski, L. M., Gebing, T. A., Anthony, J. C., & O'Brien, W. H. (1997). Meta-analysis of cognitive-behavioral treatment studies for bulimia. *Clinical Psychology Review, 17,* 703–718.

Marlatt, G. A. (1985). Lifestyle modification. In G. A. Marlatt & J. R. Gordon (Eds.), *Relapse prevention: Maintenance strategies in the treatment of addictive behaviors* (1st ed., pp. 280–348). New York: Guilford Press.

Marlatt, G. A., & Gordon, J. R. (1980). Determinants of relapse: Implications for the maintenance of behavior change. In P. O. Davidson & S. M. Davidson (Eds.), *Behavioral medicine: Changing health lifestyles* (pp. 410–452). New York: Guilford Press.

Marlatt, G. A., & Gordon, J. R. (Eds.). (1985). *Relapse prevention: Maintenance strategies in the treatment of addictive behaviors* (1st ed.). New York: Guilford Press.

Marlatt, G. A., & Kristeller, J. L. (1999). Mindfulness and meditation. In W. R. Miller (Ed.), *Integrating spirituality into treatment* (pp. 67–84). Washington, DC: American Psychological Association.

McConnaughy, E. A., Prochaska, J. O., & Velicer, W. F. (1983). States of change in psychotherapy: Measurement and sample profiles. *Psychotherapy: Theory, Research and Practice, 20,* 368–375.

Miller, W. R., & Rollnick, S. (1991). *Motivational interviewing: Preparing people for change.* New York: Guilford Press.

Miller, W. R., & Rollnick, S. (Eds.). (2002). *Motivational interviewing: Preparing people for change* (2nd ed.). New York: Guilford Press.

Mooney, J. P., Burling, T. A., Hartman, W. M., & Brenner-Liss, D. (1992). The abstinence violation effect and very low calorie diet success. *Addictive Behaviors, 17,* 319–324.

Muraven, M., & Baumeister, R. F. (2000). Self-regulation and depletion of limited resources: Does self-control resemble a muscle? *Psychological Bulletin, 126,* 247–259.

Muraven, M., Tice, D. M., & Baumeister, R. F. (1998). Self-control as a limited resource: Regulatory depletion patterns. *Journal of Personality and Social Psychology*, *74*, 774–789.

National Heart, Lung, and Blood Institute. (1998). *Clinical guidelines on the identification, evaluation, and treatment of overweight and obesity in adults.* Bethesda, MD: National Institutes of Health.

Nieman, D. C., Custer, W. F., Butterworth, D. E., Utter, A. C., & Henson, D. A. (2000). Psychological response to exercise training and/or energy restriction in obese women. *Journal of Psychosomatic Research*, *48*, 23–29.

Ogden, J., & Wardle, J. (1990). Control of eating and attributional style. *British Journal of Clinical Psychology*, *29*, 445–446.

Page, L. A., Sutherby, K., & Treasure, J. L. (2002). A preliminary description of the use of "relapse management cards" in anorexia nervosa. *European Eating Disorders Review*, *10*, 281–291.

Paxton, S. J., & Diggens, J. (1997). Avoidance coping, binge eating, and depression: An examination of the escape theory of binge eating. *International Journal of Eating Disorders*, *22*, 83–87.

Penas-Lliedo, E., Vaz Leal, F. J., & Waller, G. (2002). Excessive exercise in anorexia nervosa and bulimia nervosa: Relation to eating characteristics and general psychopathology. *International Journal of Eating Disorders*, *31*, 370–375.

Pendleton, V. R., Goodrick, G. K., Poston, W. S. C., Reeves, R. S., & Foreyt, J. P. (2002). Exercise augments the effects of cognitive-behavioral therapy in the treatment of binge eating. *International Journal of Eating Disorders*, *31*, 172–184.

Perri, M. G., Nezu, A. M., McKelvey, W. F., Shermer, R. L., Renjilian, D. A., & Viegener, B. J. (2001). Relapse prevention training and problem-solving therapy in the long-term management of obesity. *Journal of Consulting and Clinical Psychology*, *69*, 722–726.

Perri, M. G., Shapiro, R. M., Ludwig, W. W., Twentyman, C. T., & McAdoo, W. G. (1984). Maintenance strategies for the treatment of obesity: An evaluation of relapse prevention training and posttreatment contact by mail and telephone. *Journal of Consulting and Clinical Psychology*, *52*, 404–413.

Polivy, J., & Herman, C. P. (1985). Dieting and binging: A causal analysis. *American Psychologist*, *40*, 193–201.

Polivy, J., & Herman, C. P. (2002). If at first you don't succeed: False hopes of self-change. *American Psychologist*, *57*, 677–689.

Prochaska, J. O., DiClemente, C. C., & Norcross, J. C. (1992). In search of how people change. *American Psychologist*, *47*, 1102–1114.

Raynor, H. A., & Epstein, L. H. (2001). Dietary variety, energy regulation, and obesity. *Psychological Bulletin*, *127*, 325–341.

Rossi, J. S., Rossi, S. R., Velicer, W. F., & Prochaska, J. O. (1995). Motivational readiness to control weight. In D. B. Allison (Ed.), *Handbook of assessment methods for eating behaviors and weight related problems: Measures, theory, and research* (pp. 387–411). Kingston: University of Rhode Island.

Schafer, J., & Brown, S. A. (1991). Marijuana and cocaine effect expectancies and drug use patterns. *Journal of Consulting and Clinical Psychology*, *59*, 558–565.

Spangler, D. L. (1999). Cognitive behavioral therapy of bulimia nervosa: An illustration. *Journal of Clinical Psychology*, *55*, 699–713.

Stanton, A. L., Rebert, W. M., & Zinn, L. M. (1986). Self-change in bulimia: A preliminary study. *International Journal of Eating Disorders, 5*, 917–924.

Stice, E. (1999). Clinical implications of psychosocial research on bulimia nervosa
and binge-eating disorder. *Journal of Clinical Psychology, 55*, 675–683.

Sundgot-Borgen, J., Rosenvinge, J. H., Bahr, R., & Schneider, L. S. (2002). The effect
of exercise, cognitive therapy, and nutritional counseling in treating bulimia
nervosa. *Medicine and Science in Sports and Exercise, 34*, 190–195.

Teasdale, J. D., Segal, Z. V., Williams, J. M. G., Ridgeway, V. A., Soulsby, J. M., &
Lau, M. A. (2000). Prevention of relapse/recurrence in major depression by
mindfulness-based cognitive therapy. *Journal of Consulting and Clinical Psychology, 68*, 615–623.

Telch, C. F., Agras, W. S., Rossiter, E. M., Wilfley, D., & Kenardy, J. (1990). Group
cognitive-behavioral treatment for the nonpurging bulimic: An initial evaluation. *Journal of Consulting and Clinical Psychology, 58*, 629–635.

Thien, V., Thomas, A., Markin, D., & Birmingham, C. L. (2000). Pilot study of a
graded exercise program for the treatment of anorexia nervosa. *International
Journal of Eating Disorders, 28*, 101–106.

Treasure, J. L., Katzman, M., Schmidt, U., Troop, N. A., Todd, G., & de Silva, P.
(1999). Engagement and outcome in the treatment of bulimia nervosa: First
phase of a sequential design comparing motivation enhancement therapy and
cognitive behavioural therapy. *Behaviour Research and Therapy, 37*, 405–418.

Treasure, J., & Schmidt, U. (2001). Ready, willing and able to change: Motivational
aspects of the assessment and treatment of eating disorders. *European Eating
Disorders Review, 9*, 4–18.

Troop, N. A., Holbrey, A., Trowler, R., & Treasure, J. L. (1994). Ways of coping in
women with eating disorders. *Journal of Nervous and Mental Disease, 182*,
535–540.

Tuschen-Caffier, B., Pook, M., & Frank, M. (2001). Evaluation of manual-based cognitive-behavioral therapy for bulimia nervosa in a service setting. *Behaviour Research and Therapy, 39*, 299–308.

Wadden, T. A., Vogt, R. A., Foster, G. D., & Anderson, D. A. (1998). Exercise and the
maintenance of weight loss: 1-year follow-up of a controlled clinical trial. *Journal of Consulting and Clinical Psychology, 66*, 429–433.

Ward, A., Troop, N., Todd, G., & Treasure, J. (1996). To change or not to change—
"How" is the question? *British Journal of Medical Psychology, 69*, 139–146.

Ward, T., Hudson, S. M., & Bulik, C. M. (1993). The abstinence violation effect in
bulimia nervosa. *Addictive Behaviors, 18*, 671–680.

Wegner, K. E., Smyth, J. M., Crosby, R. D., Wittrock, D. A., Wonderlich, S., & Mitchell, J. E. (2002). An evaluation of the relationship between mood and binge eating in the natural environment using ecological momentary assessment. *International Journal of Eating Disorders, 32*, 352–361.

Wilson, G. T., & Fairburn, C. C. (2002). Treatments for eating disorders. In P. E. Nathan & J. M. Gorman (Eds.), *A guide to treatments that work* (2 ed., pp. 559–
592). New York: Oxford University Press.

Wilson, G. T., Fairburn, C. C., Agras, W. S., Walsh, B. T., & Kraemer, H. (2002). Cognitive-behavioral therapy for bulimia nervosa: Time course and mechanisms of
change. *Journal of Consulting and Clinical Psychology, 70*, 267–274.

Wolk, S. L., & Devlin, M. J. (2001). Stage of change as a predictor of response to psychotherapy for bulimia nervosa. *International Journal of Eating Disorders, 30,* 96–100.

Wonderlich, S., Mitchell, J. E., Peterson, C. B., & Crow, S. (2001). Integrative cognitive therapy for bulimic behavior. In R. H. Striegel-Moore & L. Smolak (Eds.), *Eating disorders: Innovative directions in research and practice* (pp. 173–195). Washington, DC: American Psychological Association.

CHAPTER 10

Treatment of Gambling Disorders

Howard J. Shaffer
Debi A. LaPlante

In order for a person to advise, even to help another, a great
deal must happen. Many different elements must coincide
harmoniously; a whole constellation of things must come
about for that to happen even once.
—RILKE (1992, p. 18)

Attempts to identify empirically validated treatments have not been met
with universal approval. There exists a continuing debate as to whether clinicians and researchers should classify treatment approaches according to
the value, quality, and quantity of empirical research supporting their use.
On one side, some suggest that without empirical exploration it is impossible to know the efficacy of treatments (Chambless & Ollendick, 2001). On
the other side, many suggest that empirical validation of treatment will result in impractical suggestions that could be used by insurance companies
to restrict treatment (Chambless & Ollendick, 2001). Although this debate
is far from being resolved and arguments on both sides have some validity,
clinicians and researchers focusing on gambling-related problems have
been taking small but steady steps toward the empirical validation of treatments for disordered gambling. This work, however, is in the most preliminary stages. Like the clinical care for many other mental illnesses, the treatment approaches for gambling disorders are many, and a substantial
amount of the evidence for success is anecdotal. Because researchers are
still devoting a significant amount of time and resources to fully understanding the nature of problem gambling and identifying the extent of
problem gambling among the general population, limited resources have

been devoted to the empirical development of treatment. Rather, treatment strategies have been "borrowed" from clinical approaches designed for similar mental health problems; these protocols have been adapted based on the many and varied models of disordered gambling.

MODELS OF DISORDERED GAMBLING

Gambling is not a risk-free activity. Although most people who gamble do so without adverse consequence, a segment of gamblers develop a range of biological, social, and psychological problems related directly or indirectly to their gambling. How healthcare providers understand excessive behaviors in general and gambling in particular determines what they will do to treat these behavior patterns. There are a variety of different perspectives on gambling disorders. These perspectives can take the form of informal but influential formulations about the nature of intemperate gambling; alternatively, the views can represent a well-developed and reasoned theory of excessive gambling. In between resides the majority of models that clinicians use to guide their treatment efforts. Despite the fact that the majority of models lie in between these ends of a continuum of views, the perspectives are varied and a considerable breadth can be observed by a brief review of these models; Table 10.1 illustrates a representative set of common perspectives that explain gambling disorders.

As Table 10.1 reveals, clinicians are likely to apply various and perhaps substantially different treatment strategies to patients seeking their treatment depending upon their theoretical perspective(s). For example, clinicians who view pathological gambling in wholly biological terms might suggest that pharmacotherapy is the best route to mental health; others who understand disordered gambling in terms of erroneous cognitions might suggest that a combination of education and cognitive-behavioral therapy represent the best path to recovery. The current chapter discusses a number of treatment approaches that have emerged from these varied perspectives. Specifically, we focus on some clinical routes to mental health for problem gamblers.

RECOVERING FROM PATHOLOGICAL GAMBLING

For those struggling with a gambling disorder, there are several pathways to recovery. Figure 10.1 illustrates varied routes to recovery. This chapter is primarily concerned with treatment-related paths to recovery. However, as Figure 10.1 illustrates, it is important to emphasize that seeking treatment is not the only means of allaying problem gambling behavior. Like many other addictive behavior patterns (e.g., Cunningham, Sobell, Sobell, &

TABLE 10.1. Common Perspectives on Gambling Disorders

Perspective	Representative	Conceptualization
Moral turpitude	Quinn (1891)	Gambling is a moral problem that requires piety and values conversion.
Behavioral excess	Seager (1970)	Social learning and reinforcement contingencies influence some gamblers, otherwise healthy, into a pattern of excessive gambling.
Bad judgment	Rosecrance (1988)	Gambling disorders represent poor gambling strategies, usually displayed by naive gamblers who do not understand the games they play.
Psychological deficiency	Jacobs (1989)	Personality and emotional vulnerabilities invite gambling or other behavioral excesses as adaptive responses to serve as an anodyne for these problems; under some conditions, these excessive behavior patterns can serve to keep people from regressing to a more primitive state.
Psychodynamic neuroticism	Linder (1950)	Gambling viewed as intrapsychic conflict that has roots in early childhood experiences.
Erroneous thought patterns	Ladouceur (1996, 1998)	Gambling viewed as a product of illogical cognition concerning laws of probability.
Impulse control disorder	DSM (American Psychiatric Association, 1980, 1994, 2000)	Gambling viewed as an inability to resist persistent impulses to engage in destructive behaviors.
Self-medication	Henry (1996)	Gambling viewed as an attempt to cope with other unrelated mental health problems, such as anxiety.
Psychosocial	Orford (1985, 2001)	Cognition and behavior pertaining to gambling is influenced by numerous moral and social factors that are responsible for its development and maintenance.
Biological vulnerability	Comings (1998); Comings et al. (1999)	Gambling disorders reflect a genetic susceptibility to impulsive and excessive behaviors.
Addiction	Gamblers Anonymous (GA)	Gambling viewed as a chronic disease for which there is no cure, save abstinence.
Public health issue	Korn & Shaffer (1999)	Gambling viewed as a multidimensional health risk for which potential biological, psychological, economic, and social costs must be considered.

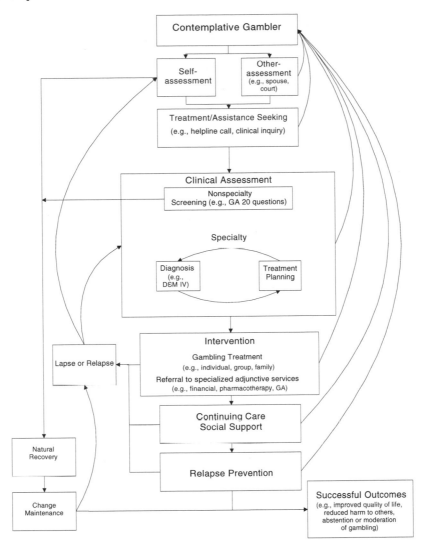

FIGURE 10.1. Pathways to recovery: The place of assessment and treatment.

Kapur, 1995; Schachter, 1982; Shaffer & Jones, 1989; Sobell, Cunning-ham, & Sobell, 1996; Sobell, Ellingstad, & Sobell, 2000; Waldorf, 1983; Waldorf & Biernacki, 1979, 1981; Waldorf, Reinarman, & Murphy, 1991; Winick, 1962), there is evidence that people with gambling disorders have the ability to change without formal treatment (e.g., Hodgins, Wynne, & Makarchuk, 1999). Similarly, treatment need not always come from experience with clinicians, since self-help recovery is also an option.

Unassisted or "Natural" Recovery

Conventional wisdom has assumed that there are only two ways out of addiction: treatment or death. However, almost every adult knows someone who has stopped smoking cigarettes without having participated in treatment (e.g., Schachter, 1982). Since Winick (1962) first described "maturing out" of narcotics use, the idea of recovery from addiction without treatment has caught the imagination of many clinical investigators. Recent research suggests that recovery from addiction without formal or informal treatment is more common than previously expected (Cunningham et al., 1995; Hodgins et al., 1999; Sobell, Cunningham, & Sobell, 1996). If gambling disorders are similar to substance use disorders, then it is likely that people without treatment recover from gambling disorders at rates similar to the rate of "natural" recovery from other addictive disorders.

Assisted Recovery

Not everyone can, or believes that he or she can, effectively evoke natural recovery processes. Consequently, although many of those who change might revise their behavior without treatment (e.g., Cunningham et al., 1995; Schachter, 1982; Shaffer & Jones, 1989; Sobell, Cunningham, & Sobell, 1996), others seek treatment and recovery via clinical pathways. However, before we turn our attention to formal treatment interventions, we provide a brief discussion of some factors that influence treatment and some typical nonclinical treatment approaches that many people use to change their gambling behavior.

Common Factors and Treatment Outcome

Easily mistaken for treatment-specific effects, nonspecific or common factors account for a considerable amount of treatment outcome (e.g., Frank, 1961; Hubble, Duncan, & Miller, 1999). Hubble et al. (1999) suggest that nonspecific treatment factors include (1) the extratherapeutic attributes that clients bring with them to treatment (e.g., education, family support, etc.), (2) relationship factors displayed by the treatment provider (e.g., empathy, caring, warmth, etc.), and (3) the hope, expectancies, and placebo effects that are often associated with the start of treatment. Estimates of specific effects for treatment programs are likely best identified via empirical research. A full discussion of the nonspecific factors that influence treatment outcome is beyond the scope and intent of this chapter. However, there are many useful resources for readers interested in the factors common to successful treatment (e.g., Frank, 1961; Havens, 1989; Hubble et al., 1999; Imhof, Hirsch, & Terenzi, 1984; Maltsberger & Buie, 1974;

Miller, 2000; Miller et al., 1995; Polanyi, 1967; Schon, 1983; Shaffer, 1994; Shaffer & Robbins, 1991, 1995). Recognizing nonspecific treatment effects within treatment episodes holds the potential to maximize treatment benefits.

Pretreatment Prevention

Researchers have suggested that disordered gambling is a public health problem in need of attention, funding, research, and prevention alternatives (Dunne, 1985). Similarly, others have suggested that in addressing this public health issue, an increased awareness among health professionals must be developed along with an examination of the problem from multiple perspectives (social, biological, financial, psychological, etc.); better recognition of associated problems; and strengthened policy, prevention, and treatment practices (Korn & Shaffer, 1999). Currently, the opportunity for youths and educators to gain information about gambling problems through school-based activities is poor (Shaffer, Forman, Scanlan, & Smith, 2000); however, some preliminary successes have been found for middle school student knowledge acquisition via video education (Ferland, Ladouceur, & Vitaro, 2002). Thus, one important avenue for reaching individuals before they develop pathological levels of gambling has not yet been adequately tapped.

Fortunately, some limited evidence suggests that public education might be beneficial. For example, despite the fact that gambling has become more socially acceptable and more readily accessible, brief interventions (e.g., pamphlets) have been found to provide individuals with new information about problems, risks, and help resources for problem gambling (Ladouceur, Vezina, Jacques, & Ferland, 2000). Hence, the accessibility of gambling is not necessarily positively related to individuals' knowledge of helpful information pertaining to gambling, but brief treatments can change this. This suggests that pre-prevention strategies might be valuable to improving public health. Research on pretreatment prevention from other addictions supports this suggestion (e.g., Brown & Miller, 1993; Walitzer, Dermen, & Connors, 1999). Unfortunately, another test–retest study of a gambling prevention program had mixed results. Specifically, educating high school adolescents about the legality of gambling, the commercial nature of the activity, automatic gambling behaviors, pathology, and coping skills did improve knowledge and coping skills over baseline measures. However, the improvement in coping skills was not maintained at follow-up and gambling behavior and attitudes were never significantly changed (Gaboury & Ladouceur, 1993). This is not to say, however, that all programs will have such mixed results, only that this one was not entirely successful. That knowledge was improved is encouraging, however, more research still is needed.

Assessment and Diagnosis

Treatment begins with assessment. A comprehensive understanding of each person seeking treatment is essential to developing a treatment plan that will guide the conduct of therapy. Treatment and assessment are knotted in an infinite feedback loop, in which each activity informs the other. Figure 10.1 illustrates this feedback loop. Thus, treatment can be understood as a succession of assessments and assessment as a sequence of interventions. Therefore, the tasks of assessment cannot be fully understood without an appreciation of treatment issues, just as understanding treatment requires an appreciation for the tasks of assessment.

Treatment Objectives and Arenas

The history of addiction treatment reveals that the consideration of treatment objectives remains one of the most controversial and contentious concerns. This situation is no different for the treatment of gambling disorders. For example, while the conventional wisdom still views abstention as the most common objective of treatment programs and providers, the goal of some treatment programs is to achieve a controlled gambling outcome. In fact, consistent with the notion of clinically significant effects (Cone, 2001), therapists increasingly have recognized the value of the alternate goal of controlled, or nonpathological gambling (e.g., Alm, 2001; Blaszczynski, McConaghy, & Frankova, 1991).

Non-abstinence-focused treatment approaches have been met with both criticism and praise. Blaszczynski et al. (1991) observed that controlled treatment outcomes can be achieved and sustained. Nevertheless, many clinicians and subscribers to the 12-step ideology remain doubtful. These concerns are not without good cause since the research on controlled gambling is sparse. Nevertheless, the existing evidence does encourage more research on the range of treatment goals since it seems that, with careful monitoring, controlled gambling is a treatment objective that might join abstinence. In addition, it is important to note that many people will not seek or enter treatment if they believe that the only treatment outcome is abstinence. Consequently, the prospect of controlled gambling often engages people in the treatment process—even if the final treatment outcome is often abstinence. Choosing to abstain is often a result of a treatment seeker learning that controlled gambling is not readily achievable.

Treatment Settings

The setting within which treatment takes place can set the tone for the entire intervention. The clinical setting can influence the development of the therapist–client relationship. Therapists care for patients in one of three settings: inpatient, outpatient, or an inpatient/outpatient hybrid. Depending on the severity of the disorder, a patient's willingness to seek help, insurance regulations, and assorted other factors, individuals are usually channeled into one or the other setting, although the patients are not usually restricted to one or the other. Obviously these settings might be used sequentially so that some patients and providers work in both settings, but only one at a time.

Treatment and Self-Help Modalities

Contemporary models of gambling treatment include a wide variety of strategies and settings. Each treatment strategy (e.g., psychodynamic, pharmacological, behavioral) and setting (e.g., inpatient, outpatient) can be distilled to three major underlying dimensions: psychological, social, and biological (Milkman & Shaffer, 1985). The following sections provide a brief review of some of the most common treatment strategies.

Brief Treatment

The use of brief treatments, such as workbooks and pamphlets has not been extensively studied among pathological gamblers. Related research for other addictive disorders, however, suggests that brief treatments might be an extremely effective treatment intervention (e.g., Fleming, 1993; Sobell, Cunningham, Sobell, et al., 1996). Preliminary work that did not include an appropriate control group has suggested that self-help workbooks reduce gambling frequency and spending (Dickerson, Hinchy, & Legg-England, 1990). Furthermore, Miller (2000) suggests that brief treatments are not significantly less effective than more intense treatments, and that empathy in single counseling sessions is predictive of treatment outcomes. Supporting this, self-help workbooks with and without motivational interviewing aided in reducing and eliminating gambling behavior among treatment seekers (Hodgins, Currie, & el-Guebaly, 2001). It seems then, that this avenue of treatment is quite promising; however, much research needs to be done. More extensive comparisons with control groups and workbooks that vary by content should be explored to determine the strength with which workbooks influence individual gambling behavior and the components of workbooks that are most influential.

Substitution/Behavioral Replacement

Conventional wisdom might suggest that occupying one's mind with other pursuits could help alleviate urges to engage in problem levels of gambling. To date, no research has explicitly investigated leisure, hobby, or activity substitution as a means of treatment. Some programs, however, integrate aspects of this approach into their treatment plan (e.g., Griffiths, Bellringer, Farrell-Roberts, & Freestone, 2001). Although researchers have yet to empirically validate replacement therapy strategies, research from other addictive disorders is suggestive. For example, with chemical substitution treatments, nicotine replacement therapies are used widely to curb cravings to smoke (e.g., Hajek et al., 1999) and methadone has been utilized successfully to curb the withdrawal symptoms associated with opioid dependence (National Consensus Development Panel on Effective Medical Treatment of Opiate Addiction, 1998).

For addictive behavior patterns that do not include the ingestion of psychoactive substances (Holden, 2001), substituting alternative thoughts and behaviors has shown promise (e.g., Blaszczynski, 1998; Federman, Drebing, & Krebs, 2000; Ladouceur & Walker, 1998; Sylvain, Ladouceur, & Boisvert, 1997). However, clinicians must apply certain cognitive strategies with great care to avoid inadvertently stimulating the very behavior that they are trying to stop. Research suggests that intentional suppression of thoughts or goals might result in an ironic rebound that ultimately causes an individual to return to unwanted thoughts quite frequently (Wenzlaff & Wegner, 2000). Much more research is needed to determine whether this treatment alternative is efficacious for pathological gambling.

Psychodynamic Psychotherapy

Psychodynamic psychotherapy and counseling have been applied widely to people with gambling problems prior to the emergence of cognitive-behavioral approaches. It is likely that this is still the most common form of psychotherapy with gambling and other addictive disorders. However, there is a paucity of psychodynamic research in the gambling field and sparse evidence in the outcome literature to support its effectiveness. The purpose of psychodynamic psychotherapy for gambling treatment seekers is to help them gain insight into the emotional origins and meaning of their gambling behavior. This perspective frames disordered gambling as a repetitive activity that exists to satisfy some need that typically remains unconscious or poorly understood. Although psychoanalytically oriented treatment can be lengthy and might be best suited for individuals with comorbid personality disorders, psychodynamically oriented treatment also offers strategies and techniques that can be used in brief treatment and supersede any particular treatment model (Bergler, 1957; Galdston, 1951; Gustafson, 1995; Khantzian, Halliday, & McAuliffe, 1990; Levin, 1987; Perry, Cooper, & Michels, 1987; Rosenthal, 1997; Rosenthal & Rugle, 1994; Weiner, 1975). Rosenthal and Rugle provide clinicians and interested readers with a comprehensive review and treatment approach for gambling problems based on psychodynamic principles (Rosenthal, 1997; Rosenthal & Rugle, 1994).

Financial Management Counseling

Financial counseling can assist people with gambling-related debt to initiate a financial plan, learn budget management, develop a payment plan, and gain an improved appreciation for the value of money (National Endowment for Financial Education & National Council on Problem Gambling, 2000). This counseling support should be made available to both the gambler and those affected by their gambling debt. Since a preoccupation with money and credit is central to the experience of an individual with a gambling disorder, it is essential to address their financial obligations and responsibilities during treatment. By diminishing these very real and pressing problems, treatment can reduce the stress and anxiety associated with financial debt. One program, "Personal Financial Strategies for the Loved Ones of Problem Gamblers," reviews several steps toward restoring financial control (National Endowment for Financial Education & National Council on Problem Gambling, 2000). Among these steps are: (1) identifying income and assets, (2) creating and maintaining a spending plan, (3) shifting all financial control to the nongambling family member, (4) repaying debts, and (5) investing wisely. This handbook also recommends that gamblers and their families consult with an attorney, tax specialist, or financial planner before enacting significant financial changes. By developing a carefully and realistically crafted financial plan, people with gambling problems can stimulate and maintain a sense of personal control and efficacy, which often stimulates the hopefulness that is integral to maintaining change and recovery. The efficacy of financial treatments that target gamblers and their loved ones requires systematic empirical testing.

Psychopharmacology

Recently, researchers have begun to explore potential biological correlates of pathological gambling (Grant & Kim, 2001; Grant, Kim, & Potenza, 2003). For example, researchers (Blanco, Orensanz-Munoz, Blanco-Jerez, & Saiz-Ruiz, 1996) have determined that low platelet monoamine oxidase activity may be a predisposing factor for impulsivity in pathological gambling. Similarly, genes and neurotransmitter systems (e.g., monoaminergic, dopamine, serotonin, and norepinephrine) have been found to be predictive of pathological gambling status (Bergh, Sodersten, & Nordin, 1997; Blanco, Ibanez, Saiz-Ruiz, Blanco-Jerez, & Nunes, 2000; Comings, 1998). Recent work by Breiter and colleagues has found that specific areas of the brain respond to the prospect of winning and losing money (Breiter, Aharon, Kahneman, Dale, & Shizgal, 2001) and neurobiology research reveals the involvement of serotonin (Moreno, Saiz-Ruiz, & Lopez-Ibor, 1991), norepinephrine (DeCaria, Begaz, & Hollander, 1998; Siever, 1987), and dopamine (Bergh et al., 1997; Blum et al., 2000; Comings, 1998) in various expressions of gambling behavior. These neurotransmitters have been associated with the expression of urges, impulsivity, risk taking and the brain's reward system. By examining such correlates, researchers seeking to utilize pharmacotherapeutic approaches will be better able to target efficacious drugs and dosages.

There is no specific pharmacotherapy protocol currently approved specifically for the treatment of disordered gambling. Since gambling typically co-occurs with other mental problems, physicians treating mental illness and addiction (e.g., psychiatrists, primary care physicians, and addiction and behavioral medicine clinicians) do prescribe various psychopharmacological agents for problem and pathological gamblers as complementary or adjunctive therapy. A variety of drug treatments, however, is being tested for application to gambling related disorders. The following discussion will review the primary drug classes and possible agents that are among the leading candidates for emerging pharmacotherapeutic protocols.

OPIOID ANTAGONISTS

Naltrexone, a competitive narcotic antagonist, blocks opioid receptors, which are the targets of both endogenous and exogenous opioids. It has been approved for the *treatment of alcohol dependence*, where it reduces both alcohol cravings and the pleasurable effects of alcohol when ingested (O'Malley et al., 1992). Similar effects are postulated for gambling-related craving (Crockford & el-Guebaly, 1998). Kim and Grant reported that naltrexone was useful in reducing gambling excursions, expenditures and urges among pathological gamblers (Kim & Grant, 2001; Kim, Grant, Adson, & Shin, 2001). It is generally well tolerated but can cause mild gastrointestinal upset. Naltrexone should be used carefully in people with any degree of liver disease, and the implementation of a monitoring protocol for hepatotoxicity is recommended.

SELECTIVE SEROTONIN REUPTAKE INHIBITORS

The class of medications known as selective serotonin reuptake inhibitors (SSRIs) is indicated for the treatment of several different but often related disorders: depression, obsessive–compulsive disorder, and other anxiety disorders (DeCaria et al., 1998; Hollander, Buchalter, & DeCaria, 2000). Members of this medication group include fluoxetine (Prozac), fluvoxamine (Luvox), paroxetine (Paxil), sertraline (Zoloft), and citalopram (Celexa). Each of these agents varies in its ability to inhibit serotonin, noradrenaline, and dopamine uptake, yielding a booster effect with these neurotransmitters. The rationale for using these medications with gamblers relates to their preoccupation with gambling and the money with which to gamble; in addition, individuals with a gambling disorder evidence a repetitive and compulsive pattern of activity. Depression or anxiety also tends to accompany treatment seekers' clinical profiles. From this perspective, clinicians are conceptualizing pathological gambling as residing toward the compulsivity end of a compulsivity–impulsivity continuum.

Research on paroxetine (Grant, Kim, Potenza, et al., 2003; Kim, Grant, Adson, Shin, & Zaninelli, 2002), fluvoxamine (Blanco, Petkova, Ibanez, & Saiz-Ruiz, 2002), and citalopram (Zimmerman, Breen, & Posternak, 2002) shows promise, but requires additional testing. For example, a study of 10 pathological gamblers demonstrated decreased gambling urges and behavior at the end of a 16-week trial (Hollander, 1998). Further research utilizing a randomized design, a larger sample, and longer periods to measure outcomes to validate these findings has begun (Hollander et al., 2000).

ANTIDEPRESSANTS AND MOOD STABILIZERS

Antidepressants and mood stabilizers used in the treatment of depression and bipolar disorder also have a theoretical rationale for use with gambling disorders. In addition to the high prevalence of depression among gamblers who present for treatment, the American Psychiatric Association considers a manic episode accounting for excessive gambling as an exclusionary criterion for the diagnosis of pathological gambling (American Psychiatric Association, 2000). Carbamazepine (Tegretol) showed significant clinical benefit during a 30-month treatment period with a single case report of a chronic pathological gambler (Haller & Hinterhuber, 1994). In a study of 14 outpatients, nefazodone (Serzone) also elicited important clinical improvements in gambling behavior, craving, depression and anxiety (Pallanti, Rossi, Sood, & Hollander, 2002). Lithium carbonate also was reported effective in treating three pathological gamblers with concurrent mood disorders (Moskowitz, 1980), and in a comparison with valproate both elicited positive outcomes (Pallanti, Quercioli, Sood, & Hollander, 2002). Since mania and depression can often co-occur among individuals with a gambling disorder (Shaffer & Korn, 2002), mood stabilizers represent a potentially important treatment resource.

OTHER MEDICATIONS

Olanzapine (Zyprexa), an atypical antipsychotic, is undergoing a clinical trial with pathological gamblers. Other drugs that theoretically might be helpful in the treatment of pathological gambling include ondansetron (Zofran), which currently is FDA-approved for the treatment of nausea associated with chemotherapy and appears to operate as a selective serotonin receptor antagonist (SSRA); recently, at much lower dosages than used to control nausea, it has demonstrated effectiveness in a randomized clinical trial during the treatment of early-onset alcohol dependence. Bupropion (Wellbutrin), a norepinephrine dopamine modulator (NDM) has demonstrated efficacy as an anticraving medication during the treatment of nicotine dependence even though the mechanism of action in smoking cessation is not well understood. Black (2004) provides preliminary results that suggest individuals who gamble problematically respond favorably clinically to bupropion. Methylphenidate (Ritalin) has been used in the treatment of attention-deficit disorder, which has impulsive characteristics similar to those of pathological gambling. Finally, there is hope that medications effective in reducing cocaine craving and urges will prove useful in reducing urges to gambling because monetary reward in a gambling-like experiment has stimulated patterns of brain activation similar to those observed in people dependent on cocaine (Breiter et al., 2001).

INTEGRATED TREATMENT STRATEGIES: COMBINING PSYCHOTHERAPY AND PHARMACOTHERAPY

Since gamblers seeking treatment often present with dysthymia and depression, clinicians should consider the potential value of a treatment strategy that addresses depression. In an important carefully conducted randomized clinical trial of three modalities, drug only (i.e., nefazodone), cognitive only, and drug plus cognitive or pharmacotherapy, Keller et al. (2000) demonstrated that the combination of pharmacotherapy and cognitive-behavioral therapy yielded meaningfully higher rates of recovery from depression than either of these treatments alone. One case study of fluoxetine and motivational interviewing showed similar promise (Kuentzel, Henderson, Zambo, Stine, & Schuster, 2003). While clinical trials of combination studies are few, this research provides strong evidence suggesting that clinicians consider the potential benefits of adjunctive treatments. Further, it is likely that other combinations of pharmacotherapy and psychotherapy also will yield improved treatment outcomes compared with each of these treatments. However, absent evidence from carefully controlled clinical trials, it is premature to recommend specific combinations of treatment.

Behavioral and Cognitive-Behavioral Therapy

There are many seminal reviews of behavioral and cognitive-behavioral treatment for addictive behaviors; some of these are now classic (e.g., Bandura, 1969; Ellis & Grieger, 1977; Ellis & Whiteley, 1979; Kendall & Hollon, 1979; Mahoney, 1974; Marlatt & Gordon, 1985; Meichenbaum, 1977). Recently, Kadden (2001) summarized the value of these strategies for alcoholism treatment. Kadden's summary also applies to gambling and the range of addictive behaviors. Behavioral strategies for the treatment of gambling assume that these disorders are learned and that the principles of learning can be applied to encourage the changes necessary to ameliorate the problem. Consequently, after a careful behavioral analysis that determines where, when, and how frequently gambling behaviors occur, behavioral treatment specialists help the gambler to determine the precise emotional and social context for their gambling and then develop and or substitute alternative behaviors. Once identified or learned, the recovering gambler can practice these alternative behaviors in real-life settings to reduce the likelihood of relapse. From its birth, when Dollard and Miller (1950) translated Freudian theory into Pavlovian stimulus–response psychology, through the Skinnerian era of contingency management (Skinner, 1969), the variety of behavioral approaches to treatment has expanded steadily and considerably (e.g., Kendall & Hollon, 1979; Meichenbaum, 1977). Gradually, psychologists came to recognize that internal cognitive events, like overt behaviors, are responsive to contextual cues. Consequently, psychologists began to consider cognitions as behaviors in their own right; from this perspective, clinicians can apply learning principles to either overt behaviors or internal cognitions (Meichenbaum, 1977).

The treatment of gambling disorders mirrors the development of behavioral and cognitive-behavioral treatment in general. For example, after some early efforts at managing cues (e.g., Barker & Miller, 1968; Seager, 1970), clinicians recognized that comorbid affective disorders were present among treatment seekers, and they began to expand their clinical strategies (e.g., McCormick, Russo, Ramirez, & Taber, 1984). Few of these treatments have been rigorously evaluated. For example, along with psychopharmacological approaches, cognitive-behavioral therapy (CBT) is one of the few treatment options that has been scientifically examined. Some argue the superiority of CBT's empirical support over other approaches (Toneatto & Ladouceur, 2003).

CBT has its roots in behavioral treatments; more specifically, CBT for problem gambling was modeled on CBT developed for substance use problems (Tavares, Zilberman, & el-Guebaly, 2003). CBT attempts to reduce individuals' maladaptive gambling by correcting erroneous perceptions about probability, skill, and luck that aid in the maintenance of problem gambling behaviors. For gambling, this approach assumes that the root of problem gambling is associated with incorrect assumptions about gambling situations. Consequently, the treatment techniques include cognitive correction, social skills training, problem-solving training, and relapse prevention (e.g., Ladouceur, Boisvert, & Dumont, 1994; Ladouceur, Sylvain, Boutin, & Doucet, 2002; Ladouceur et al., 2001; Sylvain et al., 1997). Others have added compliance interventions with significant clinical success (Milton, Crino, Hunt, & Prosser, 2002).

CBT is the only truly empirically validated psychotherapy; assessment of its efficacy has typically compared waitlist control groups to treatment groups (e.g., Ladouceur et al., 2001, 2003). Reliable reduction in gambling, urges to gamble, and the number of diagnostic criteria met have been observed at 6- and 12-month evaluations (Sylvain et al., 1997). This research also has found that patients increased their perceptions of self-efficacy and perception of control. Similarly, Ladouceur, Sylvain, Letarte, Giroux, and Jacques (1998) found that when individuals were given education about random events (i.e., chance and probability), they were able to maintain therapeutic gains (i.e., reduced problem gambling) for at least 6 months.

Other researchers have been more skeptical, however. For example, Blaszczynski and Silove (1995) suggested that conclusive statements about behavioral and cognitive treatment efficacy might be premature because of a lack of systematic empirical comparisons of these approaches. They also suggest that serious methodological limitations prevent comparison of existing treatment outcome studies.

MOTIVATIONAL ENHANCEMENT STRATEGIES

Motivational enhancement strategies (e.g., motivational counseling, resistance reduction) are cognitive-behavioral treatment approaches designed to lower resistance and enhance motivation for change. These strategies augment preexisting motivation by improving the therapeutic alliance. This is accomplished by recognizing that clients are, at best, ambivalent about experiencing personal change (Miller & Rollnick, 1991; Orford, 1985; Rollnick & Morgan, 1995; Shaffer, 1994, 1997). With improved therapeutic relationships, clients are more willing to consider and explore their ambivalence. Shaffer has suggested that painful ambivalence is responsible for stimulating denial as a defense mechanism and the appearance of intractability among people struggling with addictive disorders (Shaffer, 1992, 1994, 1997; Shaffer & Robbins, 1995). Further, attention to ambivalence improves the quality of treatment by providing a clinical context and therapeutic alliance that resonates with the client's mixed motivations.

Clinicians who utilize motivation enhancement techniques typically focus on two motivational deficiencies: (1) inadequate motivation and (2) resistance to change. For example, some have suggested that if motivation to change is inadequate, it has to be energized (charged), like a weak battery (Miller & Rollnick, 1991). If motivation to change is absent, according to enhancement strategies, clinicians need to fashion and nourish motivation during the treatment process. One way of achieving this is through systematic interviewing. Motivational interviewing strategies assume that the level of motivation necessary for change is lacking and insufficient to stimulate and sustain change, but that it can be enhanced via appropriate questioning.

Focusing on clients' resistance to change is another important way for clinicians to improve the motivational status of clients who seek treatment for addictive disorders (Shaffer & Simoneau, 2001).[1] Resistance is often considered the core of what makes it difficult for people, even the most healthy, to achieve consistently "good" mental health (Ellis, 1987; Shaffer & Simoneau, 2001). Consequently, motivational enhancement approaches devote a significant amount of time to resistance reduction. Based upon psychodynamic principles, resistance reduction assumes that internal and external obstacles dilute or weaken existing levels of motivation for change that can *already be sufficient* to drive the change process. Resistance reduction strategies encourage therapists to validate self-destructive behavior as a legitimate choice by asking clients about the perceived benefits of these activities (e.g., gambling), rather than exclusively focusing on the costs (e.g., losses). Within this safe context, clients can more freely explore *all* of the costs and benefits associated with a pattern of addictive activity. Since a resistance reduction strategy does not ask clients to give up anything, patients also have less need to resist therapeutic interventions. With little need to resist treatment, previously inhibited motivation is released for clients to use in changing seemingly intractable behavior patterns.

Resistance reduction and other motivational enhancement strategies are not mutually exclusive. Clinicians should consider employing the full range of motivational enhancement approaches to advance the treatment objectives and the health of individuals with a gambling disorder. A decision balance is the major technique used in motivational enhancement strategies. At every stage of treatment, motivational strategies ask patients to address the pros and cons of their current behavior and value of staying the same or changing.

RELAPSE PREVENTION AND RECOVERY TRAINING

Relapse prevention (RP) and recovery training are modalities designed to increase a person's ability to identify and cope with high-risk situations that commonly create problems and precipitate relapse. These strategies are most frequently associated with cognitive-behavioral treatments. The techniques have been well developed and widely used in the alcohol and drug treatment field (Annis, 1986; Annis & Davis, 1989; Marlatt & Gordon, 1985; McAulliffe & Ch'ien, 1986). More recently, these strategies have been applied to gambling treatment. The gambling risk situations identified include environmental settings (e.g., casinos, lottery outlets), intrapersonal discomfort (e.g., anger, depression, boredom, stress) and interpersonal difficulties (e.g., finances, work, family, etc.). The goal is to develop coping methods to deal effectively with these specific high-risk situations without relying on unhealthy and maladaptive gambling behavior. To date, there has been a paucity of research addressing the effectiveness of RP in the gambling field. Ladouceur and his colleagues were among the few researchers to evaluate the efficacy of RP protocols in gambling treatment programs. They helped people identify high-risk situations and the erroneous thoughts that emerge in these situations; this provided the opportunity to apply a second cognitive correction for these distortions (Ladouceur et al., 1998). Using a small sample, Ladouceur et al. found promise in this approach. Echeburua, Fernandez-Montalvo, and Baez (2000) also found fewer relapse problems when RP techniques were integrated into treatment.

A promising application of the RP model for gambling is in the late stage of development (e.g., Littman-Sharp, Turner, Stirpe, & Liu, 1999). The instrument, Inventory of Gambling Situations (IGS), builds on earlier similar tools, the Inventory of Drinking Situations (IDS) and the Inventory of Drug-Taking Situations (IDTS) (Annis, 1982, 1985). The IGS identifies an individual's high-risk situations for disordered gambling behavior by assessing the areas that have been problematic during the clients' life and that might place them at risk of relapse into unhealthy gambling during their recovery.[2] By identifying potential risk situations, this instrument can be used to teach recovering gamblers new coping strategies for use during their continuing care and aftercare experiences. In addition, this instrument can be used during the early phase of treatment to enhance awareness of the role gambling plays in maladaptive coping.[3] To date, the instrument has been validated but not published in a peer-reviewed journal.

Self-Help: Gamblers Anonymous and 12-Step Facilitation

Originally founded in 1957, Gamblers Anonymous (GA) is a widely available self-help fellowship that provides mutual support for individuals experiencing gambling problems. GamAnon is a related fellowship for family members affected by compulsive/pathological gamblers. Like Alcoholics Anonymous and Al-anon, these gambling self-help fellowships are based on 12-step principles. As fellowships, these programs are best considered to be self-help resources and not formal treatment—though participation is therapeutic for many who get involved. Because of the potential therapeutic value of self-help resources, many formal gambling treatment programs tend to include referral to GA, GamAnon, Rational Recovery, Bettors Anonymous, and Debtors Anonymous.

Deeply rooted in the GA approach is the perspective that disordered gambling (e.g., pathological, problem, compulsive) is a spiritual and medical disease. The major goal of this fellowship is to garner from its members a commitment to abstinence from gambling and a lifelong commitment to the principles of GA and participation in GA meetings. There is no professional facilitation, organizational affiliation, or fee. Despite, or perhaps because of, its status and purpose as a fellowship, there has been a paucity of research directed to evaluating its effectiveness. Outcome studies of Gamblers Anonymous have reported first-year dropout rates as high as 70% (Stewart & Brown, 1988) with abstinence rates of 8% after 1 year (Brown, 1985).

Some clinical programs make use of GA techniques. For example, 12-step facilitation is therapy based on the principles of GA. During treatment, individuals are actively encouraged to attend GA meetings and to maintain journals of their attendance and participation. During this type of treatment, clinicians place emphasis on GA steps 1–5 (see Table 10.2). Reading assignments from the GA literature also complements materials introduced during formal therapy.

MATCHING PEOPLE TO CLINICAL INTERVENTIONS

One of the principal concerns facing all clinicians is how to optimally match treatment appropriately to the clinical needs of the patient and the requirements of the treatment plan. However, matching people to the appropriate level of clinical care is more complex than it might first appear (Shaffer, 1986; Shaffer & Freed, 2005) and providing treatment is a blend of science and art (e.g., Kimberly & Minvielle, 2000; Schon, 1983). For example, the same treatment might not be the same treatment for all people. As we show later, pathological gamblers often experience their problems differently; gambling disorders take different courses for some individuals

TABLE 10.2. The 12 Steps of Gamblers Anonymous

1. We admitted we were powerless over gambling—that our lives had become unmanageable.
2. Came to believe that a Power greater than ourselves could restore us to a normal way of thinking and living.
3. Made a decision to turn our will and our lives over to the care of this Power of our own understanding.
4. Made a searching and fearless moral and financial inventory of ourselves.
5. Admitted to ourselves and to another human being the exact nature of our wrongs.
6. Were entirely ready to have these defects of character removed.
7. Humbly asked God (of our understanding) to remove our shortcomings.
8. Made a list of all persons we had harmed and became willing to make amends to them all.
9. Make direct amends to such people wherever possible, except when to do so would injure them or others.
10. Continued to take personal inventory and when we were wrong, promptly admitted it.
11. Sought through prayer and meditation to improve our conscious contact with God as we understood Him, praying only for knowledge of His will for us and the power to carry that out.
12. Having made an effort to practice these principles in all our affairs, we tried to carry this message to other compulsive gamblers.

Note. From Gamblers Anonymous (2002). Copyright 2002 by Gamblers Anonymous. Reprinted by permission.

compared with others. Similarly, individuals with a gambling disorder experience differing degrees of infirmity at different points during the development of their illness. As such, these individuals are likely to either need differing intensities of treatment or different treatment approaches altogether.

The first piece of evidence to support these ideas comes from prevalence rates. Certain groups seem to be more vulnerable to developing problem/pathological gambling than other groups. The second piece of evidence comes from research suggesting a high comorbidity rate with a number of mental illnesses. The third research thread suggests that individuals with the same diagnosis might in fact be at different stages/points in their illness and consequently need different types of treatment. These topics are discussed later in this chapter. Following this consideration is a discussion of the heuristics that clinicians can use when treatment matching.

Why Match?: Lessons from Epidemiology and Comorbidity

Psychiatric epidemiological research investigates the distribution and determinants of mental disorders in the population. The prevalence of a disorder represents the number of people with a specific disorder at a point or period in time. Since scientists first examined the prevalence of gambling in the United States, increasing numbers of people have gambled. Shaffer, Hall, and Vander Bilt demonstrated meta-analytically that an assortment of different algorithms used to calculate the rate of disordered gambling in the United States and Canada provided quite stable and similar estimates (Shaffer & Hall, 2001; Shaffer, Hall, & Vander Bilt, 1997, 1999; Table 10.3). International studies are consistent with this observation (Table 10.4).

Trends in Population Segments

A single prevalence rate cannot accurately describe all of the different demographic groups in society. Prevalence rates are most accurate when epidemiologists stratify these estimates for specific demographic groups. It is important for readers to note that avoiding one general prevalence rate is not a limitation. Fisher reminds us that studies of population segments have the major advantage of netting significantly more problem gamblers. In addition, this strategy has the potential to reveal the proportion of problem gamblers attributable to each sector (Fisher, 2000) as well as more specific insight into the nature of gambling within various population segments. Consequently, the next phase of epidemiological investigation needs to focus on more vulnerable and special-needs population segments such as women, older adults, and aboriginals, as well as selected ethnocultural and lower socioeconomic groups. Nascent research has been completed on special population segments, and the following section reviews some of these

TABLE 10.3. Mean and Trimmed Gambling Prevalence Estimates

Estimated time frame and statistic	Adult	Adolescent	College	Treatment or prison
Level 3 lifetime Mean	1.92	3.38	5.56	15.44
Median	1.80	3.00	5.00	14.29
5% trimmed mean	1.78	3.33	5.14	15.07
Andrews' wave M-estimator	1.73	2.74	4.64	13.49
Level 2 lifetime Mean	4.15	8.40	10.88	17.29
Median	3.50	8.45	6.50	15.64
5% trimmed mean	3.76	8.35	9.83	17.01
Andrews' wave M-estimator	3.31	8.22	6.51	16.59
Level 3 past year Mean	1.46	4.80	——	——
Median	1.20	4.37	——	——
5% trimmed mean	1.27	4.77	——	——
Andrews' wave M-estimator	1.10	4.65	——	——
Level 2 past year Mean	2.54	14.60	——	——
Median	2.20	11.21	——	——
5% trimmed mean	2.25	13.83	——	——
Andrews' wave M-estimator	2.15	11.26	——	——

Note. Derived from Shaffer and Korn (2002).

recent studies to illustrate the variability with which different groups are at risk for developing problem gambling behaviors.

ADOLESCENTS AND ADULTS

Most prevalence research examining special populations has been conducted on youths. Estimates of gambling disorders among young people suggest that they experience this problem at approximately 2.5–3.0 times the rate of their adult counterparts (e.g., Gupta & Derevensky, 2000; Shaffer et al., 1997; Shaffer, Hall, Vander Bilt, & George, 2003). Despite this observation, the National Research Council concluded that variation in methods, instrumentation, and conceptualization might influence these findings. Consequently, it is not yet possible to draw confident conclusions about the rate of gambling disorders among youth (National Research Council, 1999). New research supports this cautionary view. Focusing on a nationally representative sample of college students, this new research reveals unexpectedly lower rates of gambling (LaBrie, Shaffer, LaPlante, & Wechsler, 2003); prospective research on college students also reveals lower than expected rates of gambling-related problems (Slutske, Jackson, & Sher, 2003). Finally, new research suggests that South Oaks Gambling Screen (SOGS) based youthful prevalence rates might simply be inflated (Ladouceur, Bouchard, et al., 2000).

TABLE 10.4. International Estimates of Lifetime and Past-Year Disordered Gambling Prevalence Rates

	U.S./ Canada[a]	Sweden[b]	Switzerland[c]	New Zealand[d]	Britain[e]	South Africa[f]	Hong Kong[g]	Spain[b]	Norway[i]	Australia[j]
Level 3 lifetime	1.9	1.2	—	1.0	—	—	1.8	1.4–1.7	—	—
Level 2 lifetime	4.2	2.7	—	1.9	—	—	4.0	1.6–5.2	—	—
Level 1 lifetime	93.9	96.1	—	97.1	—	—	94.1	93.1–97.0	—	—
Level 3 past year	1.5	0.6	0.8	0.5	0.7	1.4	—	—	0.2	2.1
Level 2 past year	2.5	1.4	2.2	0.8	—	1.4	—	—	0.5	2.8
Level 1 past year	96.0	98.0	97.0	98.7	—	97.2	—	—	99.3	95.1

Note. Since all studies used either the SOGS or DSM criteria, cases within each study endorsing five or more criteria from those instruments were categorized as Level 3, cases endorsing three to four criteria were categorized as Level 2, and the rest of each study sample (i.e., nongamblers and nonproblem gamblers) were categorized as Level 1. Lifetime levels include results from the SOGS and DSM criteria not otherwise specified. Past-year levels include results specified as past year or within last 6 months.

[a] Shaffer and Hall (2001); [b] Volberg, Abbott, Roennberg, and Munck (2001); [c] Bondolfi, Osiek, and Ferrero (2002); [d] Abbott (2001); [e] Sproston, Erens, and Orford (2000); [f] Collins and Barr (2001); [g] Wong and So (2003); [h] Becona (1996); [i] Gotestam and Johansson (2003); [j] Productivity Commission (1999).

Researchers, however, have observed some interesting trends. Winters, Stinchfield, and Kim (1995) observed that the prevalence of Minnesota adolescents with gambling disorders did not increase despite a shift away from informal games toward more legalized games. Similarly, Wallisch (1995) observed that rate of gambling remained steady and the prevalence of gambling disorders actually diminished among Texas adolescents between 1992 and 1995. A meta-analysis revealed that the rate of disordered gambling had indeed increased during the last three decades of the twentieth century, but only among adults from the general population (Shaffer & Hall, 2001; Shaffer, Hall, & Vander Bilt, 1999). Consistent with the few local studies that had monitored young people's gambling behavior, the rate of disorder was not increasing among youth or patients with psychiatric or substance use disorders (Shaffer & Hall, 2001; Shaffer et al., 1997; Shaffer, Hall, & Vander Bilt, 1999).

SOCIOECONOMIC STATUS

Social gradients (e.g., poverty and the psychoeconomics of gambling) disproportionately influence disordered gambling patterns across population segments (Lopes, 1987). People with lower socioeconomic status experience gambling and other socioeconomically related problems at rates higher than those associated with high socioeconomic standing (Lapage, Ladouceur, & Jacques, 2000; Sebastian, 1985; Shaffer, Freed, & Healea, 2002). The homeless also evidence higher prevalence rates (Lapage et al., 2000; Sebastian, 1985; Shaffer et al., 2002).

WOMEN

Epidemiological research suggests that disordered gambling is more prevalent among men than women (National Research Council, 1999; Shaffer et al., 1997); adolescent boys are about 4 times more likely to be pathological gamblers than female adolescents. Gender differences likely reflect complex issues surrounding the attitudes and opportunities about recreational activities and the social milieu within which these occur (e.g., Bettencourt & Miller, 1996; Grant & Kim, 2002; Kiesler & Sproull, 1985).

CASINO EMPLOYEES

Casino employees have higher levels of gambling, smoking, drinking, and mood disorder compared to the general population (Shaffer, Vander Bilt, & Hall, 1999). Further, the first multiyear prospective study of casino employees (Shaffer & Hall, 2002) revealed that people troubled with gambling, drinking, or both shifted these problem behavior patterns regularly. These changes tended toward reduced levels of disorder rather than the increasingly serious problems often suggested by a traditional view of "addictive" behavior patterns (Shaffer & Hall, 2002). However, this study did not examine the pathways to recovery that casino employees experienced. This reflects a vital gap in the extant literature since it is likely that the majority of people with gambling-related problems escape this circumstance without treatment (Cunningham et al., 1995; Shaffer & Jones, 1989; Sobell, Cunningham, & Sobell, 1996; Waldorf, 1983; Winick, 1962). Prospective research designs are necessary to determine the extent of natural recovery and the determinants that influence the transition from problem to nonproblem gambling or abstinence.

OLDER ADULTS

While younger people have evidenced higher rates of gambling-related problems compared with their adult counterparts (e.g., Poulin, 2000), recently attention has shifted toward older adults and their increased risk for gambling problems. As gambling expanded and older adults sought more varied recreational activities, gambling junkets became more common. Recently, for example, investigators reported that older adults gambled to relax, pass time, get away for the day, avoid boredom and enjoy inexpensive meals (McNeilly & Burke, 2000). The prevalence of disordered gambling among this population segment is not yet determined. It is interesting to consider that the reasons for gambling among the elderly are likely very similar to the reasons for gambling among adolescents.

SELECTED ETHNOCULTURAL POPULATIONS

Though there has been no systematic evaluation of the effects of culture on gambling and problem gambling, there is evidence of cultural variation among prevalence rates. For example, higher than average rates of gambling and gambling problems are found among African American, aboriginal, and Latin American adolescents (Stinchfield, Nadav, Winter, & Latimer, 1997). Other studies identified group differences in gambling that are likely to have ethnocultural roots. In Florida, for example, problem gamblers are disproportionately Latin American (Cuadrado, 1999). Likewise, Asian groups in America have been found to show higher rates of gambling disorders compared to other groups (Zane & Huh-Kim, 1998). Gambling, including illegal gambling, continues to be popular in America's Chinese communities, with many willing to work extra shifts to afford this recreational activity (Kinkead, 1992). There is evidence of gambling's popularity in other Asian countries as well, such as, for example, in Singapore, where gambling is associated with substance abuse and other detrimental behaviors (Teck-Hong, 1992). Finally, in general, aboriginal people evidence higher rates of problem and pathological gambling, poorer mental health status as well as higher rates of substance-related problems compared with the general population (e.g., Elia & Jacobs, 1993; National Steering Committee, 1999; Office of Public Health, 1999; Volberg & Abbott, 1997; Wardman, el-Guebaly, & Hodgins, 2001). These higher rates do not necessarily reflect more psychopathology since cultural differences can influence these observations. Additional research is necessary to clarify the clinical significance of these patterns because what is (ab)normal in one culture might be normal in another.

Comorbidity

Also of concern to therapists is the comorbidity, or coexistence, of mental disorders and pathological gambling (Shaffer & Korn, 2002). Some research even suggests a genetic vulnerability (i.e., the DRD_2 gene) associated with psychiatric comorbidity among pathological gamblers (Ibanez et al., 2001). Unfortunately, most evaluations of treatment do not consider comorbid disorders (Winters & Kushner, 2003). Nevertheless, the various versions of the DSM that have included pathological gambling as a distinct disorder have drawn attention to the possibility that other disorders may coexist with pathological gambling. For example, DSM-IV notes that pathological gamblers "may be prone to developing general medical conditions that are associated with stress. . . . Increased rates of Mood Disorders, Attention-Deficit/Hyperactivity Disorder, Substance Abuse or Dependence, and Antisocial, Narcissistic, and Borderline Personality Disorders have been reported in individuals with Pathological Gambling" (American Psychiatric Association, 1994, p. 616). This coexistence can take many forms and could indicate several fundamental characteristics of the disorders involved. To illustrate, where X represents a comorbid condition, and PG represents gambling disorders, seven primary relationships can describe the association between disordered gambling and psychiatric comorbidity.

1. X contributes to, is a risk factor for, or causes PG.
2. X protects against or "treats" the occurrence of or progression to PG.
3. PG contributes to, is a risk factor for, or causes X.
4. PG protects against or "treats"[4] the occurrence of or progression to X.
5. X and PG co-occur/coexist but are coincidental and completely independent.
6. X and PG share common determinants (i.e., biological, psychological, behavioral or social).
7. X and PG combined are actually components of some "larger" entity, disorder or syndrome.

This vastly complicates the therapeutic picture. Because clinicians must deal with both primary and secondary disorders, it is vital to distinguish psychological conditions that are causal or primary from those that exist only secondary to other influences. In the following sections, we report on research that links gambling with other mental illnesses to illustrate the breadth from which the origins of pathological gambling could stem. This variety might indicate the need for some type of treatment "cocktail" that is individually tailored to the treatment seeker's individual need.

SUBSTANCE USE DISORDERS

A comprehensive review of the extant research on the comorbidity of substance use and problem gambling is beyond the scope of this chapter; we encourage interested readers to review Shaffer and Korn (2002) for a comprehensive review of comorbidity and gambling disorders. It is worth noting, however, that most gambling studies on the relationship between gambling and other psychiatric conditions have been focused on substance use and mood disorders (e.g., Feigelman, Wallisch, & Lesieur, 1998; Welte, Barnes, Wieczorek, Tidwell, & Parker, 2001). Crockford and el-Guebaly report "that between 25% and 63% of pathological gamblers meet criteria for a substance use disorder in their lifetime. . . . Correspondingly, 9% to 16% of patients with a substance use disorders are also found to be probable pathological gamblers" (Crockford & el-Guebaly, 1998, p. 44). Crockford and el-Guebaly found that alcohol is the most commonly abused substance; a high rate of nicotine use is also very common among pathological gamblers. When more than one substance is abused, the prevalence and severity of pathological gambling is increased as compared to individuals who abuse only one drug. Crockford and el-Guebaly note that there is considerable variation among study estimates of the comorbidity of substance abuse and gambling as well as the quality of these study methods, a conclusion shared by Shaffer, Hall, and Vander Bilt (1997).

MOOD DISORDERS

There is evidence to suggest that the prevalence of dysthymia, depression (unipolar and bipolar), suicidal ideation, and suicide attempts is inflated among individuals with gambling disorders (Getty, Watson, & Frisch, 2000; McCormick et al., 1984; Phillips, Welty, & Smith, 1997; Shaffer, Vander Bilt, & Hall, 1999). However, Lesieur and Blume (1990) noted that among patients treated for mood disorders, there was not an elevated prevalence of pathological gambling. This runs counter to other research (Taber, McCormick, Russo, Adkins, & Ramirez, 1987), however, that has reported that about 18% of disordered gamblers experienced continued depression "despite abstinence from gambling and improvement in their work and family lives—a percentage of depressive disorders similar to that seen in patients with substance use disorders" (Crockford & el-Guebaly, 1998, p. 46). Thus, some relationship between mood disorders and problem gambling does seem likely.

GAMBLING, SUICIDE, AND MORTALITY

The link between gambling and suicide and mortality has been quite sensationalized over time. The idea that gambling is a cause of suicide emerges primarily from (1) anecdotes about successful suicides that are preceded by episodes of losing at gambling (e.g., Lakshmanan, 1996), (2) higher rates of reported depression among individuals with gambling problems, and (3) case studies (e.g., Blaszczynski & Farrell, 1998; Jason, Taff, & Boglioli, 1990). However, between 1980 and 1997 no United States death certificate has listed gambling as the underlying cause of death (Centers for Disease Control, 2001).[5]

Investigators have explored this problem using epidemiological strategies. A retrospective analysis of patient medical charts of pathological gambling treatment seekers found that 40% had attempted suicide in their lifetime and 64% reported an attempt was related to gambling (Kausch, 2003). Alternatively, Phillips et al. (1997) suggest that there is a link between gambling and suicide by virtue of elevated suicides proximate to gambling. A study critical of this association suggests that when calculations include appropriate at-risk populations, there is no evidence to support such a link (Chew, McCleary, Merrill, & Napolitano, 2000). McCleary et al. (1998) also argue against such a link. At this point, confident conclusions about a causal link between suicide and gambling cannot be drawn (General Accounting Office, 2000).

With respect to mortality, a study of Atlantic City casino-related deaths between 1982 and 1986 showed that, of the total number of fatalities, 83% were cardiac sudden deaths. Although we can speculate that the stress of gambling activities can induce sudden cardiac death (Jason et al., 1990), scientific studies have not yet established that problem or pathological gamblers die at different rates compared with their nonproblem gambling counterparts.

ANXIETY DISORDERS

Anxiety often appears as a hallmark of gamblers who seek treatment; however, this anxiety typically is more representative of anxious depression than anxiety disorders. Clinicians have described the signs and symptoms of anxiety (e.g., fear and stress) as common prior to becoming a gambler, whereas betting and playing (e.g., gambling as escape from these unpleasant emotions) are a DSM-IV diagnostic criterion for pathological gambling; anxiety also is a common subjective state during treatment and recovery. However, clinical anxiety disorders are a complex grouping of specific mental disorders ranging from general anxiety disorder (GAD), panic attacks, obsessive–compulsive disorder (OCD) to posttraumatic stress disorder (PTSD). For these clinical conditions, "little is known about the association of anxiety disorders and problem gambling" (National Research Council, 1999, p. 138). After a careful review of the literature, Crockford and el-Guebaly concluded that "despite an increased prevalence being reported in 3 studies, there would appear to be insufficient data to support the theory that anxiety disorders are comorbid with pathological gambling. In particular, there is little support for the comorbidity with obsessive–compulsive disorder (OCD)" (Crockford & el-Guebaly, 1998, p. 47).

PERSONALITY DISORDERS

In spite of little empirical evidence to estimate the comorbidity of personality and gambling disorders, clinicians regularly describe a high level of narcissistic personality disorder among pathological gamblers. Two important general population studies found that problem gambling was associated with antisocial personality disorder (ASPD) and that pathological gambling always was secondary to ASPD (Cunningham-Williams, Cottler, Compton, & Spitznagel, 1998; Cunningham-Williams, Cottler, Compton, Spitznagel, & Ben-Abdallah, 2000). Blaszczynski and Steel (1998) concluded that "multiple overlapping personality disorders per subject [were] more the rule than the exception. . . . On average, subjects met criteria for 4.6 DSM-III personality disorders" (pp. 60, 65). In addition, the number of personality disorders was significantly related to SOGS scores in a positive direction. "The results of this study indicate that pathological gamblers as a group exhibit rates of personality disorders that are comparable to those found in general psychiatric patient populations" (p. 65). Recent research adds support for the relationship between antisocial personality and pathological gambling among treatment-seeking cohorts (Langenbucher, Bavly, Labouvie, Sanjuan, & Martin, 2001).

IMPULSE AND OTHER DISORDERS

Currently, DSM-IV-TR (American Psychiatric Association, 2000) places pathological gambling within the impulse disorders category. Kleptomania, pyromania, and trichotillomania also reside in this class of impulse disorders. It is reasonable to expect that pathological gambling would covary with these disorders of similar origin. However, despite occasionally examining impulsiveness, researchers have not comparatively investigated gambling and the other diagnoses from the DSM impulse disorders category. Instead, investigators have elected to compare and contrast gambling with substance use disorders. Consequently, there is a paucity of evidence to inform us about the comorbidity of pathological gambling and the other impulse disorders.

Crockford and el-Guebaly concluded that there is little evidence to suggest a comorbid relationship between gambling disorders and eating or sexual addiction (Crockford & el-Guebaly, 1998). However, compulsive shopping or oniomania has been identified as having etiology and comorbidity patterns similar to pathological gambling, with a very similar prevalence rate (i.e., 1.1%) (Lejoyeux, Ades, Tassain, & Solomon, 1996). Scientists have suggested that pathological gambling and other excessive behavior patterns have a common etiology that is characterized by a reward deficiency syndrome (Blum et al., 2000). This common neurobiological vulnerability also has linked the prevalence of pathological gambling to increased rates of Tourette's syndrome (Comings, 1998).

Despite a lack of concrete evidence, impulsivity should not be ignored, as it has been linked to treatment drop-out (Leblond, Ladouceur, & Blaszczynski, 2003). Neurobiological, neuropsychological, and clinical studies (e.g., Rugle & Melamed, 1993) provide growing evidence that there is an increase in attention-deficit/hyperactivity disorder (ADHD) among pathological compared to nonpathological gamblers (Comings et al., 1999; Hollander et al., 2000; National Research Council, 1999; Specker, Carlson, Christenson, & Marcotte, 1995; Wise, 1995). Research has identified preliminary evidence that noradrenaline is associated with attention problems (e.g., ADHD) and that dopamine level shifts might be associated with pathological gambling (Bergh et al., 1997). Finally, as noted previously, preliminary research suggests positive clinical outcomes on problematic gambling for individuals who take bupropion (Black, 2004).

Determining Patient Placement: Levels of Care

Guiliani and Schnoll (1985) examined the nature of clinical decision making within the context of a chemical dependence treatment program in Chicago. Guiliani and Schnoll originally noted that "numerous studies have shown that treatment works better than no treatment . . . since it is not known why treatment is effective for some patients and not for others, the focus of research has shifted to discovering which treatment or aspects of treatment work best and for whom" (Guiliani & Schnoll, 1985, p. 203). Suggesting that treatment should not be determined solely by "drug of choice," Guiliani and Schnoll argued that thorough clinical assessments should lead to assignment to the "appropriate treatment level" (p. 204). Their experience suggested that not all patients require the same level or intensity of care. Different patients are often at different points in the natural progression of a disease. Guiliani and Schnoll (1985) provided the substantive clinical and intellectual inspiration that stimulated the development of the Cleveland criteria (Hoffman, Halikas, & Mee-Lee, 1987) and the National Association of Addiction Treatment Providers (NAATP) Patient Placement Criteria (National Association of Addiction Treatment Providers, 1987). They also provided the stimulus for a clinical movement culminating in the American Society of Addiction Medicine (ASAM) patient placement criteria. Ultimately, these levels of care criteria culminated in a joint effort between NAATP and the ASAM to generate what has become known as the ASAM criteria (Hoffman, Halikas, Mee-Lee, & Weedman, 1991). Many clinicians believe that these dimensions represent an effective approach to standardize patient–treatment matching within an atmosphere of "managed care." The next section considers basic guidelines for matching treatment seekers to various levels of care.

Heuristics for Treatment-Setting Matching: Applying Patient Placement Criteria

As healthcare providers apply managed care strategies to control the costs of substance abuse treatment in the public and private sectors, identifying appropriate levels of clinical services (e.g., inpatient detoxification and residential care) requires more than simply identifying patients' wishes or desires for treatment. Patients must now meet standardized utilization management criteria. The best known and most fully developed of these criteria are the Patient Placement Criteria proposed by the American Society of Addiction Medicine. Although the ASAM criteria have important limitations (e.g., McKay et al., 1992), this system has been endorsed by a variety of organizations and states. Massachusetts, for example, uses the ASAM criteria to guide patient placement and Medicaid reimbursement.

Using criteria such as ASAM does not require one to endorse either the entire system of care or the standards (i.e., what constitutes sufficient evidence for placement at a particular level of care) represented by the ASAM placement system. To illustrate, the ASAM criteria have not included the full range of treatment options; some of the most cost-effective forms of treatment have been absent from this placement system (e.g., outpatient detoxification, methadone maintenance, and therapeutic communities). Thus, a treatment system planner could distinguish levels of care that are not included in the four levels of care that have been embraced by the ASAM criteria (i.e., outpatient treatment, intensive outpatient/partial hospitalization, medically monitored intensive inpatient, and medically managed intensive inpatient). Further, many states probably would employ more demanding standards for placing patients in a particular level of care than ASAM now requires.

Given the empirical uncertainty associated with complex patient placement criteria for substance use disorders and the absence of patient placement criteria for the treatment of gambling disorders, we suggest that clinicians judiciously apply the original patient placement criteria suggested by Guiliani and Schnoll (1985). Since comorbid psychiatric and substance use disorders are prevalent among treatment seekers with gambling disorders (Shaffer & Korn, 2002), it is important for gambling treatment specialists to note carefully the potential risks caused by these comorbid conditions on patient placement decisions. These criteria are summarized in Table 10.5.

The Clinical Art of Changing Addiction

Within each placement setting, various treatment modalities exist. Treatment interventions must shift to match each patient's current experiences and mold the shape of future understandings. These changes reflect therapeutic movement and are accomplished through therapeutic meaning making and targeted motivational strategies. These strategies are discussed, in turn, in the following sections. Movement and treatment progress stimulates hope and adherence to treatment, which, in turn, encourages more improvement.

A motion picture represents a rapid sequence of single photographic frames. When stopped, each frame of the movie depicts a moment, frozen in time. While each frame is only a cross-section of the movie experience, the meaning of this image evolves within the context of the film sequence as each frame "constructs" or revises the film narrative. Similarly, during psychotherapy each reframe shifts a client's perspective so that experience is revised. If one chooses to conceptualize psychotherapy in this way, the possibilities for clinicians and clients to use a *series* of reframes, rather than be wedded to a single approach (cf. Marlatt & Fromme, 1987), become apparent. In the following discussion, we provide a brief overview to modality matching. More comprehensive reviews are available (Shaffer & Robbins, 1991, 1995; Shaffer & Simoneau, 2001).

Many clients with addictive problems first enter treatment because of external pressures. Often, patients do not see a problem with *their* gambling or drug use. Instead, for example, they see their distress stemming from their spouse or the legal system. Many addiction treatment specialists describe these patients as "in denial," projecting their difficulties onto various aspects of their social setting. However, patient denial is often a reflection of clinical intervention or style. For example, insight-oriented treatment early in therapy can be threatening; the result often is denial or withdrawing from care.

Rather than jumping in with accusations, during the early phase of gambling treatment it is necessary for clinicians to establish a treatment alliance. To accomplish this objective, therapists need to employ a treatment

TABLE 10.5. Patient Placement Criteria

Criteria for acute inpatient hospital care

1. Failure to progress in less controlled and intense levels of treatment.
2. High-risk chemical detoxification, for example, withdrawal that might be associated with seizures or delirium tremens.
3. Chemical detoxification complicated by high levels of tolerance to multiple substances.
4. Acute exacerbation of medical and/or psychiatric problems that relate to chemical dependence (e.g., cardiomyopathy, hepatitis, severe depression).
5. Concomitant medical and/or psychiatric problems that potentially could complicate treatment (e.g., diabetes, bipolar affective disorder, hypertension).
6. Severely impaired social, familial, or occupational functioning.

Criteria for nonhospital residential care

1. Failure to progress in less intensive levels of treatment.
2. Chemical detoxification, if necessary, can proceed safely without close medical supervision.
3. The patient is psychiatrically and/or medically stable but requires daily supervision.
4. The patient's social and/or vocational level of functioning requires separation from aspects of his or her regular environment.
5. The patient's interpersonal and daily living skills are sufficiently developed to permit a satisfactory level of functioning in a milieu environment.

Criteria for partial hospitalization or day treatment care

1. Chemical detoxification, if necessary, can proceed without close medical supervision.
2. The patient is psychiatrically and/or medically stable but requires supervision daily rather than weekly or biweekly.
3. The patient's interpersonal and daily living skills are sufficiently developed to permit an autonomous level of functioning in a nonresidential environment.
4. The patient is psychiatrically stable but may need some moderate support.
5. The patient has a social system capable of providing the necessary level of support (e.g., friends, family, work).

Criteria for outpatient care

1. The patient's psychiatric/medical problems are stable (i.e., daily or weekly supervision is unnecessary).
2. The patient is capable of an autonomous level of functioning in the present social environment.
3. The patient can function effectively in individual, group, and/or family therapy environments.
4. Medical supervision is unnecessary for withdrawal.
5. The patient is willing to participate in a treatment program.

frame that is consistent with the client's view of the world. For example, though personal choice might be an obvious contributing factor to gambling problems, clinicians can use another early recovery model that externalizes the gambling "problem" by considering it as a disease process over which the client has little or no control. This understanding might more readily permit client and clinician to establish a treatment alliance. Alternatively, some clients will present for treatment with a view that suggests they are simply not thinking logically about their gambling. This circumstance might require clinicians to explain how gambling encourages a person to develop faulty logical patterns, for example, "magical thinking" or failing to remember the statistical principle of independent events. In this instance, clinicians employ a different treatment frame. In both cases, however, the clinician uses a treatment frame that resonates with the client's perspective. The patient comes to learn that he or she is not responsible for becoming addicted but does have the capacity to recover. This perspective permits the clinician and client to enter into a dialogue and to begin to move through the therapeutic process[6] (Watzlawick, 1990). As treatment continues and gambling activities abate, the recovering person's experience of personal responsibility often becomes more prominent. As this sense of accountability grows, recovering people frequently begin to look inward for any remaining sources of distress. When this aspect of recovery emerges, both clinician and patient might find insight-oriented reframes credible, effective, and comforting. As the recovery process continues to spiral, the insight clients previously gained can lead to diminished emotional distress. Now, a combination of behavioral and dynamic reframes offer useful tools for maintaining the desirable changes already accomplished.

Recall, however, that a client's understanding of his or her gambling behavior is not the only aspect of the client that is important for treatment to match. Previous discussions demonstrated that problem gamblers are also likely to differ on a number of important demographics and mental health dimensions. Thus, the clinical technique appropriate for one type of individual at a particular point in therapy may be entirely inappropriate for another. Patients with schizophrenia, for example, may never respond well to insight-oriented therapy. Consequently, therapists have the difficult task of balancing both a patient's personal understanding of him- or herself and other individuating characteristics that the patient possesses that may influence the treatment process.

Recovery from gambling disorders in particular and addictive behaviors in general is a nonlinear, iterative journey (Shaffer & Gambino, 1990). As patients pass through various aspects of this experience, different therapeutic reframes become relevant (cf. Marlatt & Fromme, 1987). Reframes change reality. New realities transform recovery. Shifts in the recovery process require novel reframes. Through this transactional process, the objects of addictive behavior recede from focus and switch from figure to background. "Once we have learned how a thing is supposed to be, we experience it differently—and never again as directly. Maturity places an obscuring veil of understanding between us and the world" (Margulies, 1989, p. 7).

Therapeutic Meaning Making[7]

One of the central questions that treatment providers confront is to consider which treatment, with which therapist, with which patient, at which point in the natural history of the patient's disorder yields the most favorable treatment outcomes. As we suggested before, accomplishing optimal treatment outcomes requires clinicians to meet patients where they "are" and then take them to a place that the patients had difficulty "finding."

To illustrate, clinicians regularly manufacture meaning during the conduct of psychotherapy (e.g., Watzlawick, 1976). For example, rather than construing "a problem" of addiction as the painful consequences of a poor adaptation to reality, or a disease process that travels relentlessly forward once set in motion, one constructivist describes it as "the painful present consequences of a specific as-if fiction . . . [that] must be replaced by the effect of a different as-if fiction which creates a more tolerable reality" (Watzlawick, 1990, p. 143). In other words, to be effective agents of change, clinicians must understand how individuals make meaning or "as-if fictions," and offer reframes that permit effective problem resolution and relief from personal distress. Consider a reframing response for a patient who presents her gambling binge "problem" as an overwhelming, out-of-control circumstance. A therapist might wonder with her whether the "problem" is also a "solution" to a more intolerable kind of distress. By so doing, clinician and client have begun to reframe, or rewrite the meaning of this experience: Now the client is a person coping rather than someone helplessly out of control. Reframes cast the proverbial glass half full or half empty depending upon which view maximizes change. The terms remain the same, but the understanding changes.[8]

Many addiction specialists already work this way. In fact, when clinicians utilize any theoretical model in their work with clients, they are using a new (i.e., new for the client) and sometimes very specific frame to reorganize or "rewrite" the client's "as-if fiction." Understanding psychotherapy this way permits therapists the freedom and flexibility to be pragmatic when choosing which model or elements of a treatment model to employ. If clinicians decide not to adopt any one model of addiction as "real" and "true," they gain the opportunity to use a treatment approach that resonates with a patient's way of creating meaning. This correspondence is what permits clinicians to meet patients where they are and then take them where they do not want to go.

Earlier in the chapter we discussed the importance of therapists' theoretical frames to the types of treatments offered and the processes of treatment. However, patients' frames can also influence this process. Kleinman (1988) and Pfifferling (1980) discussed the importance of examining a patient's perspectives for the treatment of psychiatric disorders in general. We have adapted these views, based on our clinical experience, to describe how patients might think of their gambling-related problems. For example, instead of viewing intemperate gambling as a disease or behavioral excess, there are treatment seekers who see their problems with gambling as a punishment. Some consider it a well-deserved penalty while others view it as unreasonable and unfortunate. Other patients might see their gambling disorder as an enemy and deny their capacity to resist it; alternatively, these treatment seekers might resist gambling with pronounced hostility. Still others regard pathological gambling as direct evidence of personal weakness and a moral loss of control. For some, gambling excess is a strategy by which they manage their environment and shape their identity. Gambling disorders also can provide relief from obligations and responsibilities. Quite often disordered gambling is understood as an irrevocable personal loss; this view often leads to depression. Finally, some patients seeking gambling treatment view their disorder as an opportunity, a time for personal growth and reflection.

Clinicians' understandings of gambling are similarly diverse. To illustrate, clinicians can frame gambling disorders as an excessive attachment to money or diminished cognitive capacity. Alternatively, gambling disorders can be framed as the result of deficient ego functions (e.g., ego defenses, self-esteem, affect regulation and management, self-care, and object relations; Shaffer & Jones, 1989). When clinicians and clients talk about using gambling, drugs, food, or alcohol to "numb the pain," "keep them company," "relieve anxiety," or fill up an "empty feeling," they are using "psychodynamic" language. In contrast, many clinicians use a behavioral frame to make sense of their clients' experience. When addiction treatment specialists focus on the risks that clients face by being in gambling settings, on how hard clients must work to break their "habit," or how stepping into a casino "triggers" a train of impulsive thoughts, feelings, and behaviors, clinicians are featuring a "behavioral" story to frame the problem.

Clinicians can use the disease model with those clients most familiar and comfortable with understanding their "problem" from a sickness or illness frame. Any single client–clinician pair may use different components of these or other stories during any given "treatment" encounter. This prescriptive approach recognizes that a patient's perception of his or her disorder will determine when, how, and to what treatment provider, if any, he or she will go. Understanding a patient's perception of his or her gambling problem permits the clinician to negotiate and navigate treatment interventions. Rather than use one conceptual frame, clinicians can learn how to *access* and then to *assess* the patient's view of addiction (Shaffer & Gambino, 1990). While it might be possible to impose a clinical model on some patients, most bring their own view of gambling and addiction with them when they enter treatment. When the provider and patient see things similarly, treatment can go well. However, most observers recognize that the majority of intemperate gamblers find it difficult to engage in treatment (National Research Council, 1999). Historically this has been a patient problem: Many treatment specialists blame the patient and the "disease of denial." More likely, however, this situation results when patient views do not match the therapist's opinion (Shaffer, 1994; Shaffer & Gambino, 1990).

Targeting Motivational Strategies to Stages of Change

Stages-of-change concepts have emerged as an important force in the treatment of addictive behaviors (Crowley, 1999; Prochaska, DiClemente, & Norcross, 1992; Prochaska, Norcross, & DiClemente, 1994; Quinn, 1891; Rollnick & Morgan, 1995; Shaffer, 1992, 1994, 1997; Shaffer & Robbins, 1995). Stages-of-change theory suggests that an evaluation of a gambler's readiness to change and determination of his or her stage of change are important steps to formulating treatment strategy (Shaffer & Robbins, 1995). Motivational enhancement techniques (Miller, 1996; Miller & Rollnick, 1991; Shaffer, 1997; Shaffer & Robbins, 1995; Shaffer & Simoneau, 2001) can facilitate this process and guide intervention strategies. In this following discussion, we briefly review the clinical tasks associated with matching treatment strategies with the natural history of gambling disorders to ensure that clinical interventions match appropriately to the stages of change.

Precontemplation: When Adverse Consequences Present without Awareness

Before an individual with a gambling disorder seeks treatment, he or she often experiences many problems and has little awareness that gambling is the primary cause of these problems. At this stage the gambler is not considering a change in behavior. Gambling still is viewed as a positive experience. Since this stage is characterized by lack of awareness of gambling addiction as an entity or gambling as a primary cause of distress, the major clinical challenge/themes are to enhance awareness of consequences and overcome resistance to change. In many cases, inviting or engaging gamblers into treatment is the focus of clinical efforts, since family members typically initiate contact with treatment providers. A psychoeducational strategy can help to start the change process. For example, clinicians can invite the affected family members to the office or provide them with information about gambling disorders and describe the continuum of mild, moderate, and severe gambling problems that can arise. This activity might not include the gambler, since at this point, he or she is not very interested in treatment. Consequently, family members should be instructed to take care of themselves. They should not share their treatment discussions with the gambler, and simply invite the gambler to participate in the next session or to review the available educational materials. This circumstance encourages individuals with a gambling disorder to examine their own gambling patterns, risky situations, and impact on others without alienating or coercing them to participate in treatment. Too often, family or treatment provider coercion leads to maliciousness, aversion, and ultimately abandonment; each of these experiences holds significant risk for the gambler.

Once the patient's curiosity and ambivalent feelings emerge, clinicians should request that gamblers self-monitor their gambling and document any urges to gamble. This evidence can provide the foundation for future efforts at evaluation and treatment planning. Gamblers then have the opportunity to compare their perception of their experience with that of other family members. They also have the opportunity to assess the economics of their gambling and its impact on their life objectives, both proximate and distal. During this part of treatment, gamblers also should be questioned about what gambling does for them—not just what it is doing to them. By exploring the gambler's perception of the benefits and advantages of gambling for them, clinicians are in a better position to develop realistic treatment plans that consider alternative behavior patterns that can fulfill as many of the same gambling objectives as possible without having to gamble. Taken together, these early treatment activities exercise the ambivalence associated with behavior change and gently diminish denial and resistance (Shaffer & Simoneau, 2001).

Contemplation: Adverse Consequences Enter Awareness

During this stage, treatment seekers recognize gambling as the primary cause of their gambling-related problems and evidence some receptivity to the possibility of addressing these issues. The major clinical challenge is to address the person's ambivalence about whether there is a wish to alter gambling behavior and deal with associated problems. The primary approach to stimulating the wish to want to change is to acknowledge that gambling provides positive benefits but also costs. The clinician must acknowledge that modifying the pattern of gambling that caused problems will require relinquishing some current activities. A decision balance exercise that explores the pluses and minuses of maintaining the gambling behavior and the gains and loses of changing is the major vehicle for resolving the ambivalence about the value of curbing gambling. A seminal event such as the loss of a large sum of money or job loss, often referred to as a turning point, frequently marks the treatment seeker's decision to commit to major changes.

Preparation: Turning Points and an Orientation to Change

At this stage, treatment-seeking gamblers have accepted the notion that changes are necessary and worthwhile. The major clinical challenge is to help individuals with a gambling disorder see the array of alternatives available to them; making choices is central and the key treatment activity is planning. Therapist efforts focus on goal setting and planning for treatment and life changes. Together, gambler and treatment provider explore therapeutic options and appropriate action steps. Together, patient and provider need to consider the type of treatment setting, program philosophy, level of care, kind and variety of therapeutic modalities, group or individual format, professional profile, and cost that will increase the likelihood of a favorable outcome. Treatment matching is the important principle. Success at this stage is often linked to honoring the person's preferences and validating the acceptability of the person's choices.

Active Quitting: Taking Action for Change

At this stage of gambling disorders and treatment, the major theme is active learning. The clinical strategy focuses on encouraging disordered gamblers to initiate a range of new behaviors based on the acquisition of new knowledge, insight, attitudes, and skills. This is the beginning of psychological detoxification and restoration. Identifying and substituting a different leisure activity to replace the time spent gambling is an important component of a healthy recovery. Solution-focused brief therapy for problem gamblers is being utilized and holds considerable promise. It has been implemented successfully in the substance abuse field; however, research in gambling treatment is limited (Dickerson et al., 1990). The introduction of a support program such as the fellowship of GA and more involvement in spiritually enriching experiences can be highly beneficial. However, though clinicians can suggest these support systems, almost any that recovering gamblers choose hold potential to be helpful.

Relapse Prevention and Change Maintenance

To achieve enduring treatment goals, the clinical focus at this stage of treatment is to practice the new competencies to sustain a balanced, healthy lifestyle. Adult learning theory recognizes that developing and mastering new behaviors requires training and repetition. Relapses can and often do occur; since this is a common part of recovery from gambling and other addictive behavior patterns, clinicians need to pay particular attention to situational risk as a critical component of relapse (e.g., Marlatt & Gordon, 1985; McAulliffe & Ch'ien, 1986; Svanum & Mcadoo, 1989; Vaillant, 1988).

In sum, using Prochaska and DiClemente's stages-of-change model (e.g., Prochaska et al., 1992), the clinician's tasks at each stage are specific. For example, Brosky (2001) suggests that during the precontemplation stage, the clinician should raise doubt about the current behavior. In the contemplation stage, clinicians can help gamblers to resolve ambivalence by identifying reasons to change and risks of the status quo. In the preparation stage, clinicians assist individuals to choose a best plan. In the action stage, clinicians teach skills that support the change and prevent relapse. In the maintenance stage, clients practice new behaviors and reframe relapse as learning. There is one major caveat regarding the stages-of-change model and motivational enhancement counseling. Observers often incorrectly think that changes occur in a linear and progressive fashion. In reality, the change process is recursive, with many opportunities to revisit earlier stages and successfully navigate the tasks of recovery necessary to grow as a person and rebuild one's life (Shaffer, 1992, 1997; Shaffer & Robbins, 1995).

In addition to the specific treatment tasks associated with each stage of change or stage of the disorder's natural history, stages of change also provide public health workers with the framework to develop programs strategically. This population-based view of the stages-of-change represents a shift from individually based treatment tactics to a broader set of programs designed for the community (Tucker, Donovan, & Marlatt, 1999). Although a full discussion of the public health implications for stages-of-change and program matching is beyond the scope of this chapter, Table 10.6 provides a summary of only some of the potential stage–modality matches that can be used to guide program development and implementation.

FACTORS THAT INFLUENCE TREATMENT OUTCOMES

Early in this chapter, we noted that nonspecific or common factors account for a considerable amount of treatment outcome (e.g., Frank, 1961; Hubble et al., 1999). Just as nonspecific treatment factors can increase the likelihood of positive treatment outcomes, they also can make things worse. When the relationship between clinician and treatment seeker is less than optimal, there is an increased risk of poor treatment outcomes. Arguably the most important adverse influence on the relationship factors displayed by the treatment provider (e.g., empathy, caring, warmth, etc.) is the presence of countertransference hate (Maltsberger & Buie, 1974; Shaffer, 1994). In addition to relationship issues, therapist training and experience, as well as opportunities for RP can influence treatment outcomes. We will

TABLE 10.6. Matching Stages of Change to Treatment Modalities

Stages of gambling behavior	Range of possible treatment modality matches
1. Initiation	Primary prevention (e.g., public education and information programs)
2. Positive consequences	Secondary prevention (e.g., public education, counseling)
3. Adverse consequences	Tertiary prevention (e.g., counseling), outpatient psychotherapy services, or self-help fellowships (to stimulate ambivalence, dissonance, and a readiness for change); acute inpatient services (when there is a need for medical and psychiatric crisis management)
4. Turning point(s)	Acute inpatient and outpatient services (e.g., detoxification, partial care, 12-step, and self-help programs)
5. Active quitting	Residential (only for chronic substance abusers who have little or no social support systems available), partial care, or outpatient services (e.g., chemical substitutions, counseling, 12-step, and self-help programs)
6. Relapse prevention or change maintenance	Outpatient, 12-step, self-help and residential (only for chronic substance abusers who have little or no social support systems available).

turn our attention to each of these three broadly defined areas in the following discussion.

Countertransference Hate

"When a therapist feels or acts toward a patient in ways that are neither part of the real relationship, rationally justified by the circumstances, nor part of the working alliance, appropriate to the terms of the treatment contract, he is manifesting countertransference" (Weiner, 1975, p. 244). Think about your instinctive response to someone revealing they are getting married or divorced, pregnant, detoxifying from a dependence-producing drug, or abstaining from gambling. In each case, there is a tendency to feel either congratulatory or sympathetic. When a therapist experiences one of these responses, this is countertransference. Rather than expressing either congratulations or sympathy, a more effective clinical posture would be to ask "When did you decide?" or "How did you decide?" or "What's that going to be like for you?" Congratulations leave relapsing patients in a difficult position: If they share their difficulties with their therapist in the future, there is a risk that they might disappoint the treatment provider. This may limit what patients are willing to say to their therapists.

Not only can countertransference influence patient behavior, but it can also influence therapist behavior. Maltsberger and Buie (1974) suggest that clinical hate and rage are comprised of three important elements: (1) malice, (2) aversion, and (3) a mixture of these two emotions. Malicious impulses stimulate a disgust that can make patients seems loathsome (e.g., disgust about patients who are self-indulgent). Under these circumstances, patients can become the object of punishment or torturing impulses. However, Maltsberger and Buie are quick to note that malicious impulses are less dangerous than aversive tendencies because malice allows clinicians to maintain a clinical relationship with a patient, whether he or she is abominated or loathed. Aversive impulses, in contrast, tempt the therapist to abandon the patient. Finally, unbearable malicious impulses often stimulate aversive actions. Malicious impulses are more painful to clinicians than the tendency to avoid (Maltsberger & Buie, 1974). Therefore, when patients stimulate malevolent impulses, clinicians avoid having to confront or continue working with this individual.

The Effect of Training

Clinical research has neglected the impact of treatment training on clinical outcomes (Shaffer & Costikyan, 2002). Some research has suggested that the amount of training a therapist receives is important to the success of treatment (e.g., Stein & Lambert, 1995). However, access to training for the treatment of pathological gambling is likely to be inadequate. Related work suggests that these resources are insufficient for substance abuse training (Shaffer, Hall, & Vander Bilt, 1995). Given the infancy of the study and treatment of pathological gambling, this situation is likely to be much worse for gambling. However, years of research attest to the importance of training. Specifically, meta-analytic evidence suggests that therapists with more training have relatively better treatment outcomes, such as fewer dropouts and greater satisfaction, than therapists with less training (Stein & Lambert, 1995). Taking this one step further, given the influence of individuating characteristics on the therapeutic process, others have argued for the inclusion of ethnic and cultural diversity education in professional psychology training (Yutrzenka, 1995).

However, more research is needed to explore the link between treatment training and treatment outcomes. Several primary questions remain to be answered. What skills specifically influence these outcomes? What types of training are most effective? How can we best care for patients while providing therapy experience to "new" therapists? Although much remains to be determined, at a minimum these findings suggest the need for common training standards, greater supervision of therapists in training, and an increase in mandatory continuing education.

Relapse Prevention Strategies: Toward Treatment Integration

RP strategies are most often associated with cognitive-behavioral treatment approaches (Kadden, 2001; Marlatt & Gordon, 1985; McAulliffe & Ch'ien, 1986; Shaffer, 1997; Sylvain et al., 1997; Washton, 1989). However, since relapse is common among gamblers who enter recovery, and not all treatment providers employ cognitive-behavioral treatment methods, it is important to integrate these strategies into other treatment approaches. RP strategies are consistent with the work of dynamically oriented and psychoeducational treatment providers; however, behavioral treatment approaches and psychoanalysis have been the object of important clinical strategies (e.g., Wachtel, 1977). One step that is important for all therapists to take is to identify individuals who are at the highest risk for relapse and individuals' unique triggers. Doing so allows for the development and practice of adequate coping strategies. For example McCormick and Taber (1991) found that an increased relapse rate was related to cognitive dysfunction. Similarly, individuals who demonstrate high levels of neuroticism prior to treatment also are at increased risk for relapse (Echeburua, Fernandez-Montalvo, & Baez, 2001). In contrast, contrary to what conventional wisdom might suggest, locus of control, as measured by the Rotter I-E scales did not prove to be a good predictor of relapse (Johnson, Nora, & Bustos, 1992). More recently, Hodgins and el-Guebaly (2004) reported relapse rates among individuals with a gambling disorder (92%) at a 12-month follow-up that were very similar to the rates associated with patients treated for substance dependence. Hodgins et al. identified relapse risk factors that related to time of day, thinking about winning, and feeling the need to make money. More research is needed to determine the extent of overlap between the risk factors for relapse to gambling and the risk factors for relapse to excessive eating and substance abuse (e.g., Brownell, Marlatt, Lichtenstein, & Wilson, 1986). Developing coping skills for these triggers can change the likelihood of relapse. Consequently, throughout the course of treatment, therapists should be particularly attendant to the risks associated with relapse because this experience is very common (Hunt, Barnett, & Branch, 1971; Marlatt, Baer, Donovan, & Kivlahan, 1988; Marlatt & Gordon, 1985).

CONCLUSIONS

Research pertaining to the treatment of gambling disorders is in its infancy. This circumstance has neither prevented an increasing demand for treatment nor a growing interest among providers in delivering such treatment. However, because the study of treatment for gambling-related problems is still very young, there exist many opportunities to for scientists and clinicians to advance the field. At this point, there is a continuing and persistent need for rigorous research that utilizes sufficient follow-up periods (i.e., no less than 5 years). With few exceptions (e.g., Sylvain et al., 1997), little treatment outcome research has been conducted. Furthermore, researchers need to begin focusing on questions that pertain to individual treatment needs. For example, is the nature of adolescent gambling problems the same or different from adult gambling disorders? We can ask similar questions for other population segments and ethnic groups that are at increased risk for gambling disorders. If the experience of pathological gambling is different for different individuals or varies significantly for identifiable segments of the population, then it might be necessary to develop more sector-oriented treatments than are now available.

It is likely that there is not a single best treatment for gambling disorders. Shaffer and Korn (2002) suggest that the symptoms associated with pathological gambling reflect a complex syndrome instead of single disorder. Our current understanding of the comorbidity and co-occurrence of pathological gambling with other diagnostic entities probably is an artifact of DSM-IV, misdirecting observers away from the likelihood that it is a syndrome. Overlapping symptoms can represent a common underlying factor. However, when a variety of symptoms are associated with a disorder, but not all the symptoms are always present, a syndrome is evident. Since syndromes have unique components (e.g., betting) and elements that are shared with other disorders (e.g., anxiety and depression), assessment is complex and the treatment of gambling disorders is multifaceted. For example, like HIV, we expect that the most effective treatments for gambling problems will reflect a multimodal "cocktail" approach combined with patient–treatment matching. These multidimensional treatments will include various combinations of psychopharmacology, psychotherapy, financial, educational and self-help interventions; these various treatment elements are both additive and interactive, a circumstance necessary to deal with the multidimensional nature of gambling disorders (Shaffer & Korn, 2002).

Treatment for gambling disorders is promising. The treatment strategies that are widely used often have their roots in other addictive disorders. However, the clinical practice of other addictive disorders also might be informed by the techniques that have evolved for treating gambling. Treatments for other addictive disorders often focus too much on drug influences and ignore important psychosocial aspects. Since the study of gambling and gambling treatment permit scientists to distinguish chemical from behavioral influences, this area of inquiry holds the potential to advance the understanding of all addictive behaviors. Further, improved treatments for gambling problems can lead to strategies that focus on the often disregarded nondrug dimensions of addiction that are inherent in drug use disorders.

ACKNOWLEDGMENTS

We extend thanks to Richard LaBrie, Chris Reilly, Chrissy Thurmond, Laura van der Leeden, Christopher Freed, and Katie Witkiewitz for their advice regarding earlier versions of this chapter. We also extend special thanks to Mark Albanese and David Korn for their guidance and contributions to the psychopharmacology sections of this chapter and for their collaboration on related works that helped to establish the foundation for portions of this chapter. Preparation of this chapter was supported, in part, by funding from the Institute for Research on Pathological Gambling and Related Disorders and the National Center for Responsible Gaming.

NOTES

1. Although this chapter focuses primarily on addictive behaviors, the discussion and its application are not limited exclusively to the addictions. Many of the treatment strategies and techniques described in this chapter also will apply to other clinical problems.
2. The Inventory of Gambling Situations includes 11 items: Negative Affective Situations (negative emotions, conflict with others), Temptation Situations (urges and temptations, testing personal control), Positive Affect Situations (pleasant emotions, social pressure, and need for excitement), and Gambling Cycle Situations (worried about debt, winning and chasing loses, confidence in skill, need to be in control).
3. An electronic version of the Inventory of Gambling Situations is available from the Centre for Addiction and Mental Health; phone: 800-661-1111 or e-mail: marketing@camh.net.
4. When pathological gambling "treats" the occurrence of a coexisting disorder or the progression of these problems, gambling serves as a "self-medication" (e.g., Khantzian, 1985).
5. The absence of pathological gambling as the underlying cause of death on the death certificate does not mean that no one has died of factors associated with pathological gambling. Medical examiners, who must identify the immediate cause and contributing causes of death on the death certificate, for any number of reasons, might be unaware of pathological gambling or unwilling to list it as a cause of death.
6. Consider the lines spoken by Lilly Tomlin in her one-woman play *The Search for Signs of Intelligent Life in the Universe*: "After all, what is reality anyway? Nothin' but a collective hunch. . . . reality is the leading cause of stress amongst those in touch with it. I can take it in small doses, but as a lifestyle I found it too confining. It was just too needful; it expected me to be there for it all the time" (Wagner, 1986, p. 18).
7. This section is adapted from Shaffer and Robbins (1991).
8. Barker (1985) and Marlatt and Fromme (1987) provide and analyze a selection of metaphorical reframes for use during psychotherapy in general and the addictions in particular.

REFERENCES

Abbott, M. W. (2001). *Problem and non-problem gamblers in New Zealand: A report on phase two of the 1999 National Prevalence Survey* (Report number six of the New Zealand Gaming Survey). Wellington: New Zealand Department of Internal Affairs.

Alm, R. (2001, August 7). "Harm reduction" best for some gamblers. Kansas City Star, p. D5.

American Psychiatric Association. (1980). *Diagnostic and statistical manual of mental disorders* (3rd ed.). Washington, DC: Author.

American Psychiatric Association. (1994). *Diagnostic and statistical manual of mental disorders* (4th ed.). Washington, DC: Author.

American Psychiatric Association. (2000). *Diagnostic and statistical manual of mental disorders* (4th ed., text rev.). Washington, DC: Author.

Annis, H. M. (1982). *Inventory of Drinking Situations.* Toronto: Addiction Research Foundation.

Annis, H. M. (1985). *Inventory of Drug-Taking Situations.* Toronto: Addiction Research Foundation.

Annis, H. (1986). A relapse prevention model for treatment of alcoholics. In W. R. Miller & N. Heather (Eds.), *Treating addictive behaviors: Processes of change* (pp. 407–433). New York: Plenum.

Annis, H. M., & Davis, C. S. (1989). Relapse prevention. In R. K. Hester & W. R. Miller (Eds.), *Handbook of alcoholism treatment approaches: Effective alternatives* (pp. 170–182). New York: Pergamon.

Bandura, A. (1969). *Principles of behavior modification.* New York: Holt, Rinehart & Winston.

Barker, J. C., & Miller, M. (1968). Aversion therapy for compulsive gambling. *Journal of Nervous and Mental Illness, 146,* 285–302.

Barker, P. (1985). *Using metaphors in psychotherapy.* New York: Brunner/Mazel.

Becona, E. (1996). Prevalence surveys of problem and pathological gambling in Europe: The cases of Germany, Holland and Spain. *Journal of Gambling Studies, 12*(2), 179–192.

Bergh, C., Sodersten, E. P., & Nordin, C. (1997). Altered dopamine function in pathological gambling. *Psychological Medicine, 27,* 473–475.

Bergler, E. (1957). *The psychology of gambling.* New York: Hill & Wang.

Bettencourt, B. A., & Miller, N. (1996). Gender differences in aggression as a function of provocation: A meta-analysis. *Psychological Bulletin, 119*(3), 422–447.

Black, D. W. (2004). An open-label trial of bupropion in the treatment of pathologic gambling. *Journal of Clinical Psychopharmacology, 24*(1), 108–110.

Blanco, C., Ibanez, A., Saiz-Ruiz, J., Blanco-Jerez, C., & Nunes, E. V. (2000). Epidemiology, pathophysiology and treatment of pathological gambling. *CNS Drugs, 13*(6), 397–407.

Blanco, C., Orensanz-Munoz, L., Blanco-Jerez, C., & Saiz-Ruiz, J. (1996). Pathological gambling and platelet MAO activity: A psychobiological study. *American Journal of Psychiatry, 153*(1), 119–121.

Blanco, C., Petkova, E., Ibanez, A., & Saiz-Ruiz, J. (2002). A pilot placebo-controlled study of fluvoxamine for pathological gambling. *Annals of Clinical Psychiatry, 14*(1), 9–15.

Blaszczynski, A. (1998). *Overcoming compulsive gambling: A self-help guide using cognitive behavioral techniques.* London: Robinson.

Blaszczynski, A., & Farrell, E. (1998). A case series of 44 completed gambling-related suicides. *Journal of Gambling Studies, 14*(2), 93–109.

Blaszczynski, A., McConaghy, N., & Frankova, A. (1991). Control versus abstinence in the treatment of pathological gambling: A two to nine year follow-up. *British Journal of Addiction, 86,* 299–306.

Blaszczynski, A., & Silove, D. (1995). Cognitive and behavioral therapies for pathological gambling. *Journal of Gambling Studies, 11*(2), 195–220.

Blaszczynski, A., & Steel, Z. (1998). Personality disorders among pathological gamblers. *Journal of Gambling Studies, 14*(1), 51–71.

Blum, K., Braverman, E. R., Holder, M. M., Lubar, J. F., Monastra, V. J., Miller, D., et al. (2000). Reward deficiency syndrome: A biogenetic model for the diagnosis and treatment of impulsive, addictive, and compulsive behaviors. *Journal of Psychoactive Drugs, 32*(Suppl.), 1–112.

Bondolfi, G., Osiek, C., & Ferrero, F. (2002). Pathological gambling: An increasing and underestimated disorder. *Schweizer Archiv für Neurologie und Psychiatrie, 153*(3), 116–122.

Breiter, H. C., Aharon, I., Kahneman, D., Dale, A., & Shizgal, P. (2001). Functional imaging of neural responses to expectancy and experience of monetary gains and losses. *Neuron, 30,* 619–639.

Brosky, G. (2001). Update on methods for patient behavior change. *Canadian Journal of CME,* 135–145.

Brown, J. M., & Miller, W. R. (1993). Impact of motivational interviewing on participation and outcome in residential alcoholism treatment. *Psychology of Addictive Behaviors, 7*(4), 211–218.

Brown, R. I. F. (1985). The effectiveness of Gamblers Anonymous. In W. R. Eadington (Ed.), *The gambling studies: Proceedings of the Sixth National Conference on Gambling and Risk Taking* (Vol. 5, pp. 258–284). Reno: University of Nevada.

Brownell, K. D., Marlatt, G. A., Lichtenstein, E., & Wilson, G. T. (1986). Understanding and preventing relapse. *American Psychologist, 41*(7), 765–782.

Centers for Disease Control. (2001). *Compressed mortality database.* Retrieved March 9, 2001, from wonder.cdc.gov.

Chambless, D. L., & Ollendick, T. H. (2001). Empirically supported psychological interventions: Controversies and evidence. *Annual Review of Psychology, 52*(1), 685–716.

Chew, K. S. Y., McCleary, R., Merrill, V., & Napolitano, C. (2000). Visitor suicide risk in casino resort areas. *Population Research and Policy Review, 19,* 551–570.

Collins, P., & Barr, G. (2001). *Gambling and problem gambling in South Africa: A national study.* National Center for the Study of Gambling. Capetown, South Africa: University of Capetown.

Comings, D. E. (1998). The molecular genetics of pathological gambling. *CNS Spectrums, 3*(6), 20–37.

Comings, D. E., Gonzalez, N., Wu, S., Gade, R., Muhleman, D., Saucier, G., et al. (1999). Studies of the 48 bp repeat polymorphism of the DRD4 gene in impulsive, compulsive, addictive behaviors: Tourette syndrome, ADHD, pathological gambling, and substance abuse. *American Journal of Medical Genetics Neuropsychiatric Genetics, 88*(4), 358–368.

Cone, J. D. (2001). *Evaluating outcomes: Empirical tools for effective practice.* Washington, DC: American Psychological Association.

Crockford, D. N., & el-Guebaly, N. (1998). Psychiatric comorbidity in pathological gambling: A critical review. *Canadian Journal of Psychiatry—Revue Canadienne de Psychiatrie, 43*(1), 43–50.

Crowley, J. W. (Ed.). (1999). *The drunkard's progress: Narratives of addiction, despair, and recovery.* Baltimore, MD: John Hopkins University Press.

Cuadrado, M. (1999). A comparison of Hispanic and Anglo calls to a gambling help hotline. *Journal of Gambling Studies, 15*(1), 71–81.

Cunningham, J. A., Sobell, L. C., Sobell, M. B., & Kapur, G. (1995). Resolution from alcohol problems with and without treatment: Reasons for change. *Journal of Substance Abuse, 7*(3), 365–372.

Cunningham-Williams, R. M., Cottler, L. B., Compton, W. M., & Spitznagel, E. L. (1998). Taking chances: Problem gamblers and mental health disorders. Results from the St. Louis epidemiologic catchment area study. *American Journal of Public Health, 88,* 1093–1096.

Cunningham-Williams, R. M., Cottler, L. B., Compton, W. M., Spitznagel, E. L., & Ben-Abdallah, A. (2000). Problem gambling and comorbid psychiatric and substance use disorders among drug users recruited from drug treatment and community settings. *Journal of Gambling Studies, 16*(4), 347–376.

DeCaria, C. M., Begaz, T., & Hollander, E. (1998). Serotonergic and noradrenergic function in pathological gambling. *CNS Spectrums, 3*(6), 38–47.

Dickerson, M., Hinchy, J., & Legg-England, S. (1990). Minimal treatments and problem gamblers: A preliminary investigation. *Journal of Gambling Studies, 6*(1), 87–102.

Dollard, J., & Miller, N. E. (1950). *Personality and psychotherapy: An analysis in terms of learning, thinking, and culture.* New York: McGraw Hill.

Dunne, J. A. (1985). Increasing public awareness of pathological gambling: A history of the National Council on Compulsive Gambling. *Journal of Gambling Behavior, 1*(1), 8–16.

Echeburua, E., Fernandez-Montalvo, J., & Baez, C. (2000). Relapse prevention in the treatment of slot-machine pathological gambling: Long-term outcome. *Behavior Therapy, 31,* 351–364.

Echeburua, E., Fernandez-Montalvo, J., & Baez, C. (2001). Predictors of therapeutic failure in slot-machine pathological gamblers following behavioural treatment. *Behavioural and Cognitive Psychotherapy, 29,* 379–383.

Elia, C., & Jacobs, D. F. (1993). The incidence of pathological gambling among Native Americans treated for alcohol dependence. *International Journal of the Addictions, 28*(7), 659–666.

Ellis, A. (1987). The impossibility of achieving consistently good mental health. *American Psychologist, 42,* 364–375.

Ellis, A., & Grieger, R. (1977). *Handbook of rational-emotive therapy.* New York: Springer.

Ellis, A., & Whiteley, J. M. (1979). *Theoretical and empirical foundations of rational-emotive therapy.* Monterey, CA: Brooks/Cole.

Federman, E. J., Drebing, C. E., & Krebs, C. (2000). *Don't leave it to chance.* Oakland, CA: New Harbinger.

Feigelman, W., Wallisch, L. S., & Lesieur, H. R. (1998). Problem gamblers, problem substance users, and dual problem individuals: An epidemiological study. *American Journal of Public Health, 88*(3), 467–470.

Ferland, F., Ladouceur, R., & Vitaro, F. (2002). Prevention of problem gambling: Modifying misconceptions and increasing knowledge. *Journal of Gambling Studies, 18*(1), 19–29.

Fisher, S. (2000). Measuring the prevalence of sector-specific problem gambling: A study of casino patrons. *Journal of Gambling Studies, 16*(1), 25–51.

Fleming, M. F. (1993). Screening and brief intervention for alcohol disorders. *Journal of Family Practice, 37*(3), 231–234.

Frank, J. D. (1961). *Persuasion and healing.* Baltimore, MD: Johns Hopkins University Press.

Gaboury, A., & Ladouceur, R. (1993). Evaluation of a prevention program for pathological gambling among adolescents. *Journal of Primary Prevention, 14*(1), 21–28.

Galdston, I. (1951). The psychodynamics of the triad, alcoholism, gambling, and superstition. *Mental Hygiene, 35,* 589–598.

Gamblers Anonymous. (2002). *12 step program.* Retrieved January 26, 2002, from www.gamblersanonymous.org/recovery/html.

Getty, H. A., Watson, J., & Frisch, G. R. (2000). A comparison of depression and styles of coping in male and female GA members and controls. *Journal of Gambling Studies, 16*(4), 377–391.

Giuliani, D., & Schnoll, S. H. (1985). Clinical decision making in chemical dependence treatment: A programmatic model. *Journal of Substance Abuse Treatment, 2*(4), 203–208.

Gotestam, K. G., & Johansson, A. (2003). Characteristics of gambling and problematic gambling in the Norwegian context: A DSM-IV-based telephone interview study. *Addictive Behaviors, 28,* 189–197.

Govoni, R., Rupcich, N., & Frisch, G. (1996). Gambling behavior of adolescent gamblers. *Journal of Gambling Studies, 12*(3), 305–317.

Grant, J. E., & Kim, S. W. (2001). Pharmacotherapy of pathological gambling disorder. *Psychiatric Annals, 32,* 161–170.

Grant, J. E., & Kim, S. W. (2002). Gender differences in pathological gamblers seeking medication treatment. *Comprehensive Psychiatry, 43*(1), 56–62.

Grant, J. E., Kim, S. W., & Potenza, M. N. (2003). Advances in the pharmacological treatment of pathological gambling. *Journal of Gambling Studies, 19*(1), 85–109.

Grant, J. E., Kim, S. W., Potenza, M. N., Blanco, C., Ibanez, A., Stevens, L., et al. (2003). Paroxetine treatment of pathological gambling: A multi-centre randomized controlled trial. *International Clinical Psychopharmacology, 18*(4), 243–249.

Griffiths, M., Bellringer, P., Farrell-Roberts, K., & Freestone, F. (2001). Treating problem gamblers: A residential therapy approach. *Journal of Gambling Studies, 17*(2), 161–169.

Gupta, R., & Derevensky, J. L. (Eds.). (2000). Youth gambling [Special Issue]. *Journal of Gambling Studies, 16*(2–3).

Gustafson, J. P. (1995). *The dilemmas of brief psychotherapy.* New York: Plenum.

Hajek, P., West, R., Foulds, J., Nilsson, F., Burrows, S., & Meadow, A. (1999). Randomized comparative trial of nicotine polacrilex, a transdermal patch, nasal spray, and an inhaler. *Archives of Internal Medicine, 159*(17), 2033–2038.

Haller, R., & Hinterhuber, H. (1994). Treatment of pathological gambling with carbamazepine. *Pharmacopsychiatry, 27,* 129.

Havens, L. (1989). *A safe place: Laying the groundwork of psychotherapy.* Cambridge, MA: Harvard University Press.

Henry, S. L. (1996). Pathological gambling: Etiologic considerations and treatment efficacy of eye movement desensitization/reprocessing. *Journal of Gambling Studies, 12*(4), 395–405.

Hodgins, D. C., Currie, S. R., & el-Guebaly, N. (2001). Motivational enhancement and self-help treatments for problem gambling. *Journal of Consulting and Clinical Psychology, 69*(1), 50–57.

Hodgins, D. C., & el-Guebaly, N. (2004). Retrospective and prospective reports of precipitants to relapse in pathological gambling. *Journal of Consulting and Clinical Psychololgy, 72*(1), 72–80.

Hodgins, D. C., Wynne, H., & Makarchuk, K. (1999). Pathways to recovery from gambling problems: Follow-up from a general population survey. *Journal of Gambling Studies, 15*(2), 93–104.

Hoffman, N. G., Halikas, J. A., & Mee-Lee, D. (1987). *The Cleveland admission, discharge, and transfer criteria: Model for chemical dependency treatment programs.* Cleveland: Northern Ohio Chemical Dependency Treatment Directors Association.

Hoffman, N. G., Halikas, J. A., Mee-Lee, D., & Weedman, R. D. (1991). *ASAM patient placement criteria for the treatment of psychoactive substance use disorders.* Washington, DC: American Society of Addiction Medicine.

Holden, C. (2001). Behavioral addictions: Do they exist? *Science, 294*, 980–982.

Hollander, E. (1998). Treatment of obsessive–compulsive spectrum disorders with SSRIs. *British Journal of Psychiatry, 173*(Suppl. 35), 7–12.

Hollander, E., Buchalter, A. J., & DeCaria, C. M. (2000). Pathological gambling. *Psychiatric Clinics of North America, 23*(3), 629–642.

Hubble, M. L., Duncan, B. L., & Miller, S. D. (1999). *The heart and soul of change: What works in therapy.* Washington, DC: American Psychological Association.

Hunt, W. A., Barnett, L. W., & Branch, L. G. (1971). Relapse rates in addiction programs. *Journal of Clinical Psychology, 27*(4), 455–456.

Ibanez, A., Blanco, C., Donahue, E., Lesieur, H. R., Perez de Castro, I., Fernandez-Piqueras, J., et al. (2001). Psychiatric comorbidity in pathological gamblers seeking treatment. *American Journal of Psychiatry, 158*(10), 1733–1735.

Imhof, J. E., Hirsch, R., & Terenzi, R. E. (1984). Countertransferential and attitudinal considerations in the treatment of drug abuse and addiction. *Journal of Substance Abuse Treatment, 1*(1), 21–30.

Jacobs, D. F. (1989). A general theory of addictions: Rationale for and evidence supporting a new approach for understanding and treating addictive behaviors. In H. J. Shaffer, S. Stein, B. Gambino, & T. N. Cummings (Eds.), *Compulsive gambling: Theory, research and practice* (pp. 35–64). Lexington, MA: Lexington Books.

Jason, J. R., Taff, M. L., & Boglioli, L. R. (1990). Casino-related deaths in Atlantic City, New Jersey: 1982–1986. *American Journal of Forensic Medicine and Pathology, 11*(2), 112–123.

Johnson, E. E., Nora, R. M., & Bustos, N. (1992). The Rotter I-E Scale as a predictor of relapse in a population of compulsive gamblers. *Psychological Reports, 70*, 691–696.

Kadden, R. M. (2001). Behavioral and cognitive-behavioral treatments for alcoholism: Research opportunities. *Addictive Behaviors, 26*(4), 489–507.

Kausch, O. (2003). Suicide attempts among veterans seeking treatment for pathological gambling. *Journal of Clinical Psychiatry, 64*(9), 1031–1038.

Keller, M. B., McCullough, J. P., Klein, D. N., Arnow, B., Dunner, D. L., Gelenberg, A. J., et al. (2000). A comparison of nefazodone, the cognitive behavioral-analysis system of psychotherapy, and their combination for the treatment of chronic depression. *New England Journal of Medicine, 342*(20), 1462–1470.

Kendall, P. C., & Hollon, D. S. (Eds.). (1979). *Cognitive behavioral interventions: Theory, research, and procedures.* New York: Academic Press.

Khantzian, E. J. (1985). The self-medication hypothesis of addictive disorders: Focus on heroin and cocaine dependence. *American Journal of Psychiatry, 142*(11), 1259–1264.

Khantzian, E. J., Halliday, K. S., & McAuliffe, W. E. (1990). *Addiction and the vulnerable self: Modified dynamic group therapy for substance abusers.* New York: Guilford Press.

Kiesler, S., & Sproull, L. (1985). Pool halls, chips, and war games: Women in the culture of computing. *Psychology of Women Quarterly, 9*(4), 451–462.

Kim, S. W., & Grant, J. E. (2001). An open naltrexone treatment study in pathological gambling disorder. *International Clinical Psychopharmacology, 16*(5), 285–289.

Kim, S. W., Grant, J. E., Adson, D. E., & Shin, Y. C. (2001). Double-blind naltrexone and placebo comparison study in the treatment of pathological gambling. *Biological Psychiatry, 49,* 914–921.

Kim, S. W., Grant, J. E., Adson, D. E., Shin, Y. C., & Zaninelli, R. (2002). A double-blind placebo-controlled study of the efficacy and safety of paroxetine in the treatment of pathological gambling. *Journal of Clinical Psychiatry, 63*(6), 501–507.

Kimberly, J. R., & Minvielle, E. (2000). Introduction: The quality imperative—Origins and challenges. In J. R. Kimberly & E. Minvielle (Eds.), *The quality imperative* (pp. 1–12). London: Imperial College Press.

Kinkead, G. (1992). *Chinatown: Portrait of a closed society.* New York: HarperCollins.

Kleinman, A. (1988). *The illness narratives: Suffering, healing and the human condition.* New York: Basic Books.

Korn, D. A., & Shaffer, H. J. (1999). Gambling and the health of the public: Adopting a public health perspective. *Journal of Gambling Studies, 15*(4), 289–365.

Kuentzel, J. G., Henderson, M. J., Zambo, J. J., Stine, S. M., & Schuster, C. R. (2003). Motivational interviewing and fluoxetine for pathological gambling disorder: A single case study. *North American Journal of Psychology, 5*(2), 229–248.

LaBrie, R. A., Shaffer, H. J., LaPlante, D. A., & Wechsler, H. (2003). Correlates of college student gambling in the United States. *Journal of American College Health, 52*(2), 53–62.

Ladouceur, R., Boisvert, J. M., & Dumont, J. (1994). Cognitive-behavioral treatment for adolescent pathological gamblers. *Behavior Modification, 18*(2), 230–242.

Ladouceur, R., Bouchard, C., Rheaume, N., Jacques, C., Ferland, F., Leblond, J., et al. (2000). Is the SOGS an accurate measure of pathological gambling among children, adolescents and adults? *Journal of Gambling Studies, 16*(1), 1–24.

Ladouceur, R., Paquet, C., & Dube, D. (1996). Erroneous perceptions in generating sequences of random events. *Journal of Applied Social Psychology, 26*(24), 2157–2166.

Ladouceur, R., Sylvain, C., Boutin, C., & Doucet, C. (2002). *Understanding and treating the pathological gambler.* West Sussex, England: Wiley.

Ladouceur, R., Sylvain, C., Boutin, C., Lachance, S., Doucet, C., & Leblond, J.

(2003). Group therapy for pathological gamblers: A cognitive approach. *Behaviour Research and Therapy, 41*(5), 587–596.

Ladouceur, R., Sylvain, C., Boutin, C., Lachance, S., Doucet, C., Leblond, J., et al. (2001). Cognitive treatment of pathological gambling. *Journal of Nervous and Mental Disorders, 189*(11), 774–780.

Ladouceur, R., Sylvain, C., Letarte, H., Giroux, I., & Jacques, C. (1998). Cognitive treatment of pathological gamblers. *Behaviour Research and Therapy, 36*(12), 1111–1119.

Ladouceur, R., Vezina, L., Jacques, C., & Ferland, F. (2000). Does a brochure about pathological gambling provide new information? *Journal of Gambling Studies, 16*(1), 103–107.

Ladouceur, R., & Walker, M. (1998). The cognitive approach to understanding and treating pathological gambling. In A. S. Bellack & M. Hersen (Eds.), *Comprehensive clinical psychology* (pp. 588–601). New York: Pergamon.

Lakshmanan, I. A. R. (1996, March 9). A woman's life lost to gambling: Suicide highlights betting's dark side. *Boston Globe*, pp. 13, 20.

Langenbucher, J., Bavly, L., Labouvie, E., Sanjuan, P. M., & Martin, C. S. (2001). Clinical features of pathological gambling in an addictions treatment cohort. *Psychology of Addictive Behaviors, 15*(1), 77–79.

Lapage, C., Ladouceur, R., & Jacques, C. (2000). Prevalence of problem gambling among community service users. *Community Mental Health Journal, 36*(6), 597–601.

Leblond, J., Ladouceur, R., & Blaszczynski, A. (2003). Which pathological gamblers will complete treatment? *British Journal of Clinical Psychology, 42*(Pt 2), 205–209.

Lejoyeux, M., Ades, J., Tassain, V., & Solomon, J. (1996). Phenomenology and psychopathology of uncontrolled buying. *American Journal of Psychiatry, 153*(12), 1524–1529.

Lesieur, H. R., & Blume, S. B. (1990). Characteristics of pathological gamblers identified among patients on a psychiatric admissions service. *Hospital and Community Psychiatry, 41*, 1009–1012.

Levin, J. D. (1987). *Treatment of alcoholism and other addictions*. Northvale, NJ: Aronson.

Lindner, R. M. (1950). The psychodynamics of gambling. *Annals of the American Academy of Political and Social Science, 269*, 93–107.

Littman-Sharp, N., Turner, N., Stirpe, T., & Liu, E. (1999, April). *The Inventory of Gambling Situations: A newly revised instrument for the identification of problem gamblers' high risk situations*. Paper presented at the Canadian Foundation on Compulsive Gambling Annual Conference, Ottawa.

Lopes, L. L. (1987). Between hope and fear: The psychology of risk. In L. Berkowitz (Ed.), *Advances in experimental social psychology* (Vol. 20, pp. 255–295). San Diego: Academic Press.

Mahoney, M. J. (1974). *Cognition and behavior modification*. Cambridge, MA: Ballinger.

Maltsberger, J. T., & Buie, D. (1974). Countertransference hate in the treatment of suicidal patients. *Archives of General Psychiatry, 30*, 625–633.

Margulies, A. (1989). *The empathic imagination*. New York: Norton.

Marlatt, G. A., Baer, J. S., Donovan, D. M., & Kivlahan, D. R. (1988). Addictive behaviors: Etiology and treatment. *Annual Review of Psychology, 39,* 223–252.

Marlatt, G. A., & Fromme, K. (1987). Metaphors for addiction. *Journal of Drug Issues, 17,* 9–28.

Marlatt, G. A., & Gordon, J. (Eds.). (1985). *Relapse prevention* (1st ed.). New York: Guilford Press.

McAulliffe, W. E., & Ch'ien, J. M. N. (1986). Recovery training and self help: A relapse-prevention program for treated opiate addicts. *Journal of Substance Abuse Treatment, 3,* 9–20.

McCleary, R., Chew, K., Feng, W., Merrill, V., Napolitano, C., Males, M., et al. (1998). *Suicide and gambling: An analysis of suicide rates in U.S. counties and metropolitan areas.* Irvine: University of California Irvine, School of Social Ecology.

McCormick, R. A., Russo, A. M., Ramirez, L. F., & Taber, J. I. (1984). Affective disorders among pathological gamblers seeking treatment. *American Journal of Psychiatry, 141,* 215–218.

McCormick, R. A., & Taber, J. I. (1991). Follow-up of male pathological gamblers after treatment: The relationship of intellectual variables to relapse. *Journal of Gambling Studies, 7*(2), 99–108.

McKay, J. R., McLellan, A. T., & Alterman, A. I. (1992). An evaluation of the Cleveland criteria for inpatient treatment of substance abuse. *American Journal of Psychiatry, 149,* 1212–1218.

McNeilly, D. P., & Burke, W. J. (2000). Late life gambling: The attitudes and behaviors of older adults. *Journal of Gambling Studies, 16*(4), 393–415.

Meichenbaum, D. (1977). *Cognitive-behavior modification: An integrative approach.* New York: Plenum.

Milkman, H. B., & Shaffer, H. J. (Eds.). (1985). *The addictions: Multidisciplinary perspectives and treatments.* Lexington, MA: Lexington Books.

Miller, W. R. (1996). Motivational interviewing: Research, practice, and puzzles. *Addictive Behaviors, 21*(6), 835–842.

Miller, W. R. (2000). Rediscovering fire: Small interventions, large effects. *Psychology of Addictive Behaviors, 14*(1), 6–18.

Miller, W. R., Brown, J. M., Simpson, T. L., Handmaker, N. S., Bein, T. H., Luckie, L. F., et al. (1995). What works? A methodological analysis of the alcohol treatment outcome literature. In R. K. Hester & W. R. Miller (Eds.), *Handbook of alcoholism treatment approaches: Effective alternatives* (2nd ed., pp. 12–44). Boston: Allyn & Bacon.

Miller, W. R., & Rollnick, S. (Eds.). (1991). *Motivational interviewing: Preparing people to change addictive behavior.* New York: Guilford Press.

Milton, S., Crino, R., Hunt, C., & Prosser, E. (2002). The effect of compliance-improving interventions on the cognitive-behavioural treatment of pathological gambling. *Journal of Gambling Studies, 18*(2), 207–229.

Moreno, I., Saiz-Ruiz, J. Y., & Lopez-Ibor, J. J. (1991). Serotonin and gambling dependence. *Human Psychopharmacology, 6,* 6–9.

Moskowitz, J. (1980). Lithium and lady luck: Use of lithium carbonate in compulsive gambling. *New York State Journal of Medicine, 89,* 785–788.

National Association of Addiction Treatment Providers. (1987). *Adult and adoles-*

cent alcohol and drug dependence admission, continued stay, and discharge criteria. Lancaster, PA: Author.

National Consensus Development Panel on Effective Medical Treatment of Opiate Addiction. (1998). Effective medical treatment of opiate addiction. *Journal of the American Medical Association, 280,* 1936–1943.

National Endowment for Financial Education, & National Council on Problem Gambling. (2000). *Personal financial strategies for the loved ones of problem gamblers.* National Endowment for Financial Education. Greenwood Village, CO.

National Research Council. (1999). *Pathological gambling: A critical review.* Washington, DC: National Academy Press.

National Steering Committee. (1999). *First Nations and Inuit Regional Health Survey.* St. Regis, Quebec: First Nations and Inuit Regional Health Survey.

Office of Public Health. (1999). *Trends in Indian health.* Rockville, MD: Indian Health Services.

O'Malley, S. S., Jaffe, A. J., Chang, G., Schottenfeld, R. S., Meyer, R. E., & Rounsaville, B. J. (1992). Naltrexone and coping skills therapy for alcohol dependence: A controlled study. *Archives of General Psychiatry, 49*(11), 881–887.

Orford, J. (1985). *Excessive appetites: A psychological view of addictions.* New York: Wiley.

Orford, J. (2001). *Excessive appetites: A psychological view of addictions* (2nd ed.). New York: Wiley.

Pallanti, S., Quercioli, L., Sood, E., & Hollander, E. (2002). Lithium and valproate treatment of pathological gambling: A randomized single-blind study. *Journal of Clinical Psychiatry, 63*(7), 559–564.

Pallanti, S., Rossi, B. N., Sood, E., & Hollander, E. (2002). Nefazodone treatment of pathological gambling: A prospective open-label controlled trial. *Journal of Clinical Psychiatry, 63*(11), 1034–1039.

Perry, S., Cooper, A. M., & Michels, R. (1987). The psychodynamic formulation: Its purpose, structure, and clinical application. *American Journal of Psychiatry, 144,* 543–550.

Pfifferling, J. H. (1980). A cultural prescription for medicocentrism. In L. Eisenberg & A. Kleinman (Eds.), *The relevance of social science for medicine* (pp. 197–222). Boston: Reidel.

Phillips, D. P., Welty, W. R., & Smith, M. M. (1997). Elevated suicide levels associated with legalized gambling. *Suicide and Life-Threatening Behavior, 27*(4), 373–378.

Polanyi, M. (1967). *The tacit dimension.* New York: Doubleday.

Poulin, C. (2000). Problem gambling among adolescent students in the Atlantic provinces of Canada. *Journal of Gambling Studies, 16*(1), 53–78.

Prochaska, J. O., DiClemente, C. C., & Norcross, J. C. (1992). In search of how people change: Applications to addictive behaviors. *American Psychologist, 47,* 1102–1114.

Prochaska, J. O., Norcross, J. C., & DiClemente, C. C. (1994). *Changing for good: A revolutionary six-stage program for overcoming bad habits and moving your life positively forward.* New York: Avon.

Productivity Commission. (1999). *Australia's Gambling Industries: Final Report* (No. 10). Canberra: AusInfo.

Quinn, J. P. (1891). *Fools of fortune*. Chicago: Anti-Gambling Association.

Rilke, R. M. (1992). *Letters to a young poet* (J. M. Burnham, Trans.). San Rafael, CA: New World Library.

Rollnick, S., & Morgan, M. (1995). Motivational interviewing: Increasing readiness for change. In A. M. Washton (Ed.), *Psychotherapy and substance abuse: A practitioner's handbook* (pp. 179–191). New York: Guilford Press.

Rosecrance, J. (1988). *Gambling without guilt: The legitimation of an American pastime*. Pacific Grove: Books/Cole.

Rosenthal, R. J. (1997). The psychodynamics of pathological gambling: A review of the literature. In D. L. Yalisove (Ed.), *Essential papers on addiction* (pp. 184–212). New York: New York University Press.

Rosenthal, R. J., & Rugle, L. J. (1994). A psychodynamic approach to the treatment of pathological gambling: I. Achieving abstinence. *Journal of Gambling Studies, 10*(1), 21–42.

Rugle, L., & Melamed, L. (1993). Neuropsychological assessment of attention problems in pathological gamblers. *Journal of Nervous and Mental Disorders, 18*(2), 107–112.

Schachter, S. (1982). Recidivism and self-cure of smoking and obesity. *American Psychologist, 37*, 436–444.

Schon, D. A. (1983). *The reflective practitioner*. New York: Basic Books.

Seager, C. P. (1970). Treatment of compulsive gamblers by electrical aversion. *British Journal of Psychiatry, 117*, 545–553.

Sebastian, J. G. (1985). Homelessness: A state of vulnerability. *Family and Community Health, 8*(3), 11–24.

Shaffer, H. J. (1986). Assessment of addictive disorders: The use of clinical reflection and hypotheses testing. *Psychiatric Clinics of North America, 9*(3), 385–398.

Shaffer, H. J. (1992). The psychology of stage change: The transition from addiction to recovery. In J. H. Lowinson, P. Ruiz, R. B. Millman, & J. G. Langrod (Eds.), *Substance abuse: A comprehensive textbook* (2nd ed., pp. 100–105). Baltimore, MD: Williams & Wilkins.

Shaffer, H. J. (1994). Denial, ambivalence and countertransference hate. In J. D. Levin & R. Weiss (Eds.), *Alcoholism: Dynamics and treatment* (pp. 421–437). Northdale, NJ: Jason Aronson.

Shaffer, H. J. (1997). The psychology of stage change. In J. H. Lowinson, P. Ruiz, R. B. Millman, & J. G. Langrod (Eds.), *Substance abuse: A comprehensive textbook* (3rd ed., pp. 100–106). Baltimore, MD: Williams & Wilkins.

Shaffer, H. J., & Costikyan, N. (2002). *Treatment for substance use disorders: Exploring the relationship between treatment training and treatment outcomes*. Boston: Robert Wood Johnson Foundation & Join Together.

Shaffer, H. J., Forman, D. P., Scanlan, K. M., & Smith, F. (2000). Awareness of gambling-related problems, policies and educational programs among high school and college administrators. *Journal of Gambling Studies, 16*(1), 93–101.

Shaffer, H. J., & Freed, C. R. (2005). The assessment of gambling related disorders. In D. M. Donovan & G. A. Marlatt (Eds.), *Assessment of addictive behaviors* (2nd ed.). New York: Guilford Press.

Shaffer, H. J., Freed, C. R., & Healea, D. (2002). Gambling disorders among homeless persons with substance use disorders seeking treatment at a community center. *Psychiatric Services, 55*(9), 1112–1117.

Shaffer, H. J., & Gambino, B. (1990). Epilogue: Integrating treatment choices. In H. B. Milkman & L. I. Sederer (Eds.), *Treatment choices for alcoholism and substance abuse* (pp. 351–375). Lexington, MA: Lexington Books.

Shaffer, H. J., & Hall, M. N. (2001b). Updating and refining prevalence estimates of disordered gambling behaviour in the United States and Canada. *Canadian Journal of Public Health*, 92(3), 168–172.

Shaffer, H. J., & Hall, M. N. (2002). The natural history of gambling and drinking problems among casino employees. *Journal of Social Psychology*, 142(4), 405–424.

Shaffer, H. J., Hall, M. N., & Vander Bilt, J. (1995). *Training needs among New England substance abuse treatment providers* (No. ATCNE Technical Report No. 040395–NA100). Boston: Harvard Medical School, Division on Addictions, and Brown University, Addiction Training Center of New England.

Shaffer, H. J., Hall, M. N., & Vander Bilt, J. (1997). *Estimating the prevalence of disordered gambling behavior in the United States and Canada: A meta-analysis.* Boston: Presidents and Fellows of Harvard College.

Shaffer, H. J., Hall, M. N., & Vander Bilt, J. (1999). Estimating the prevalence of disordered gambling behavior in the United States and Canada: A research synthesis. *American Journal of Public Health*, 89, 1369–1376.

Shaffer, H. J., Hall, M. N., Vander Bilt, J., & George, E. (Eds.). (2003). *Youth, gambling and society: Futures at stake.* Reno: University of Nevada Press.

Shaffer, H. J., & Jones, S. B. (1989). *Quitting cocaine: The struggle against impulse.* Lexington, MA.: Lexington Books.

Shaffer, H. J., & Korn, D. A. (2002). Gambling and related mental disorders: A public health analysis. In *Annual Review of Public Health*, 23, 171–212.

Shaffer, H. J., & Robbins, M. (1991). Manufacturing multiple meanings of addiction: Time-limited realities. *Contemporary Family Therapy*, 13, 387–404.

Shaffer, H. J., & Robbins, M. (1995). Psychotherapy for addictive behavior: A stage-change approach to meaning making. In A. M. Washton (Ed.), *Psychotherapy and substance abuse: A practitioner's handbook* (pp. 103–123). New York: Guilford Press.

Shaffer, H. J., & Simoneau, G. (2001). Reducing resistance and denial by exercising ambivalence during the treatment of addiction. *Journal of Substance Abuse Treatment*, 20(1), 99–105.

Shaffer, H. J., Vander Bilt, J., & Hall, M. N. (1999). Gambling, drinking, smoking and other health risk activities among casino employees. *American Journal of Industrial Medicine*, 36(3), 365–378.

Siever, L. J. (1987). Role of noradrenergic mechanisms in the etiology of the affective disorders. In H. Y. Meltzer (Ed.), *Psychopharmacology: Third generation of progress* (pp. 493–504). New York: Raven.

Skinner, B. F. (1969). *Contingencies of reinforcement: A theoretical analysis.* Englewood Cliffs, NJ: Prentice-Hall

Slutske, W. S., Jackson, K. M., & Sher, K. J. (2003). The natural history of problem gambling from age 18 to 29. *Journal of Abnormal Psychology*, 112(2), 263–274.

Sobell, L. C., Cunningham, J. A., & Sobell, M. B. (1996). Recovery from alcohol problems with and without treatment: Prevalence in two population surveys. *American Journal of Public Health*, 86(7), 966–972.

Sobell, L. C., Cunningham, J. A., Sobell, M. B., Agrawal, S., Gavin, D. R., Leo, G. I., et al. (1996). Fostering self-change among problem drinkers: A proactive community intervention. *Addictive Behaviors, 21*(6), 817–833.

Sobell, L. C., Ellingstad, T. P., & Sobell, M. B. (2000). Natural recovery from alcohol and drug problems: Methodological review of the research with suggestions for future directions. *Addiction, 95*(5), 749–764.

Specker, S. M., Carlson, G. A., Christenson, G. A., & Marcotte, M. (1995). Impulse control disorders and attention deficit disorder in pathological gamblers. *Annals of Clinical Psychiatry, 7*(4), 175–179.

Sproston, K., Erens, B., & Orford, J. (2000). *Gambling behaviour in Britain: Results from the British gambling prevalence survey.* London: National Centre for Social Research.

Stein, D. M., & Lambert, M. J. (1995). Graduate training in psychotherapy: Are therapy outcomes enhanced? *Journal of Consulting and Clinical Psychology, 63*(2), 182–196.

Stewart, R. M., & Brown, R. I. F. (1988). An outcome study of Gamblers Anonymous. *British Journal of Psychiatry, 152,* 284–288.

Stinchfield, R., Nadav, C., Winter, K., & Latimer, W. (1997). Prevalence of gambling among Minnesota public school students in 1992 and 1995. *Journal of Gambling Studies, 13*(1), 25–48.

Svanum, S., & Mcadoo, W. G. (1989). Predicting rapid relapse following treatment for chemical dependence: A matched-subjects design. *Journal of Consulting and Clinical Psychology, 57,* 222–226.

Sylvain, C., Ladouceur, R., & Boisvert, J. M. (1997). Cognitive and behavioral treatment of pathological gambling: A controlled study. *Journal of Consulting and Clinical Psychology, 65*(5), 727–732.

Taber, J. I., McCormick, R. A., Russo, A. M., Adkins, B. J., & Ramirez, I. F. (1987). Follow-up of pathological gamblers after treatment. *American Journal of Psychiatry, 144,* 757–761.

Tavares, H., Zilberman, M. L., & el-Guebaly, N. (2003). Are there cognitive and behavioural approaches specific to the treatment of pathological gambling? *Canadian Journal of Psychiatry, 48*(1), 22–27.

Teck-Hong, O. (1992). The behavioral characteristics and health conditions of drug abusers: Some implications for workers in drug addiction. *International Social Work, 35*(1), 7–17.

Toneatto, T., & Ladouceur, R. (2003). Treatment of pathological gambling: A critical review of the literature. *Psychology of Addictive Behaviors, 17*(4), 284–292.

Tucker, J. A., Donovan, D. M., & Marlatt, G. A. (Eds.). (1999). *Changing addictive behavior.* New York: Guilford Press.

U.S. General Accounting Office. (2000). *Impact of gambling: Economic effects more measurable than social effects* (Report to the Honorable Frank R. Wolf No. GGD-00-78). Washington, DC: Author.

Vagge, L. M. (1996). *The development of youth gambling* (Unpublished honors thesis). Cambridge: Harvard-Radcliffe Colleges.

Vaillant, G. E. (1988). What can long-term follow-up teach us about relapse and prevention of relapse in addiction? *British Journal of Addiction, 83,* 1147–1157.

Volberg, R. A., & Abbott, M. W. (1997). Gambling and problem gambling among indigenous peoples. *Substance Use and Misuse, 32*(11), 1525–1538.

Volberg, R. A., Abbott, M. W., Roennberg, S., & Munck, I. M. (2001). Prevalence and risks of pathological gambling in Sweden. *Acta Psychiatrica Scandinavica, 104*(4), 250–256.

Wachtel, P. L. (1977). *Psychoanalysis and behavior therapy: Toward an integration.* New York: Basic Books.

Wagner, J. (1986). *The search for signs of intelligent life in the universe.* New York: Harper & Row.

Waldorf, D. (1983). Natural recovery from opiate addiction: Some social-psychological processes of untreated recovery. *Journal of Drug Issues, 13,* 237–280.

Waldorf, D., & Biernacki, P. (1979). Natural recovery from heroin addiction: A review of the incidence literature. *Journal of Drug Issues, 9*(2), 282–289.

Waldorf, D., & Biernacki, P. (1981). The natural recovery from opiate addiction: some preliminary findings. *Journal of Drug Issues, 11*(1), 61–74.

Waldorf, D., Reinarman, C., & Murphy, S. (1991). *Cocaine changes: The experience of using and quitting.* Philadelphia: Temple University Press.

Walitzer, K. S., Dermen, K. H., & Connors, G. J. (1999). Strategies for preparing clients for treatment. A review. *Behavior Modification, 23*(1), 129–151.

Wallisch, L. S. (1993). *Gambling in Texas: 1993 Texas survey of adolescent gambling behavior.* Austin: Texas Commission on Alcohol and Drug Abuse.

Wallisch, L. S. (1996). *Gambling in Texas: 1995 Texas survey of adult and adolescent gambling behavior.* Austin: Texas Commission on Alcohol and Drug Abuse.

Wardman, D., el-Guebaly, N., & Hodgins, D. (2001). Problem and pathological gambling in North American Aboriginal populations: A review of the empirical literature. *Journal of Gambling Studies, 17*(2), 81–100.

Washton, A. M. (1989). *Cocaine addiction: Treatment, recovery, and relapse prevention.* New York: Norton.

Watzlawick, P. (1976). *How real is real?* New York: Random House.

Watzlawick, P. (1990). *Munchhausen's pigtail, or psychotherapy and "reality": Essays and lectures.* New York: Norton.

Weiner, I. B. (1975). *Principles of psychotherapy.* New York: Wiley.

Welte, J., Barnes, G., Wieczorek, W., Tidwell, M.-C., & Parker, J. (2001). Alcohol and gambling pathology among U.S. adults: Prevalence, demographic patterns and comorbidity. *Journal of Studies on Alcohol, 62,* 706–712.

Wenzlaff, R. M., & Wegner, D. M. (2000). Thought suppression. In S. T. Fiske, D. L. Schacter & C. Zahn-Waxler (Eds.), *Annual Review of Psychology, 51,* 59–91.

Winick, C. (1962). Maturing out of narcotic addiction. *United Nations Bulletin on Narcotics, 14,* 1–7.

Winters, K. C., & Kushner, M. G. (2003). Treatment issues pertaining to pathological gamblers with a comorbid disorder. *Journal of Gambling Studies, 19*(3), 261–277.

Winters, K. C., Stinchfield, R. D., & Kim, L. G. (1995). Monitoring adolescent gambling in Minnesota. *Journal of Gambling Studies, 11*(2), 165–183.

Wise, R. A. (1995). Addictive drugs and brain stimulation reward. In *Annual Review of Neuroscience, 18,* 319–340.

Wong, I. L. K., & So, E. M. T. (2003). Prevalence estimates of problem and pathological gambling in Hong Kong. *American Journal of Psychiatry, 160*(7), 1353–1354.

Yutrzenka, B. A. (1995). Making a case for training in ethnic and cultural diversity in

increasing treatment efficacy. *Journal of Consulting and Clinical Psychology,*
63(2), 197–206.

Zane, N. W. S., & Huh-Kim, J. (1998). Addictive behaviors. In L. C. Lee & N. W. S.
Zane (Eds.), *Handbook of Asian American psychology* (pp. 527–554). South
Oaks, CA: Sage.

Zimmerman, M., Breen, R. B., & Posternak, M. A. (2002). An open-label study of
citalopram in the treatment of pathological gambling. *Journal of Clinical Psy-*
chiatry, 63(1), 44–48.

CHAPTER 11

Enhancing the Relapse Prevention Model for Sex Offenders

Adding Recidivism Risk Reduction Therapy to Target Offenders' Dynamic Risk Needs

Jennifer G. Wheeler
William H. George
Susan A. Stoner

Longitudinal follow-up studies indicate that without treatment approximately 10–42% of known sex offenders will commit another sexual offense (Alexander, 1999; Marques, Day, Nelson, & West, 1994; Marshall & Barbaree, 1988; Nicholaichuk, Gordon, Gu, & Wong, 2000). These rates vary, depending on factors such as an offender's conviction history, the nature of his sexual offense, and the length of time that he is followed after release (Hanson & Bussiere, 1998). However, offenders who receive treatment appear to reoffend at significantly lower rates, between 7 and 13% (Alexander, 1999; Hanson et al., 2002; Marques et al., 1994; Marshall, Jones, Ward, Johnston, & Barbaree, 1991; Nicholaichuk et al., 2000). Research has also demonstrated that cognitive-behavioral approaches appear to be the most effective treatments for incarcerated sexual offenders (Alexander, 1999; Antonowicz & Ross, 1994; Hanson et al., 2002; Marshall et al., 1991), with sex offense recidivism rates reported between 3 and 13% (Hanson et al., 2002; Marques et al., 1994; Marshall & Barbaree, 1988; Pithers & Cumming, 1989), compared to the 17–36% recidivism rates associated with other treatment approaches (e.g., psychosurgery; pharmacology, nonbehavioral therapy; see Marshall et al., 1991, for review). Although further treatment outcome studies are needed to obtain a more accurate picture of the relationship between sex offender treatment and recidivism, cognitive-behavioral treatment has earned recognition as the treatment of choice for sexual offenders (Laws, Hudson, & Ward, 2000; Marshall et al., 1991).

Relapse prevention (RP) is currently the most popular cognitive-behavioral approach to treating sex offenders (Laws et al., 2000). This transfer of theory and techniques from the addictions field provides a fresh way to conceptualize sex offender treatment, posttreatment recovery, and postincarceration adjustment. Despite its popularity, RP sex offender treatment has also been subject to considerable scrutiny and debate (e.g., Hanson, 2000; Laws, 1996, 1999a, 1999b, 2003; Thornton, 1997), including theory- and evidence-based criticisms (e.g., Hanson, 2000; Laws, 1995a; Thornton, 1997; Ward & Hudson, 1996a; see Laws, 2003, for review), and revisions or reformulations (Hudson, Ward, & Marshall, 1992; Ward & Hudson, 1996b, 1998, 2000; Ward, Louden, Hudson, & Marshall, 1995; see Laws, 2003 for review).

The overarching goal of this chapter and Chapter 12 in *Assessment of Addictive Behaviors, Second Edition* (Wheeler, 2005) is to review the application of RP to the treatment of sexual offenders and some of its inherent limitations. We then describe an approach to enhance the RP model for sex offender treatment that will "update" it with some recent and important developments in the field. One key development is the emergence of "risk assessment" as a dominant conceptual framework for managing sex offenders in correctional, treatment, and community settings. Another important development has been the migration of other cognitive-behavioral techniques into sex offender treatment. For instance, the skills training "modules" of dialectical behavior therapy (Linehan, 1993b) have received attention for their potential application to sexual offending (e.g., Hover, 1999; Hover & Packard, 1998, 1999; Quigley, 2000; Shingler, 2004). In the context of these two developments, we propose an approach called recidivism risk reduction therapy (3RT), which integrates the problem/need-targeting advantages of the risk assessment paradigm with the skills training/treatment-module advantages of RP and other cognitive-behavioral strategies. We believe that this integration of risk assessment with strategically applied treatment modules offers an updated approach and an enhanced model of RP for sexual offenders.

Elsewhere (Wheeler, 2003; Wheeler, George, & Marlatt, in press; Wheeler et al., 2005), we provide an overview of the application of RP terminology to sexual offending, including a discussion of some of the challenges to effectively assessing the "relapse cycle" in sexual offenders. We describe actuarial risk assessment and some of the recently identified "dynamic risk factors" for sexual offense recidivism. Finally, we provide suggestions and recommendations for how to approach the assessment of these factors in the context of sex offender treatment.

In this chapter, we review approaches to RP-based sex offender treatment, describe how the 3RT model conceptualizes dynamic risk factors as treatment needs, and suggest techniques and interventions to specifically target those needs. We conclude with a brief discussion about the controversial concept of applying a "harm reduction" perspective to the treatment of sexual offenders.

THE APPLICATION OF RELAPSE PREVENTION TO SEXUAL OFFENDING

Although RP was adapted from the addictions field, the rationale for its application to sex offenders is based on the shared problem of maintaining successful abstinence following treatment. It is this struggle to maintain the success of treatment, that is, to remain successfully abstinent from the problem behavior, that makes RP relevant to the treatment of sexual offenders. As with addiction, the desired outcome of sexual offender treatment goes beyond the point of stopping the problematic behavior in the present, by teaching skills and techniques for preventing the problem behavior from recurring in the future.

Interrupting the "Relapse Cycle" in Sexual Offenders

For any given offender, the offending behavior is understood to follow a prototypical progression; this is referred to as his relapse "cycle." When an offender's characteristic pattern of thoughts and behaviors has been identified and understood in terms of the relapse cycle, then interventions are developed to interrupt this pattern and prevent the offender progression from a "lapse" to a "relapse" (see Chapter 11 in Donovan & Marlatt, 2005, for a discussion of RP terminology as it is applied to sexual offenders).

The Identification of Points for Intervention in the Sexual Offense Cycle: A Hypothetical Example

> Joe Offender had a fight with his girlfriend, Lucy. Lucy stormed out of the house, and Joe continued thinking about their fight (e.g., "Who is she to treat me like that?" and "I deserve a break from all of her sh**"). He soon left the house to seek out his friends at the local tavern, where he spent several hours drinking and exchanging negative stories about their wives and girlfriends. After returning home from the tavern, Joe learned that Lucy wasn't due home for a few hours, leaving him home alone with her 12-year-old daughter, Tina. Intoxicated, he went to Tina's room to see if she needed help with her home-

work. He found Tina lying on her bed wearing a t-shirt and under-
wear, and Joe found himself sexually aroused. He entered Tina's
room, sat next to her on the bed, and said he needed to talk with her
about something important. He proceeded to tell her about the fight
he had earlier with Lucy, including details about Joe and Lucy's sexual
relationship. Joe told Tina how sad and lonely he felt, and suggested
that a hug would make him feel better. During the hug, Joe told Tina
how much he cared about her, what a pretty girl she was, and how
good it felt to hug her. He then touched her genitals.

In this example, several RP constructs and potential points for intervention are easily identified. First, Joe would be taught to identify the various events of his cycle and label these in context of RP terminology (see
Chapter 12 in Donovan & Marlatt, 2005, for a description of how these
events are defined using RP terminology). Next, Joe would learn to identify
various points in his relapse cycle where his choice facilitated the progression and escalation of his offense cycle (e.g., ruminating about his conflict
with Lucy; seeking out friends at a local tavern when he was in a state of
distress; facilitating a negative conversation about Lucy and women in general; facilitating an interaction with Tina when he was alone in the house
with her; entering Tina's room when he was sexually aroused; engaging
Tina in an intimate, adult conversation). Joe would then learn alternative
responses to these maladaptive thoughts and behaviors (e.g., using more
effective coping methods after he has a conflict with Lucy; implementing
preplanned interventions when he is alone in the house with Tina; self-
monitoring his sexual arousal and more effectively regulating his thoughts
and decisions when he is sexually aroused). In this way, the RP model
draws upon the offender's past experiences and his historical patterns of
thoughts, feelings, and behaviors in order to help him identify this pattern
and interrupt it in the future.

Equally important but "unobservable" points for intervention in this
cycle would include Joe's cognitive and affective responses to a lapse (defined for a sexual offender as "offense precursor activities," such as indulg-
ing deviant fantasies or cruising for potential victims; see Laws, 2003).
One such cognitive/emotional event in the relapse cycle is the "abstinence
violation effect" (AVE), which is presumed to occur when the individual
recognizes that he or she has broken a self-imposed rule; that is, by engaging in a single act of prohibited behavior, his or her commitment to abstinence has been violated.[1] According to the RP model, an individual's
response to this violation can determine whether the lapse turns into a full-
blown relapse (Marlatt & George, 1984; Marlatt & Gordon, 1980, 1985),
and therefore plays a critical role in the relapse cycle.

In the preceding example, depending on which event is defined as the
"lapse" (see discussion in the following section), Joe's response may have

been to feel ashamed and hopeless about his inability to regulate his thoughts and actions and to attribute these responses to factors that are internal (e.g., he has a "natural" sexual attraction to Tina) and uncontrollable (e.g., his sexual attraction to young girls is never going to change). According to the RP model, such a response will increase the likelihood that a lapse will progress to a relapse. Therefore, an important point for intervention would be to help Joe identify the point at which he experienced the AVE and learn more adaptive responses to the "lapse" that might interrupt this progression.

Another important but unobservable cognitive/affective event in the relapse cycle is the problem of immediate gratification (PIG). The PIG refers to the process of attending only to the positive aspects of a prohibited behavior, while ignoring the negative consequences. The PIG can occur before or after a lapse; therefore it can increase the risk of a high-risk situation leading to a lapse, in addition to increasing the risk of a lapse becoming a full-blown relapse (see Marlatt, 1989).

In the preceding example, Joe's progression from hugging to fondling Tina might be conceptualized as a function of the PIG, since it is likely that Joe was focused only on the positive aspects of sexual contact with Tina and ignoring the negative aspects of this behavior. Therefore, an important point for intervention would be to help Joe identify when he is experiencing the PIG, and to challenge his positive expectancies with considerations for the negative outcomes of his behavior (e.g., harming his victim, getting caught and sent to prison). It would also be important to help Joe identify and more effectively regulate his sexual thoughts, interests, and arousal, and to learn more adaptive/less harmful responses to them.

Limitations of Relapse Prevention Treatment for Sexual Offenders

Elsewhere (Wheeler et al., 2005), we described some of the limitations of using RP terminology to identify and define the events of the sexual offense "cycle." One such limitation is the necessary but perhaps confusing semantic redesignation of the terms "lapse" and relapse," and the questions that this redesignation raises about the role of the AVE in facilitating the progression of a lapse to a relapse. In the example, it is not clear which event in the offense cycle Joe would experience as a "lapse" (e.g., entering Tina's room? Sitting with her on the bed? Talking about sex and intimacy with her? Asking for a hug? Hugging her?) To develop an effective intervention for Joe, it is imperative to accurately identify the point at which he feels he has "violated" his commitment to abstaining from harmful behavior. Joe may need some treatment specifically to help him understand how his behavior is harmful to Tina, so that he learns to understand certain behaviors as "lapses." Alternatively, Joe's therapist may need to conduct an ideographic assessment to learn from which behaviors Joe has committed to abstain. Without consideration for Joe's commitment to abstinence from particular behaviors, efforts to impose a prototypical RP treatment paradigm on this individual might be met with notable resistance, resulting in a loss of credibility for the therapist if not the therapy itself.

Another concern about RP for sex offenders is whether the PIG is being adequately emphasized in RP's current format, given the apparent conflict between the PIG that is inherent to sexual fantasizing/arousal, and the negative affective response that is putatively associated with the AVE (see Hudson et al., 1992; Ward & Hudson, 1996a; Ward, Hudson, & Siegert, 1995). There is some evidence to suggest that for sexual offenders, the progression from lapse to relapse may be more influenced by the PIG than by other factors (e.g., the AVE; see Wheeler, 2003), suggesting that the PIG may need to assume a more prominent role in sex offender RP treatment programs.

Summary

In the last two decades, RP has become the most popular and perhaps most effective approach to the treatment of sexual offenders (e.g., Hanson et al., 2002; Knopp, Freeman-Longo, & Stevenson, 1992; Laws et al., 2000; Marques et al., 1994). The sex offender RP application has also undergone important criticism and associated reformulations (Laws, 2003; Ward & Hudson, 1996a, 1996b; Ward et al., 1995) to address some of the limitations of applying RP to the sex offender population.

In addition to these specific concerns, a broader critique of RP for sex offenders is that it is not being implemented as an *adjunct* to successful treatment (as it was originally implemented with addictive disorders), but has become the primary treatment itself. Although incarceration may force some individuals to abstain from sexual offending, incarceration is not equivalent to committed abstinence, nor does it preclude an offender from engaging in other offense-related behaviors (e.g., masturbating to offense fantasies). If an offender has not yet discontinued certain prohibited behaviors, it may be premature to teach him techniques for preventing a "relapse" of those behaviors. For this reason, RP has been criticized as a necessary but insufficient approach to the treatment of sexual offenders.

RECENT DEVELOPMENTS IN SEX OFFENSE RESEARCH: RISK ASSESSMENT

RP originally developed and applied to sexual offenders without the benefit of our current knowledge about risk factors for sexual offense recidivism. Risk assessment is a fast-growing area in the criminal justice system and forensic mental health settings. In the second edition of *Assessment of*

Addictive Behaviors (Donovan & Marlatt, 2005), we summarize issues associated with actuarial risk assessment and discuss differences between static and dynamic risk factors. Although research on dynamic factors is ongoing, preliminary findings have identified several promising dynamic risk factors for recidivism. In the current chapter, we focus specifically on dynamic risk factors for sexual offense recidivism, and how the application of extant treatment approaches might be used to target these factors in the treatment setting.

A variable is identified as a dynamic risk factor if any change in this variable is associated with an increase or decrease in recidivism risk. Therefore, dynamic risk factors are increasingly being regarded as signifying *treatment needs*, high-priority targets for treatment interventions. With regard to sexual offenders, dynamic risk factors for sexual offense recidivism appear to be associated with one of two broad categories: deviant sexual interests and an antisocial orientation (Hanson & Bussiere, 1998; Hanson & Harris, 2000, 2001; Hanson & Morton-Bourgon, 2004; Hudson, Wales, Bakker, & Ward, 2002; Quinsey, Lalumiere, Rice, & Harris, 1995; Roberts, Doren, & Thornton, 2002). For example, a recent meta-analysis found that certain measures of sexual deviancy (e.g., sexual interests and preferences, sexual preoccupations) and/or an antisocial orientation (e.g., antisocial personality disorder, general self-regulation problems, substance abuse, rule violations) significantly predicted sexual offense recidivism (Hanson & Harris, 2000; Hanson & Morton-Bourgon, 2004). Other significant dynamic risk factors in this analysis included intimacy deficits (e.g., emotional identification with children, conflicts in an intimate relationship) and attitudes tolerant of sexual offending (Hanson & Harris, 2000; Hanson & Morton-Bourgon, 2004). These preliminary findings provide a basic framework for integrating dynamic risk factors into extant approaches to sex offender treatment.

INCORPORATING RISK ASSESSMENT INTO SEX OFFENDER TREATMENT: RECIDIVISM RISK REDUCTION THERAPY

As described previously, an important criticism of RP for sex offenders is that it has evolved from being considered as an *adjunct* to cessation treatment (as it was originally proposed with addictions) to becoming the primary treatment itself. Although RP may be useful for identifying problematic thoughts and behaviors and possible points of intervention, it was not intended to be the primary approach to change those aspects of an offender's lifestyle that result in his sexual offense cycle (i.e., his maladaptive coping skills, self-regulation deficits, problematic thinking styles, and/or ineffective interpersonal skills). An obvious response to this criticism is to implement a primary cessation-oriented approach to sex offender treatment to target these long-term treatment needs, in conjunction with RP treatment to target the sexual offense cycle itself.

Based on the preceding review of trends in risk assessment, a new primary treatment approach for sexual offenders should incorporate risk-based treatment principles (Andrews, 1989) to target sex offenders' dynamic risk factors for recidivism (e.g., Hanson & Harris, 2000; Hanson & Morton-Bourgon, 2004). Specifically, RP could be enhanced by integrating dynamic risk factors into the treatment paradigm and generally approaching sex offender treatment from a more risk-based perspective (Andrews, 1989).[2] Therefore, we propose an enhanced treatment model that is grounded in the RP approach, but incorporates an emphasis on directly identifying offenders' dynamic risk factors and targeting these in treatment.

With these considerations in mind, we propose that sex offender treatment providers and programs (henceforth referred to as SOTPs) adopt a new risk-based, primary approach to the assessment and treatment of sexual offenders that we will refer to as *recidivism risk reduction therapy* (3RT). 3RT can include a variety of group-format approaches, and draw upon extant techniques to target stable dynamic risk factors in conjunction with their RP treatment. In their RP groups, offenders will have the opportunity to practice new 3RT skills, while specifically addressing the more acute risk areas that are associated with their sexual offense cycle. Consistent with risk-based treatment principles (Andrews, 1989) and with recommendations that treatment plans should be based on ideographic rather than prototypical techniques (e.g., Heilbrun, Nezu, Keeney, Chung, & Waserman, 1998), 3RT treatment plans are developed based on an assessment of each individual offender's risk-based treatment needs (see Wheeler et al., 2005), for suggested techniques to assess dynamic risk factors in the context of treatment).

An important question to address is how 3RT and RP might coexist with one another. One way of considering how the 3RT approach would be integrated with extant RP treatment approaches is to consider "stable" versus "acute" risk factors for recidivism (Hanson & Harris, 2001). The goal of 3RT is to reduce maladaptive thoughts and behaviors that are associated with risk to sexually reoffend and to replace these with more adaptive skills and behaviors. Thus, 3RT might be conceptualized as a treatment for "stable" dynamic risk factors, with a goal of facilitating longer-term changes in offenders' behavior. RP techniques give primary consideration to the offender's thoughts and behaviors in the days, hours, or even minutes preceding a sexual offense. Thus, RP might be conceptualized as a treatment approach to managing offender's "acute" dynamic risk factors.

The following section provides suggestions for designing 3RT groups to target sex offenders' risk needs. This is not meant to be an exhaustive nor an exclusive list of dynamic risk factors or possible treatment approaches; rather, it is provided to illustrate how extant treatment approaches might be applied to our current knowledge of sex offenders' dynamic risk factors for recidivism. As our knowledge of risk factors and treatment efficacy develops, 3RT protocols can be enhanced and modified accordingly.

Targeting Dynamic Risk Factors as "Treatment Needs": A Skills Training Approach

An initial consideration for developing a treatment model to address sexual offenders' dynamic risk needs was how to conceptualize "dynamic risk factors" as "treatment needs" such that appropriate interventions could be developed to specifically target those needs. Toward that end, we reviewed the risk need areas that had been identified empirically (e.g., Hanson & Harris, 1998, 2000; Hanson & Morton-Bourgon, 2004) and approached these from a basic behavioral perspective. Specifically, we conducted a "functional analysis" of each risk need area (What is the problem behavior? In what context does it usually occur? How is it maintained/reinforced?) and considered what alternative responses would result in a less harmful/ more effective outcome (following the basic behavioral principle that it is ineffective to try to change a maladaptive behavior without learning an alternative response).

This process (i.e., identifying a problem behavior, stopping it, and replacing it with a more effective response) is best characterized as "skills training," and as such we have conceptualized dynamic risk needs as "skills deficits." By conceptualizing risk needs as skill deficits, the 3RT model lends itself to numerous extant approaches to target problem behaviors. Specifically, there are many available cognitive-behavioral skills training techniques that were developed for managing behaviors that are similar to, if not the same as, many of the risk need areas that have been identified for sexual offenders.

One promising set of skills training techniques are those provided in the *Skills Training Manual for Treating Borderline Personality Disorder* (Linehan, 1993b). Dialectical behavior therapy (DBT) has demonstrated empirical success in reducing the maladaptive behaviors of individuals with borderline personality disorder (Linehan, Armstrong, Suarez, Allmon, & Heard, 1991), and has since been implemented for use with other client populations (e.g., Hoffman, Fruzzetti, & Swenson, 1999; Linehan et al., 1999; Miller, Wyman, Huppert, Glassman, & Rathus, 2001; Safer, Telch, & Argas, 2001; Telch, Argas, & Linehan, 2000; Wolpow, Porter, & Hermanos, 2000). More recently, the applicability of DBT skills to the treatment of sexual offenders has been considered (e.g., Hover, 1999; Hover & Packard, 1998, 1999; Quigley, 2000; Shingler, 2004).

DBT skills training addresses four important areas, each of which has potential relevance for targeting the risk needs of sexual offenders:

1. The "mindfulness" module addresses maladaptive thought processes and teaches skills for improved self-monitoring and regulation.
2. The "emotion regulation" module addresses mood lability and affective dysregulation and teaches skills for effectively identifying and managing emotions.
3. The "distress tolerance" module addresses maladaptive coping behaviors and teaches skills for managing impulsive/harmful behaviors in the face of inevitable life stressors.
4. The "interpersonal effectiveness" module addresses interactions with others and teaches skills for more effectively getting needs/goals met without violating the rights/needs of others.

Given the apparent compatibility between these skills training modules and sexual offenders' risk needs (described in the following section), the 3RT model draws heavily on DBT techniques to target offenders' dynamic risk needs. Although the efficacy of DBT skills training has not yet been empirically validated for its application to forensic populations, it was developed to target many of the skills deficits that have also been empirically associated with sex offenders' recidivism risk. Because of its consistency with risk-based treatment principles, DBT skills training modules are provided in this chapter as specific examples of extant approaches that could be implemented in the context of the 3RT model.

In addition to the apparent utility of the DBT skills training modules for sex offender treatment, there are other compelling reasons for considering the application of DBT techniques to this population (see Quigley, 2000, and Shingler, 2004, for a review of the theoretical and practical compatibilities between DBT and sexual offender treatment needs). Among these reasons is the fact that DBT techniques are comprised of many of the "greatest hits" of cognitive-behavioral techniques; therefore, the theories and approaches that are described in the manual are likely to be familiar to therapists who have a background in cognitive-behavioral treatment (i.e., SOTPs using RP). In addition, the manual itself is "user friendly" and includes handouts and homework assignments that can be photocopied for repeated use (permission is explicitly given by the author for this purpose). Furthermore, the techniques themselves are not necessarily "population-specific," but can be applied to problem behaviors in any client population. If needed, the techniques can be easily modified to meet the treatment needs of a particular client population (e.g., adolescents; Wheeler & Schafer, 2000).

In addition to these practical reasons for considering DBT skills training techniques for sexual offenders, DBT is a cognitive-behavioral approach that was developed for the specific purpose of treating a population of clients whose problematic and often harmful behaviors were long-standing, pervasive, and highly resistant to change. Furthermore, the specific demands these clients placed on their therapists appeared to be associated with therapist "burnout" and high turnover rates among treatment providers (see Linehan, 1993a, for a description of the development of DBT). Accordingly, the DBT approach includes specific suggestions and techniques for managing the process of conducting therapy with "difficult-to-treat" clients, in addition to providing numerous and useful suggestions for targeting these clients' problem behaviors. DBT specifically considers important aspects of the therapist–client relationship that might enhance or impede treatment progress, and includes techniques for keeping clients and therapists committed to and involved in the treatment process. Given the empirically demonstrated relationship between treatment dropout and sexual offense recidivism (e.g., Hanson & Harris, 1998; Hanson & Morton-Bourgon, 2004), this aspect of DBT appears to have particular utility in the context of sex offender treatment.

In the following sections, we outline the general risk domains that have been identified as significant predictors of sexual offense recidivism (Hanson & Harris, 1998, 2000; Hanson & Morton-Bourgon, 2004). For each domain, we identify its features (the "risk needs") and conceptualize these as "skill deficits." We then provide examples of extant techniques that might be used to specifically target those maladaptive thoughts and behaviors and replace them with more effective, adaptive responses.

Antisocial Risk Needs

This problem area reflects a generally unstable life that facilitates and indulges the use of the deception, manipulation, and secrecy; fosters resentment of others and a sense of entitlement and self-indulgence; supports noncompliance with rules and authority; and provides opportunities and reinforcement for behavioral disinhibition. Although not unique to sex offenders, some or all of these factors may be necessary preconditions to the perpetration of a sexual offense. Conversely, the development of a stable lifestyle that supports individual responsibility and accountability, prosocial attitudes and relationships, and compliance with rules and structure could serve to curtail such antisocial behaviors, attitudes, and relationships.

For the purposes of this chapter, the dynamic risk factors that are associated with the development and maintenance of an imbalanced, non-"mainstream," defiant, or otherwise antisocial lifestyle, will collectively be referred to as the sex offender's *antisocial risk needs*. Offenders who endorse risk needs in this area (see Wheeler et al., 2005, for specific approaches to evaluating offenders' dynamic risk needs) would be assigned to a 3RT–Antisocial Risk Needs group (or 3RT-A) to target those problem areas. The goal of 3RT-A is to help offenders identify their antisocial risk needs; monitor and self-regulate their antisocial thoughts, behaviors, and relationships; and develop alternative approaches to functioning more effectively in a prosocial environment.

According to Hanson and Morton-Bourgon's recent meta-analysis (2004), the following "antisocial" dynamic factors were associated with increased risk for sexual reoffending: "antisocial personality," "antisocial traits," and/or a "history of rule violations." According to the *Diagnostic and Statistical Manual of Mental Disorders* (4th edition) (DSM-IV) criteria for antisocial personality disorder[3] (American Psychiatric Association, 1994), antisocial personality features include the following (items marked with an asterisk indicate specific antisocial traits that were significantly associated with recidivism; Hanson & Morton-Bourgon, 2004):

- Failure to conform to social norms with respect to lawful behaviors, as indicated by repeatedly engaging in behaviors that are grounds for arrest.
- Deceitfulness, as indicated by repeated lying, use of aliases, conning others for personal gain.
- Impulsivity or failure to plan ahead.*
- Irritability or aggressiveness, as indicated by repeated fights or assaults.*
- Reckless disregard for the safety of self or others.
- Consistent irresponsibility, as indicated by failure to sustain consistent work or to financial obligations.*
- Lack of remorse, as indicated by being indifferent to or rationalizing having hurt, mistreated, or violated the rights of another.

In addition to these general antisocial personality features, other significant dynamic risk factors identified as part of an "antisocial orientation" (Hanson & Morton-Bourgon, 2004) include the following:

- Substance abuse (including any substance abuse and being intoxicated at the time of the offense).
- History of rule violations (including noncompliance with supervision and violations of conditional release).

The authors described many of these factors as "general self-regulation problems" (i.e., impulsivity, hostility, employment instability, substance abuse), which is consistent with the 3RT conceptualization of these risk needs as skill deficits. Problems with self-regulation can result from skill deficits in many areas, such as misinterpreting environmental cues (e.g., mislabeling another person's behavior as hostile or threatening), being unable to recognize internal processes and to label accurately emotions (e.g., misidentifying fear as anger), responding to distress with ineffective or even harmful behavior (e.g., getting in a fight; substance abuse), and/or failing to consider the effect of his own behavior on the rights/needs of others (e.g., impulsive/reckless acting out; criminal activity). If an offender endorses any risk factors in this area, he will need to develop skills to (1) increase self-monitoring and accurately observe cues in his environment, (2) improve his emotional regulation, (3) replace his maladaptive coping responses with effective coping strategies; and (4) learn effective ways to get his needs met without violating the rights and needs of others, and generally increase prosocial relationships and activities. Accordingly, 3RT-A groups would target an offenders antisocial risk needs using several skills training approaches, depending on the needs of a particular offender or of the group as a whole.[4]

1. To improve their general self-monitoring skills, 3RT-A group members would first learn skills for observing and describing their own internal processes (e.g., thoughts and beliefs, sensory perceptions, physical sensations) and for objectively perceiving stimuli in their external environment (e.g., observing and describing without interpretation or judgment). These skills should target the antisocial thought patterns (e.g., attitudes, beliefs, distortions) that generally contribute to offenders' maladaptive self-regulation, and replace these maladaptive cognitions with more effective methods for self-monitoring and regulation.

Skills training approach: The mindfulness module of DBT skills training teaches techniques for learning to observe and describe one's internal and external environment from a nonjudgmental stance, monitoring one's own thoughts and thinking errors, practicing radical acceptance, and balancing factors that influence our thoughts and behavior processes (i.e., logic and emotion). Other mindfulness training approaches incorporate general techniques to improve self-awareness, which might include meditation, yoga, exercise, and/or spiritually or culturally focused activities (e.g., Kumar, 1995; Marlatt, 2002).

2. To decrease "antisocial" emotional difficulties (e.g., irritability, hostility) and improve their overall emotion regulation skills, 3RT-A group members would learn skills to identify, label, monitor, and control their feelings and emotional responses. These skills should be addressed by including a psychoeducational component to help group members understand the relationship between physiology and emotions. Group members can learn to monitor their physiological reactions, and to label the physiological responses accordingly. They can also learn to differentiate emotional responses and to label them accurately. Finally, they would learn to develop skills to deescalate their emotions as indicated.

Skills training approach: The emotion regulation (ER) module of DBT skills training teaches individuals to monitor the quality and quantity of their emotional responses, and to identify, label, and regulate a wide array of both positive and negative emotional responses.

3. To decrease maladaptive coping strategies (e.g., substance abuse, violence) and improve distress tolerance and coping skills, 3RT-A groups must first identify group members' maladaptive coping strategies and replace these with more effective coping techniques. Initially, a functional analysis of coping strategies can provide valuable information about how certain problem behaviors (e.g., violence, substance use) are fostered and maintained with positive reinforcement (e.g., getting one's way) and/or negative reinforcement (e.g., avoiding painful emotions).[5] When the function of a maladaptive coping strategy is understood, skills training interventions can then be developed to replace these problem behaviors with more effective coping techniques.

Skills training approach: The distress tolerance (DT) module of DBT skills training includes many specific techniques for replacing maladaptive coping behavior with more effective responses to stress. In addition to developing skills for acute coping responses, DT skills include a broader emphasis on how to reduce the overall distress in one's life by increasing the adaptive behaviors that the individual finds comforting, relaxing, and/or pleasurable.

4. To decrease their antisocial interactions, relationships and activities, and replace these with prosocial interactions, relationships and activities, 3RT-A group members would learn and practice skills to engage in prosocial interactions and to generally function more effectively in a prosocial environment. Initially, a *functional analysis* of group members' antisocial interactions (e.g., use of manipulation or coercion to get goals met), family/peer relationships (e.g., criminal contacts), and activities (e.g., drug use, criminal activity) can provide valuable information about how antisocial attitudes, behavior, and relationships are fostered and maintained with positive reinforcement (e.g., financial or emotional support) and/or negative reinforcement (e.g., avoiding failure or responsibility). It is important to identify not only observable maladaptive behavior (e.g., socializing with a drug-dealing friend), but also any antisocial attitudes, thinking errors, or other cognitive distortions that may be reinforced by antisocial peer influences (e.g., "Why should I get a 'mainstream' job when I make more money selling drugs with my friend?"). When the function of negative peer interactions, relationships, and activities are understood, skills training interventions can then be developed to replace these with more prosocial behaviors, relationships, and activities. These skills are modeled and rehearsed in group (in role plays), and *in vivo* (through homework assignments or group outings).

As part of their 3RT-A treatment, group members should also have increased involvement in prosocial activities (e.g., employment, joining an athletic team, developing a hobby) because these activities will increase contacts with prosocial peer groups. Group members' skills and interests should be assessed in order to identify appropriate prosocial activities that will (a) meet their skill level and (b) provide some intrinsic reward. In addition, token economies can be established so that group members receive incentives and reinforcement for engaging in prosocial activities.

Skills training approach: The interpersonal effectiveness (IE) module of DBT skills training emphasizes specific techniques for teaching prosocial skills. [6] *Specifically, the IE module teaches general and specific techniques for effective communication, problem solving, assertiveness, and conflict resolution, with an emphasis on learning to interact with others in a mutually respectful way. IE skills are designed to help individuals identify their goal(s) in a given interaction and to effectively address these needs while attending to the wants/needs of the other person in the interaction, without violating the rights/needs of others.*

5. Another area that has received attention in risk assessment research is offenders' cooperation with treatment and/or postrelease supervision. Issues such as therapeutic alliance and readiness to change are receiving increased attention in recent literature (see Derrickson, 2000; Sarran, Fernandez, & Marshall, 2003; Tiernay & McCabe, 2002, 2004). Given the potential association between treatment-cooperation and recidivism risk, it seems prudent to address this problem area as part of any approach to sex offender treatment.[7] Similar to other risk factors in the antisocial risk need area, problems cooperating with treatment can be conceptualized as deficits in particular skills (e.g., time management, decision making). However, unlike other risk factors, this risk area may result from an interaction between the offenders' skills deficits and therapist behavior (e.g., failing to provide reinforcement for group attendance and treatment progress).

As soon as problems cooperating with treatment are detected, a functional analysis of the behavior should be conducted. Specifically, SOTPs should consider ways in which these behaviors are reinforced for the offender (e.g., missing group to avoid feelings of guilt and shame) *and* for the therapist (e.g., not having to manage "difficult" offenders during group). Interventions should be considered for the offender to increase his cooperation with treatment, and for the therapist to facilitate this behavior. Finally, ongoing peer-consultation/group supervision would be implemented to help therapists identify and manage factors associated with their therapy-interfering behaviors and to generally enhance treatment effectiveness.

Skills training approach: Linehan (1993b) specifically addresses this problem area, referred to as "therapy-interfering behavior." Specific techniques are used to identify and understand the function of the problem behavior, and interventions for both the client and therapist are implemented.

There is also evidence to indicate that IE skills training may enhance of-
fenders' collaboration with their therapists (Hover & Packard, 1998).

Erotopathic Risk Needs

In addition to sex offenders' antisocial risk needs, risk assessment research
has also identified other dynamic risk factors that have particular salience
for sexual offenders. As described previously, these sex offender-specific
dynamic risk factors include problems in forming adaptive sexual interests
and preferences, regulating their sexual thoughts and behaviors, maintaining attitudes tolerant of sexual offending, and problems with their inti-
mate/love relationships (e.g., Hanson & Morton-Bourgon, 2004). When
examined together, these dynamic risk factors appear to be broadly associated with the confluence of two inter- and intrapersonal behavioral trajectories: (1) the offender's failure to successfully develop and maintain stable,
intimate relationships with appropriate partners, and (2) his development
and maintenance of deviant sexual interests, attitudes, preferences, and behaviors.

For the purposes of 3RT, we have clustered these two trajectories and
labeled them collectively as an offender's *"erotopathic" risk needs*. This
problem area refers to the offender's maladaptive sexual/love "schema"
and its associated behaviors and relationships. Examples of an "erotopathic"
orientation include the development/maintenance of emotionally detached
and/or abusive relationships and avoidance of relationships/interactions
that threaten his detachment; a preference for "relationships" with partners whom he can control (e.g., with minors, or through the use of force),
and avoidance of relationships/partners that challenge his control; and/or
his paired-association between his sexual gratification with real or imag-
ined situations in which he is in ultimate control, and avoidance of situations in which his "sexual ideal" is threatened. Conversely, the development of satisfying and prosocial intimate/sexual relationships could serve
to curtail future acts of sexual offending. Offenders who endorse risk
needs in this area (see Wheeler et al., 2005, for specific approaches to
assessing offenders' dynamic risk factors) would be assigned to a 3RT–
Erotopathic Risk Needs group (or 3RT-E) to target those problem areas.
The goal of 3RT-E is to help offenders' identify their erotopathic risk
needs; monitor and self-regulate their maladaptive sexual thoughts, behaviors, and relationships; and develop alternative, approaches to functioning
more effectively in satisfying, intimate relationships with appropriate partners.

According to Hanson and Morton-Bourgon's (2004) recent meta-
analysis the following "erotopathic" dynamic factors were associated with
increased risk for sexual reoffending: "deviant sexual interests" (including
a sexual interest in children, any paraphiliac interest, and sexual preoccu-

pation), and/or a phallometric assessment indicating "deviant sexual preferences" (including any deviant sexual preference and a sexual preference for children), "intimacy deficits" (including emotional identification with children and conflicts with intimate partners), and "attitudes supportive of sexual crimes."

Risk factors associated with sexual deviancy have been described as "sexual self-regulation problems" (e.g., Hanson & Harris, 2002), which is consistent with the 3RT conceptualization of dynamic risk needs as skills deficits. Problems with sexual self-regulation can result from skill deficits in many areas, such as misinterpreting environmental cues (e.g., mislabeling a child's behavior as "seductive"), being unable to recognize internal processes and accurately label emotions (e.g., misidentifying anger as sexual arousal), responding to distress with ineffective or even harmful behavior (e.g., masturbating to a deviant fantasy), and/or failing to consider the effect of one's own behavior on the rights/needs of others (e.g., committing a sexual offense). If an offender endorses any risk factors in this area, he will need to develop skills to (1) increase his sexual self-monitoring and accurately observe cues in his environment, (2) improve his sexual/emotional regulation, (3) replace his maladaptive sexual coping responses with effective coping strategies, and (4) learn effective ways to get his sexual/intimacy needs met without violating the rights and needs of others. Accordingly, 3RT-E groups would target an offender's antisocial risk needs using several skills training approaches, depending on the needs of a particular offender or of the group as a whole.[8]

Many of the skills that are addressed by 3RT-A groups are applicable to 3RT-E groups; however, 3RT-E groups should have a particular emphasis on developing interpersonal and self-regulation skills for the specific purpose of decreasing sexually deviant attitudes and behavior and developing satisfying, prosocial love relationships. [9]

1. To improve their sexual self-monitoring skills, 3RT-E group members would first learn skills for monitoring their own arousal processes (e.g., sexual thoughts, subjective arousal, sensory perceptions, and physical sensations) and for objectively perceiving stimuli in their environment (e.g., describing sexual stimuli without interpreting or judging it). These skills should target the maladaptive patterns of sexualized thoughts and behaviors (e.g., an assumption that sexual arousal = entitlement to engage in sexual activity; an expectation that sexual activity will eliminate subjective feelings of distress) that contribute to offenders' maladaptive sexual self-regulation (e.g., preoccupation), and replace these maladaptive patterns with more effective methods for sexual self-monitoring and regulation.

Skills training approach: The mindfulness module of DBT skills training teaches techniques for learning to observe and to describe one's internal and external environment from a nonjudgmental stance, monitoring one's own thoughts and thinking errors, practicing radical acceptance, and balancing factors that influence our thoughts and behavior processes (i.e., logic and emotion). Other mindfulness training approaches incorporate general techniques to improve self-awareness, which might include meditation, yoga, exercise, and/or spiritually or culturally focused activities (e.g., Kumar, 1995; Marlatt, 2002). Specifically, mindfulness skills would teach offenders to "observe" sexual thoughts and fantasies, but not to act on them.

2. To improve their sexual/emotion regulation skills, 3RT-E group members would learn skills to identify, label, monitor, and control their sexual feelings and emotional responses. These skills should be addressed by including a psychoeducational component to help group members understand the relationship between physiology and emotions (data from their phallometric assessments might be very useful here). Group members learn to monitor their sexual arousal and other physiological reactions, and label the physiological responses accordingly. For example, 3RT-E would teach offenders skills to effectively identify and manage the emotions that can either facilitate or impede the development of a healthy relationship (e.g., lust, love, jealousy, rejection). They can also learn to differentiate levels of arousal and other emotional responses and to label these accurately. Finally, they would learn to develop skills to deescalate their arousal and/or emotions as indicated.

Skills training approach: The emotion regulation (ER) module of DBT skills training teaches individuals to monitor the quality and quantity of their emotional responses, and to identify, label, and regulate a wide array of both positive and negative emotional responses (specific recommendations for addressing deviant sexual preferences are described in a later paragraph).

3. To reduce their maladaptive use of certain sexual thoughts or behaviors as a coping response, 3RT-E groups must identify group members' pattern of maladaptive sexual coping strategies and replace these with more effective coping techniques. Initially, a functional analysis of coping strategies can provide valuable information about how certain sexual thoughts and behaviors are fostered and maintained with positive reinforcement (e.g., positive outcome expectancies, sexual gratification) and/or negative reinforcement (e.g., avoiding feared stimuli, such as interacting with potential adult partners).[10] When the function of a maladaptive sexual coping strategy is understood, skills training interventions can then be developed to replace these problem behaviors with more effective coping techniques.

Skills training approach: The distress tolerance (DT) module of DBT skills training includes many specific techniques for replacing maladaptive coping behavior with more effective responses to stress. In addition to developing skills for acute coping responses, DT skills include a broader em-

phasis on how to reduce the overall distress in one's life by increasing the adaptive behaviors that the individual finds comforting, relaxing, and/or pleasurable.

4. To decrease their maladaptive romantic/sexual relationships and interactions, 3RT-E group members would learn and practice skills to engage in prosocial intimate interactions and relationships. Initially, a *functional analysis* of group members' maladaptive sexual/romantic interactions and relationships can provide valuable information about how an offender's attitudes (e.g., about women or sex), behaviors (e.g., adversarial/ conflictual, avoidant, or manipulative/controlling), and relationships (e.g., with minors or vulnerable partners) are fostered and maintained with positive reinforcement (e.g., fulfilling intimacy needs; fostering feelings of power and control) and/or negative reinforcement (e.g., avoiding feared stimuli, such as being rejected by an "equal" partner). It is important to identify not only observable maladaptive behavior (e.g., the use of threats or violence to control the partner), but also any maladaptive sexual/romantic attitudes, thinking errors, or other cognitive distortions that may be reinforced by having relationships with vulnerable partners (e.g., "She stays with me, so my behavior can't be that bad"; "she doesn't tell me to stop so she must like what I'm doing"). When the function of maladaptive relationship interactions are understood, skills training interventions can then be developed to replace these with more prosocial behaviors and intimate/ sexual relationships. Ideally, these prosocial skills would directly target those skills necessary for forming and maintaining healthy romantic relationships (e.g., dating, terminating relationships) and facilitating responsible sexual interactions (e.g., intimacy building, acquiring mutual consent). These skills are modeled and rehearsed in group (in role plays), and *in vivo* (through homework assignments or group outings).

Skills training approach: The interpersonal effectiveness (IE) module of DBT skills training emphasizes specific techniques for teaching prosocial skills. [11] *Specifically, the IE module teaches general and specific techniques for effective communication, problem solving, assertiveness, and conflict resolution, with an emphasis on learning to interact with others in a mutually respectful way. IE skills are designed to help individuals identify their goal(s) in a given interaction and to effectively address these needs while attending to the wants/needs of the other person in the interaction, without violating the rights/needs of others.*

Other treatment considerations: Another aspect of 3RT-E to be considered is the use male and female coleaders. Coed group leader dyads can provide a constant source for modeling effective male/female interactions, open communication, and mutual respect (in role plays and in general group dynamics). 3RT-E groups might be further enhanced by the addition of couple therapy (e.g., Christensen & Jacobson, 2000) for offenders and their partners and/or support groups for nonoffending partners.

5. An important consideration for developing 3RT-E groups is the fact that some groups of offenders may have a clear sexual preference that is regarded as "deviant" (defined in the dominant culture as sexual relations that are victimizing and therefore illegal). These include (but are not limited to) sexual preferences for prepubescent children, postpubescent adolescents who are below the age of consent, and adults who resist or do not consent to sexual activity. Offenders who show evidence of possessing deviant sexual preferences (via subjective self-report or objective plethysmographic assessment) represent a particular challenge for SOTPs. Unlike offenders with general erotopathic risk needs, these offenders may be averse to the basic prosocial treatment goal of developing healthy adult sexual relations. For this reason, these offenders may require interventions that explicitly target deviant preferences. Currently, deviant sexual preferences are targeted through the use of behavioral conditioning techniques.

Established approaches: There is a long history of applying behavioral conditioning techniques to treat deviant sexual arousal (e.g., Hallam & Rachman, 1972). Some of these techniques, such as aversion therapy and covert sensitization, were based on aversion learning principles and were developed to reduce deviant sexual arousal. Covert sensitization, which has received the most research attention, involves pairing deviant arousal fantasies with exposure to images of noxious stimuli. There is evidence that when used alone (Hayes, Brownell, & Barlow, 1983) and in conjunction with methods to intensify noxious stimuli (Weinrott, Riggan, & Frothingham, 1997), covert sensitization can be effective in reducing deviant arousal. In contrast, therapies such as verbal satiation (e.g., Laws, 1995b) and masturbatory satiation (e.g., Gray, 1995), which are based on extinction principles, have also been effective at reducing deviant arousal. Occasionally such approaches are coupled with orgasmic reconditioning techniques designed to redirect arousal to nondeviant sources of stimulation (e.g., Enright, 1989). The effectiveness of these techniques in reducing deviant arousal can be assessed physiologically. Additionally, these techniques can be used modularly in conjunction with other cognitive-behavioral interventions.

3RT Treatment Planning and Implementation: A Hypothetical Example

We return to our hypothetical example of Joe to demonstrate how the process of 3RT treatment planning and implementation. Based on a review of Joe's assessment summary (see Chapter 12 in Donovan & Marlatt, 2005), Joe's therapist decided that Joe had significant erotopathic risk needs that would need to be targeted in his sex offender treatment program. Therefore, she assigned Joe to an adjunct 3RT-E group, in addition to his usual RP group. Specifically, she recommended that Joe participate in skills training modules to target his sexual self-monitoring skills (to develop increased awareness of problematic attitudes and beliefs about women, and to more effectively monitor his sexual thoughts and feelings), sexual and emotional regulation skills (to help him more effectively manage his feelings of anger at his partner, and not confuse his negative emotions such as rejection and betrayal with sexual/emotional "needs"), sexual coping skills (to teach him more effective methods for self-soothing when he is in distress), and interpersonal effectiveness skills (to enhance his prosocial interactions and relationships with appropriate intimate partners).

In addition to Joe's erotopathic risk needs, Joe's therapist determined that he had some antisocial risk needs that would benefit from treatment. Specifically, she recommended that he participate in at least a 3RT-A skills training module to target his maladaptive distress tolerance/coping skills (to help him find alternatives to drinking and seeking out negative peer contacts when he is in distress). However, within 3 months of RP treatment it became apparent to Joe's therapist that he had deficits managing his emotions in group, as indicated by his frequent temper tantrums and outbursts directed at other group members. Therefore, she assigned him to additional 3RT-A modules, to help him develop general self-regulation and affective management skills.

Summary of Treatment Considerations for 3RT

In this section we have proposed 3RT, a new primary treatment approach that refers to any combination of techniques for targeting sex offenders' dynamic risk factors for recidivism. Structured according to risk-based treatment principles (Andrews, 1989), 3RT is a flexible approach that is compatible with current RP-based sex offender treatment programs. 3RT assumes a cognitive-behavioral skills training model to target offenders' risk needs and replaces maladaptive behaviors with more adaptive, prosocial skills. In the current chapter, we have given extensive consideration to the applicability of DBT skills training techniques to the treatment of antisocial and erotopathic risk factors; however, 3RT can be continually modified and enhanced as we increase our understanding about sex offenders' dynamic risk factors for recidivism.

Before implementing a new primary treatment for sex offenders, an important consideration is the additional demand that any such approach might place on already limited SOTP resources. As proposed in this chapter, 3RT should place minimal demand on SOTP resources. For example, ideographic assessments are typically conducted as part of an SOTP intake protocol (e.g., file review, individual interview, questionnaire administration, and/or plethysmographic assessment); therefore, this aspect of 3RT should provide no additional burden on SOTP evaluators or therapists. 3RT should be theoretically and functionally compatible with RP (i.e., cognitive-behaviorally based, administered in a group format); therefore, current RP therapists would need minimal training beyond that which is already required to conduct RP with sex offenders. 3RT could also employ extant manualized treatment protocols, further minimizing therapist workload. Finally, if 3RT groups replaced some proportion of current RP groups (to reduce overlap between theoretically similar groups), they would place no demand on an SOTP's allocated group therapy time.

RELAPSE PREVENTION AND 3RT EXTENDED: PUBLIC HEALTH, HARM REDUCTION, AND SEX OFFENDER RECIDIVISM

In the sex offender treatment arena, the primary goal is to minimize the likelihood that a perpetrator will offend again. Despite ongoing vociferous demands from some members of the community seeking to lock up sexual predators for life, for most offenders in most jurisdictions, jail terms ultimately do come to an end, and offenders must be prepared for that eventuality. It is with this in mind that we consider the merits of adopting a harm reduction philosophy.

Harm reduction (HR) is a controversial philosophy that, like RP, was born in the addictions treatment field. It emerged primarily out of frustration with narrowly defined treatment goals for dealing with problem behaviors that are highly resistant to change. Drug and alcohol dependence are notoriously difficult to overcome. Historically, treatment programs demanded that clients remain abstinent to remain in treatment. Because relapse was forbidden, the stakes were high, and those who did relapse frequently found themselves essentially abandoned by their treatment providers, who would not accept successive approximations of sobriety. Due to the relative intractability of addiction and the persistent likelihood of relapse, treatment providers began to think about "damage control." If primary prevention of relapse seemed at times doomed to fail despite the best of interventions, why not consider taking steps to minimize the damage that relapse could cause? From an HR perspective, this is a fundamental question (Stoner & George, 2000).

On a basic level, HR seeks to do precisely that: reduce harm. As a public health alternative to the moral and the medical/disease models of addictions, the HR philosophy suggests a more pragmatic focus on the consequences or effects of the addictive behavior rather than on the behavior itself (Marlatt, 1996, 1998). Those who adopt such a philosophy do not get caught up in the moral debate of whether a behavior is right or wrong; rather, they focus on the harmful effects of the problematic behavior and strive to minimize that harm with a practical approach. Examples of HR interventions in the substance abuse field include changing the route of drug administration from a more damaging one (e.g., injecting) to a less damaging one (e.g., smoking), using a safer drug (e.g., methadone) rather than a more dangerous one (e.g., heroin), and using clean needles. It is important to note that abstinence is the *ultimate* HR.

Some may bristle at the notion of attempting to translate the HR philosophy from the addictions treatment field to the sex offender treatment field. In adopting such a philosophy for sex offender treatment, one is *not* saying that "a little bit of sex offending is okay" or that "victimizing in this way is less damaging than victimizing in that way." Victimization in any form is abhorrent. Thus, bearing in mind that most sex offenders will eventually return to society, a critical concern is minimizing the likelihood that any new victims will be created and that any existing victims will be further victimized. On the surface, locking sex offenders up for life may seem like the safest intervention from an HR perspective, but such a draconian approach is also likely to create harm by driving "free" sex offenders further underground, increasing the number of victims they create before being caught, increasing the financial burden on society and the strain on the prisons, and so on.

An HR philosophy in the sex offender treatment field should inspire treatment providers and innovators to determine how treatment and follow-up can be improved to minimize victimization. In the treatment context, combating the AVE is paramount, and in particular the AVE that is likely to occur following relapse, that is, the commission of a sexual offense. Although of course it is hoped and expected that relapse will never occur, failing to prepare for such a possibility could have dire consequences. Without knowing how to deal with relapse, offenders would be particularly vulnerable to the AVE. Thus, important topics in treatment are not only what to do if offenders find themselves in a High Risk Situation (HRS), but also what to do if they find themselves having succumbed to an HRS and committed a sexual offense. From an HR perspective, it is critical for offenders to know whom to call or what to do in such a case and to challenge the AVE that would impel them to create more victims. Preparation of a postrelapse action plan would ensure that offenders do know how to get help to regain abstinence as soon as possible. Offenders should learn and be encouraged to "catch" themselves and return to treatment voluntarily. If they do not, and they continue to victimize until law enforcement catches up with them, much more harm is likely be done.

Opponents to an HR approach may express concern that preparing a postrelapse plan "sends the wrong message," that it may be perceived as tacit permission to relapse. However, postrelapse planning can be framed in such a way as to prevent sending the message that a brief foray back into the world of sexual offending would be acceptable. In fact, it is so *unacceptable* that, in addition to being taught how to prevent it from happening, offenders are prepared to change their course immediately if it does indeed happen despite their best efforts. This type of approach has been advocated for over a decade. As Marshall, Hudson, and Ward (1992) have stated:

> It is important to have the client understand that a single offense after treatment does not necessarily have to lead to a full return to prior rates of offending, while at the same time emphasizing the importance of avoiding even a single offense. . . . we do not want clients to view reoffending as an all-or-none phenomenon. If they do reoffend, we want them to stop the process there and not let it escalate to more victims and perhaps more aggressive and intrusive behaviors. (pp. 241–242)

Such an approach is consistent with a model in which clients are strongly encouraged to take responsibility for their behavior. Offenders are expected to maintain their own abstinence. DBT uses commitment strategies to engage clients in treatment and to encourage them to become invested in their own treatment (Linehan, 1993a). Such strategies could be adapted and used in conjunction with 3RT and RP.

Adopting an HR perspective also affects the way treatments are evaluated. Outcomes are considered in terms of whether harm is reduced and, if so, by how much (Stoner & George, 2000). Consider a hypothetical study of treatment outcomes, in which offenders who underwent Treatment A and Treatment B are compared to untreated offenders. At 1-year follow-up, all 50 offenders in the control (untreated) group reoffended with five victims each, for a total of 250 victims. Of 50 offenders who received Treatment A, all reoffended with one victim each, for a total of 50 victims. Of 50 offenders in Treatment B, 49 offenders remained abstinent for the year, but one offender created 50 victims. If the goal was to prevent relapse, Treatment A was clearly a failure because 100% of the subjects relapsed, and Treatment B was a phenomenal success because 98% of the subjects remained abstinent. From an HR perspective, the bottom line is that the number of new victims was reduced by 80% in each case, compared to the control group.

Thus, in summary, adopting an HR perspective helps keep the focus on the bottom line: reducing the harm to the individual, the community, and society in general. It provides an objective measure of whether treatment works, and suggests other avenues where it may be improved. In the addictions field, cognitive-behavioral approaches such as RP have coincided with a movement away from the essentially medical concept of "addiction" to a focus on the more general and pragmatic question of what can be done to improve dysfunctional or problematic behavior. Since RP has been and continues to be adapted successfully to sex offender treatment, and cognitive-behavioral treatments in general are the treatments of choice with sex offenders, perhaps the field can again profit from looking toward pioneering work in the addictions arena. Perhaps, like RP, HR philosophy can be successfully adapted to an even greater extent in sex offender treatment.

CONCLUDING REMARKS AND FUTURE DIRECTIONS

Much has changed in the 20 years since the first application of RP to sex offenders (Marshall & Laws, 2003). RP has become a very popular treatment approach in SOTPs and there is evidence to support its effectiveness (e.g., Hanson et al., 2002; Marques et al., 1994; Nicholaichuk et al., 2000). However, as critics have noted, its popularity has been problematic because many SOTPs now rely on RP as the primary treatment strategy rather than as being adjunctive to offense cessation intervention.

Professionals responsible for managing and treating sex offenders have come to embrace the importance of actuarial risk assessment as a central pivot point in predicting reoffense, prioritizing treatment access, and tailoring treatment protocols. Moreover, just as RP was "adopted" from the addictions field 20 years ago, other cognitive-behavioral approaches (e.g., DBT) have begun to be incorporated into the sex offender treatment domain.

In response to these trends, we have offered an enhanced and updated RP approach for sex offenders. Based on maximizing reoffense prevention, we have described a recidivism risk reduction therapy. This approach incorporates risk assessment principles for selecting from a broad range of RP, DBT, and other cognitive-behavioral techniques to tailor intervention protocols to the precise recidivism reduction focal points for each offender. This approach can be employed sequentially or concurrently with traditional RP sex offender protocols. It is expected that, like RP, this approach will be subjected to future empirical evaluation.

ACKNOWLEDGMENTS

Preparation of this chapter was supported in part by a grant from the National Institute on Alcohol Abuse and Alcoholism (No. AA13565) to William H. George. Gratitude is expressed to Kenneth Schafer and Rebecca Schacht for their assistance.

NOTES

1. The "rule" that has been broken is not necessarily abstinence. Moderation is also considered a legitimate goal within the RP model for substance use.
2. Andrews (1989) has enumerated three risk-based treatment principles for working with criminal offenders. These principles provide a structure for prioritizing treatment candidates and tailoring the treatment process.

3. Note that the Hanson and Morton-Bourgon (2004) meta-analysis did not use a DSM-IV "diagnosis" of antisocial personality disorder (ASPD) as the exclusive indicator for "antisocial personality." These criteria are provided as guidelines for conceptualizing various features characteristic of an antisocial personality.
4. Note that if many offenders endorse a particular risk factor and/or if a particular risk factor demands more in-depth therapeutic attention (e.g., substance abuse), specialized 3RT-A subgroups could be implemented to target those particular risk needs.
5. 3RT-E groups can address sexual offending as a maladaptive coping strategy, so 3RT-A groups can focus on other maladaptive coping strategies.
6. Some modifications may be indicated for its application to special populations; for example, for teaching interpersonal effectiveness skills to juveniles/juvenile sex offenders, see Wheeler and Schafer (2000).
7. Although this chapter is focused on SOTP-based interventions, these techniques could also be implemented by other types of supervisors in the community.
8. Note that if many offenders endorse a particular risk factor and/or if a particular risk factor demands more in-depth therapeutic attention (e.g., conflicts with intimate partners), specialized 3RT-E subgroups could be implemented to target those particular risk needs.
9. Although the vast majority of sexual offenders are self-identified as heterosexually oriented, some offenders self-identify as bisexually or homosexually oriented. Since most 3RT-E groups will be predominantly comprised of heterosexually oriented offenders, separate 3RT-E groups might be developed to address the specific needs of bisexually and/or homosexually oriented offenders.
10. 3RT-E groups can address sexual offending as a maladaptive coping strategy, so 3RT-A groups can focus on other maladaptive coping strategies.
11. Some modifications may be indicated for its application to special populations; for example, for teaching interpersonal effectiveness skills to juveniles/juvenile sex offenders, see Wheeler and Schafer (2000).

REFERENCES

Alexander, M. A. (1999). Sexual offender treatment efficacy revisited. *Sexual Abuse: A Journal of Research and Treatment, 11*, 101–117.
American Psychiatric Association. (1994). *Diagnostic and statistical manual of mental disorders* (4th ed.). Washington, DC: Author.
Andrews, D. A. (1989). Recidivism is predictable and can be influenced: Using risk assessments to reduce recidivism. *Forum on Corrections Research, 1*, 11–18.
Antonowicz, D. H., & Ross, R. R. (1994). Essential components of successful rehabilitation programs for offenders. *International Journal of Offender Therapy and Comparative Criminology, 38*, 97–104.
Christensen, A., & Jacobson, N. S. (2000). *Reconcilable differences*. New York: Guilford Press.
Derrickson, D. L. (2000). Working alliance and readiness to change in incarcerated sex offenders. *Dissertation Abstracts International, 60*(8-B), 4215.
Donovan, D. M., & Marlatt, G. A. (Eds.). (2005). *Assessment of addictive behaviors* (2nd ed.). New York: Guilford Press.
Enright, S. J. (1989). Paedophilia: A cognitive/behavioural treatment approach in a single case. *British Journal of Psychiatry, 155*, 399–401.
Gray, S. R. (1995). A comparison of verbal satiation and minimal arousal condition-

ing to reduce deviant arousal in the laboratory. *Sexual Abuse: Journal of Research and Treatment*, 7, 143–153.

Hallam, R. S., & Rachman, S. (1972). Some effects of aversion therapy on patients with sexual disorders. *Behaviour Research and Therapy*, 10, 171–180.

Hanson, R. K. (2000). What is so special about relapse prevention? In D. R. Laws, S. M. Hudson, & T. Ward (Eds.), *Remaking relapse prevention with sex offenders: A sourcebook* (pp. 27–38). Thousand Oaks, CA: Sage.

Hanson, R. K., & Bussiere, M. T. (1998). Predicting relapse: A meta-analysis of sexual offender recidivism studies. *Journal of Consulting and Clinical Psychology*, 66, 348–362.

Hanson, R. K., Gordon, A., Harris, A. J., Marques, J. K., Murphy, W., Quinsey, V. L., & Seto, M. C. (2002). First report of the Collaborative Outcome Data Project on the effectiveness of psychological treatment for sex offenders. *Sexual Abuse: A Journal of Research and Treatment*, 14, 169–194.

Hanson, R. K., & Harris, A. J. R. (1998). *Dynamic predictors of sexual recidivism* (User Report 1998–01). Ottawa: Department of the Solicitor General of Canada.

Hanson, R. K., & Harris, A. J. R. (2000). Where should we intervene? Dynamic predictors of sexual offense recidivism. *Criminal Justice and Behavior*, 27(1), 6–35.

Hanson, R. K., & Harris, A. J. R. (2001). A structured approach to evaluating change among sexual offenders. *Sexual abuse: A Journal of Research and Treatment*, 13, 105–122.

Hanson, R. K., & Harris, A. (2002). *STABLE and ACUTE Scoring Guides: Developed for the Dynamic Supervision Project: A collaborative initiative on the community supervision of sexual offenders* (May 30, 2002 Version). Ottawa: Department of the Solicitor General of Canada.

Hanson, R. K., & Morton-Bourgon, K. (2004). *Predictors of sexual recidivism: An updated meta-analysis* (User Report 2004-02). Ottawa: Public Safety and Emergency Preparedness Canada. Available at www.psepc.gc.ca.

Hayes, S. C., Brownell, K. D., & Barlow, D. H. (1983). Heterosocial-skills training and covert sensitization: Effects on social skills and sexual arousal in sexual deviants. *Behaviour, Research, and Therapy*, 21, 383–392.

Heilbrun, K., Nezu, C. M., Keeney, M., Chung, S., & Wasserman, A. L. (1998). Sexual offending: Linking assessment, intervention, and decision making. *Psychology, Public Policy, and Law*, 4, 138–174.

Hoffman, P. D., Fruzzetti, A. E., & Swenson, C. R. (1999). Dialectical behavior therapy—Family skills training. *Family Process*, 38, 399–414.

Hover, G. (1999). Using DBT Skills with incarcerated sex offenders. *ATSA Forum*, 11(3).

Hover, G. R., & Packard, R. L. (1998, October). *The effects of skills training on incarcerated sex offenders and their ability to get along with their therapist*. Poster presented at the annual convention of the Association for the Treatment of Sexual Abusers.

Hover, G. R., & Packard, R. L. (1999, September). *The treatment effects of dialectical behavior therapy with sex offenders*. Paper presented at the annual convention of the Association for the Treatment of Sex Offenders Convention.

Hudson, S. M., Wales, D. S., Bakker, L., & Ward, T. (2002). Dynamic risk factors:

The Kia Marama evaluation. *Sexual Abuse: A Journal of Research and Treatment, 14,* 103–119.

Hudson, S. M., Ward, T., & Marshall, W. L. (1992). The abstinence violation effect in sex offenders: A reformulation. *Behaviour Research and Therapy, 30,* 435–441.

Knopp, F. H., Freeman-Longo, R., & Stevenson, W. F. (1992). *Nationwide survey of juvenile and adult sex offender treatment programs and models.* Brandon, VT: Safer Society.

Kumar, T. (1995). Vipassana meditation courses in Tihar jail. In *Vipassana: Its relevance to the present world: An international seminar.* Maharashtra, India: Vipassana Research Institute.

Laws, D. R. (1995a). Central elements in relapse prevention procedures with sex offenders. *Psychology, Crime, and Law, 2,* 41–53.

Laws, D. R. (1995b). Verbal satiation: Notes on procedure, with speculations on its mechanism of effect. *Sexual Abuse: A Journal of Research and Treatment, 7,* 155–166.

Laws, D. R. (1996). Relapse prevention or harm reduction? *Sexual Abuse: A Journal of Research and Treatment, 8,* 243–247.

Laws, D. R. (1999a). Harm reduction or harm facilitation? A reply to Maletzky. *Sexual Abuse: A Journal of Research and Treatment, 11,* 233–241.

Laws, D. R. (1999b). Relapse prevention: The state of the art. *Journal of Interpersonal Violence, 14,* 285–302.

Laws, D. R. (2003). The rise and fall of relapse prevention. *Australian Psychologist, 38,* 22–30.

Laws, D. R., Hudson, S. M., & Ward, T. (2000). The original model of relapse prevention with sex offenders. In D. R. Laws, S. M. Hudson, & T. Ward (Eds.), *Remaking relapse prevention with sex offenders: A sourcebook* (pp. 2–24). Thousand Oaks, CA: Sage.

Linehan, M. M. (1993a). *Cognitive-behavioral treatment of borderline personality disorder.* New York: Guilford Press.

Linehan, M. M. (1993b). *Skills training manual for treating borderline personality disorder.* New York: Guilford Press.

Linehan, M. M., Armstrong, H. E., Suarez, A., Allmon, D., & Heard, H. L. (1991). Cognitive-behavioral treatment of chronically parasuicidal borderline patients. *Archives of General Psychiatry, 48,* 1060–1064.

Linehan, M. M., Schmidt, H., Dimeff, L. A., Craft, J. C., Kanter, J., & Comtois, K. A. (1999). Dialectical behavior therapy for patients with borderline personality disorder and drug-dependence. *American Journal on Addictions, 8,* 279–292.

Marlatt, G. A. (1989). Feeding the PIG: The problem of immediate gratification. In D. R. Laws (Ed.), *Relapse prevention with sex offenders.* New York: Guilford Press.

Marlatt, G. A. (1996). Harm reduction: Come as you are. *Addictive Behaviors, 21,* 779–788.

Marlatt, G. A. (Ed.). (1998). *Harm reduction: Pragmatic strategies for managing high-risk behaviors.* New York: Guilford Press.

Marlatt, G. A. (2002). Buddhist philosophy and the treatment of addictive behavior. *Cognitive and Behavioral Practice, 9,* 44–49.

Marlatt, G. A., & George, W. H. (1984). Relapse prevention: Introduction and overview of the model. *British Journal of Addictions, 79,* 261–273.

Marlatt, G. A., & Gordon, J. R. (1980). Determinant of relapse: Implications for the maintenance of behavior change. In P. O. Davidson & S. M. Davidson (Eds.), *Behavioral medicine: Changing health lifestyles*. New York: Brunner/Mazel.

Marlatt, G. A., & Gordon, J. R. (1985). *Relapse prevention: Maintenance strategies in the treatment of addictive behavior* (1st ed.). New York: Guilford Press.

Marques, J. K., Day, D. M., Nelson, C., & West, M. A. (1994). Effects of cognitive-behavioral treatment on sex offender recidivism. *Criminal Justice and Behavior, 21*, 28–54.

Marshall, W. L., & Barbaree, H. E. (1988). The long-term evaluation of a behavioral treatment program for child molesters. *Behaviour Research and Therapy, 26*, 499–511.

Marshall, W. L., Hudson, S. M., & Ward, T. (1992). Sexual deviance. In P. H. Wilson (Ed.), *Principles and practice of relapse prevention* (pp. 235–254). New York: Guilford Press.

Marshall, W. L., Jones, R., Ward, T., Johnston, P., & Barbaree, H. E. (1991). Treatment outcome with sex offenders. *Clinical Psychology Review, 11*, 465–485.

Marshall, W. L., & Laws, D. R. (2003). A brief history of behavioral and cognitive-behavioral approaches to sexual offender treatment: Part 2. The modern era. *Sexual Abuse: A Journal of Research and Treatment, 15*, 93–120.

Miller, A. L., Wyman, S. E., Huppert, J. D., Glassman, S. L., & Rathus, J. H. (2001). Analysis of behavioral skills utilized by suicidal adolescents receiving dialectical behavior therapy. *Cognitive and Behavioral Practice, 7*, 183–187.

Nicholaichuk, T., Gordon, A., Gu, D., & Wong, S. (2000). Outcome of an institutional sexual offender treatment program: A comparison between treated and matched untreated offenders. *Sexual Abuse: A Journal of Research and Treatment, 12*, 139–153.

Pithers, W. D., & Cumming, G. F. (1989). Can relapse be prevented? Initial outcome data from the Vermont Treatment Program for Sexual Aggressors. In D. R. Laws (Ed.), *Relapse prevention with sex offenders* (pp. 313–325). New York: Guilford Press.

Quigley, S. M. (2000). Dialectical behavior therapy and sex offender treatment: An integrative model. *Dissertation Abstracts International, 60*, 4904B.

Quinsey, V. L., Lalumiere, M. L., Rice, M. E., & Harris, G. T. (1995). Predicting sexual offenses. In J. C. Campbell (Ed.), *Assessing dangerousness: Violence by sexual offenders, batterers, and child abusers* (pp. 114–137). Thousand Oaks, CA: Sage.

Roberts, C. F., Doren, D. M., & Thornton, D. (2002). Dimensions associated with assessments of sex offender recidivism risk. *Criminal Justice and Behavior, 29*, 569–589.

Safer, D. L., Telch, C. F., & Argas, W. S. (2001). Dialectical behavior therapy for bulimia nervosa. *American Journal of Psychiatry, 158*, 632–634.

Shingler, J. (2004). A process of cross-fertilization: What sex offender treatment can learn from Dialectical Behavior Therapy. *Journal of Sexual Aggression, 10*(2), 171–180.

Stoner, S. A., & George, W. H. (2000). Relapse prevention and harm reduction: Areas of overlap. In D. R. Laws, S. M. Hudson, & T. Ward (Eds.), *Remaking relapse prevention with sex offenders: A sourcebook* (pp. 56–75). Thousand Oaks, CA: Sage.

Telch, C. F., Argas, W. S., & Linehan, M. M. (2000). Group dialectical behavior therapy for binge-eating disorder: A preliminary, uncontrolled trial. *Behavior Therapy, 31,* 569–582.

Thornton, D. (1997). *Is relapse prevention really necessary?* Paper presented at the meeting of the Association of the Treatment of Sexual Abusers, Arlington, VA.

Tierney, D. W., & McCabe, M. (2002). Motivation for behavior change among sex offenders: A review of the literature. *Clinical Psychology Review, 22*(1), 113–129.

Tierney, D. W., & McCabe, M. P. (2004). The assessment of motivation for behaviour change among sex offenders against children: An investigation of the utility of the Stages of Change Questionnaire. *Journal of Sexual Aggression, 10*(2), 237–249.

Ward, T., & Hudson, S. M. (1996a). Relapse prevention: A critical analysis. *Sexual Abuse: A Journal of Research and Treatment, 8,* 177–200.

Ward, T., & Hudson, S. M. (1996b). Relapse prevention: Future directions. *Sexual Abuse: A Journal of Research and Treatment, 8,* 249–256.

Ward, T., & Hudson, S. M. (1998). A model of the relapse process in sexual offenders. *Journal of Interpersonal Violence, 13,* 700–725.

Ward, T., & Hudson, S. M. (2000). A self-regulation model of relapse prevention. In D. R. Laws, S. M. Hudson, & T. Ward (Eds.), *Remaking relapse prevention with sex offenders: A sourcebook* (pp. 79–101). Thousand Oaks, CA: Sage.

Ward, T., Hudson, S. M., & Siegert, R. J. (1995). A critical comment of Pither's relapse prevention model. *Sexual Abuse: A Journal of Research and Treatment, 7,* 167–175.

Ward, T., Louden, K., Hudson, S. M., & Marshall, W. L. (1995). A descriptive model of the offense chain for child molesters. *Journal of Interpersonal Violence, 10,* 452–472.

Weinrott, M. R., Riggan, M., & Frothingham, S. (1997). Reducing deviant arousal in juvenile sex offenders using vicarious sensitization. *Journal of Interpersonal Violence, 12,* 704–728.

Wheeler, J. G. (2003). The abstinence violation effect in a sample of incarcerated sexual offenders: A reconsideration of the terms lapse and relapse. *Dissertation Abstracts International, 63,* 3946B.

Wheeler, J. G., George, W. H., & Marlatt, G. A. (in press). The Abstinence Violation Effect: A reconsideration of the terms Lapse and Relapse for Sexual Offenders. *Sexual Abuse: Journal of Research and Treatment.*

Wheeler, J. G., George, W. H., & Stephens, K. A. (2005). Assessment of sexual offenders: A model for integrating dynamic risk assessment and relapse prevention approaches. In D. M. Donovan & G. A. Marlatt (Eds.), *Assessment of addictive behaviors* (2nd ed., pp. 392–424). New York: Guilford Press.

Wheeler, J. G., & Schafer, K. D. (2000). *Social skills training for juvenile sexual offenders.* Unpublished treatment manual. (Available from the authors. Requests may be sent to dr.wheeler@comcast.net.)

Wolpow, S., Porter, M., & Hermanos, E. (2000). Adapting a dialectical behavior therapy (DBT) group for use in a residential program. *Psychiatric Rehabilitation Journal, 24,* 135–141.

Relapse Prevention for Sexually Risky Behaviors

Tina M. Zawacki
Susan A. Stoner
William H. George

The AIDS epidemic continues seemingly unabated. Around the globe in 2003, 5 million people were newly infected, 3 million people died, and 40 million people were living with the human immunodeficiency virus (HIV) and Acquired Immune Deficiency Syndrome (AIDS). Sexual transmission is the chief route to new infections (Centers for Disease Control and Prevention, 2004). Consequently, until a successful vaccine is developed, the primary way to prevent further spread of the virus is to reduce the occurrence of sexually risky behaviors (SRBs). Recent evidence from Uganda shows that societalwide reductions in SRBs can have the "similar . . . impact of a vaccine of 80% effectiveness" (Stoneburner & Low-Beer, 2004, p. 714). Conversely, failure to maintain reductions in SRBs carries grave health consequences not only for individuals but also for the communities in which they (and we) live. Thus, although HIV/AIDS-related morbidity and mortality make for high stakes when developing and applying behavioral interventions, the prospective public health benefits are enormous.

Relapse prevention (RP), with its emphasis on initiating and maintaining behavior change, provides apt theory and technology for affecting reductions in SRBs. Some RP-oriented intervention programs have emerged for reducing SRBs (e.g., Roffman et al., 1998). However, compared to RP applications in another sexual domain, sex offending, RP applications to

SRBs have not become as popular and widespread, nor have they been as extensively developed and investigated. Nevertheless, RP encompasses a conceptual model and a system of assessment and intervention techniques that together continue to hold promise for applications to SRBs. RP may offer unique insights about reduction efforts for SRBs and can inform strategies for maintaining such reduction. Most intervention programs aimed at reduction of SRBs are—like RP—psychosocial in nature, based on cognitive-behavioral therapy concepts, and incorporate cognitive-behavioral treatment techniques. The scholarly literature about such programs is copious and far exceeds the scope of this chapter (see reviews by Kalichman, 1998; Kelly & Kalichman, 2002; Perloff, 2001). Our objective in the current chapter is to provide a brief overview of RP-based formulations about SRBs and their potential contributions in this behavioral domain. Within this limited objective, we consider illustrative empirical investigations that either examine an RP-based construct or treatment component or evaluate a comprehensive RP application. The plan for this chapter is that we first discuss the relevance of RP for the reduction of SRBs, then we outline how the RP conceptual model applies, and finally we describe existing comprehensive applications of RP treatment techniques.

SEXUAL RISK TAKING AND THE RELEVANCE OF RELAPSE PREVENTION

For the purposes of this chapter, SRBs are defined as behaviors that allow for an exchange of bodily fluids sufficient for transmitting HIV. Blood, semen, and vaginal secretions are the only bodily fluids—besides breast milk—that can contain a concentration of HIV sufficient for transmission. Thus, SRBs targeted for reduction primarily include the following:

1. *Unprotected (i.e., condomless) anal intercourse.* Penetrative anal sex incurs risk by exposing penile mucous membranes—as well as small lacerations that may exist on the penis—to HIV potentially contained in a receptive partner's rectal blood. Receptive anal sex partners run the risk of absorbing potentially HIV-infected semen through the vascular anal cavity.

2. *Unprotected vaginal intercourse.* Generally speaking, vaginal intercourse is considered somewhat less risky than anal intercourse because it typically involves less bleeding. Nonetheless, as with anal sex, both penetrative and receptive vaginal intercourse partners are potentially exposed to HIV, either via semen through vaginal walls or via vaginal fluids through the genital tissue of the penis. Women are 2–4 times more likely to contract HIV through vaginal sex than are their male partners (Haverkos & Battjes, 1992).

3. *Unprotected oral (without condom or, in the case of female-receptive oral sex, dental dam) intercourse.* Debate continues about the risk level of oral sex (e.g., oral–genital receptive sex), although it is biologically tenable that oral mucous membranes can absorb HIV (Page-Shafer et al., 2002). Relatively stronger support—although extremely mixed and controversial— has been found for penile–oral transmission compared to vaginal–oral transmission. In sum, reduction programs for SRBs typically target prevention of unprotected anal, vaginal, and receptive penile–oral intercourse.

It is the focus on maintenance that makes RP so relevant to SRBs. Although RP was adapted from the addictions field, the rationale for its application to the reduction of SRBs is not based on the idea that risky sex is an "addiction." Instead, the rationale for this application is based on the shared problem of maintaining successful abstinence or moderation following a self-initiated behavior change. Maintaining HIV-seronegativity on an individual level and controlling the spread of HIV on a societal level is not only a matter of avoiding SRBs for a circumscribed amount of time, it requires consistent risk avoidance into the foreseeable future. Because HIV is communicable and eventually fatal, even infrequent risk-reduction lapses carry more grave consequences at an individual and community level than do other behaviors to which RP has been applied, such as alcohol use, overeating, and gambling. In no other health behavior area can even infrequent engagement in the behavior carry such grave consequences. In particular, the high prevalence of HIV infection in some populations, such as men who have sex with men (MSM), means that each lapse into SRBs has a relatively high risk of transmission, making reduction maintenance for SRBs especially crucial. The MSM community has been one of the hardest hit by the AIDS epidemic, and thus has received the most attention in terms of epidemiological research and prevention programming. Research during the 1990s suggested that on the whole, the MSM community had achieved tremendous reductions in HIV risk-taking behaviors and transmission. Nonetheless, studies also revealed that, on an individual level, many men continued to report sporadic or consistent engagement in SRBs (Catania et al., 2001; Kelly, Kalichman, et al., 1991; Stall, Hays, Waldo, Ekstrand, & McFarland, 2000). Researchers began highlighting the importance of maintenance in eradicating the disease, and acknowledged that little theory had been developed to guide intervention efforts to maintain safer-sex behavior changes over the long term and to address the issue of "relapse" to high-risk behavior (Stall & Ekstrand, 1994; Stall, Ekstrand, Pollack, McKusick, & Coates, 1990). Thus, the RP model can provide enormous guidance to reduction efforts for SRBs because of its explicit focus on addressing maintenance challenges in behavior change (Brownell, Marlatt, Lichtenstein, & Wilson, 1986).

KEY BACKGROUND CONSIDERATIONS IN APPLYING
RELAPSE PREVENTION TO SEXUALLY RISKY BEHAVIORS

Definitions of Relapse and Lapse in Relapse Prevention and Sexually Risky Behaviors

A fundamental aspect of applying RP approaches to the reduction of SRBs is establishing what "relapse" means when translated to the domain of SRB. There has been controversy regarding the use of the term "relapse" to refer to SRBs (Donovan, Mearns, McEwan, & Sugden, 1994; Hart, Boulton, Fitzpatrick, McLean, & Dawson, 1992; Stall & Ekstrand, 1994), likely because of lingering connotations with medical-disease models of addiction. Prior to the advent of the RP model in the addictions field, it was standard practice to define relapse as any return to the target behavior, no matter how minor. For example, having one drink constituted a relapse to alcoholism. Relapse carried with it a negative construal as an all-or-nothing function of a disease that is internally, biologically driven and thus beyond the person's conscious control (George & Marlatt, 1989). The RP model actively countered the medical-disease model, and reformulated the concept of relapse as a violation of a self-imposed rule or set of rules governing the rate or pattern of a selected behavior. In this way, behavior change and maintenance were placed squarely within the conscious control of the individual.

Furthermore, the RP model focused on relapse as a process rather than as a dichotomous outcome (relapsed/not relapsed) by developing the idea of a "lapse." A lapse is a less extreme or temporary return to the target behavior. In terms of treatment outcomes, a lapse is commonly defined as a single instance of the target behavior (e.g., smoking one cigarette), whereas a relapse is defined as a return to pretreatment levels of the behavior (e.g., smoking two packs of cigarettes a day, again). A lapse is viewed as a transitional state that can lead to relapse, but that can also lead to a return to abstinence or moderation. The cognitive-behavioral processes governing the progression from lapse to relapse are the focus of the RP model and are discussed later in this chapter.

Although engaging in high-risk sex is sometimes labeled as "lapse" or "relapse" in the SRBs literature, considerable variance exists in the definitions and operationalizations of these terms, and they are rarely applied according to the definitions suggested by the RP model. Many of these studies do not claim to incorporate the RP definitions of lapse and relapse; therefore we are not implying that their definitions and operationalizations are incorrect or inadequate in any way. Rather, they are presented as examples of how the terms have been used in the SRBs literature. The label of relapse has been used to describe both the episodic failure to engage in safer-sex practices (Adib, Joseph, Ostrow, Tal, & Schwartz, 1991; Stall et al., 1990) and the complete discontinuation of safer-sex practices (e.g., condom use) by those who have routinely used them in the past (Donovan, Mearns, McEwan, & Sugden, 1994; Williams, Elwood, & Bowen, 2000). In this way, what the RP model considers a lapse (episodic behavior) often is not discriminated from relapse (consistent behavior). Others have defined relapse as a prolonged return to risky sex, so as to distinguish it from a lapse (de Wit, van Griensven, Kok, & Sandfort, 1993; Kippax, Crawford, Davis, Rodden, & Dowsett, 1993). The role of intention to reduce risk taking—a key component of the RP definitions of lapse and relapse— is often unclear in studies of SRBs. Engagement in SRBs has been referred to as a lapse or relapse when there was no treatment involved, and when it was not clear that participants intended to reduce their SRBs (de Wit et al., 1993; Kelly, Kalichman, et al., 1991; Stall et al., 1990). Because of the life-threatening consequences of HIV infection, it is often an implicit assumption among researchers that participants want to reduce their HIV risk.

The preceding definitions were drawn from studies in which SRBs often were measured on an aggregate level among a large group of participants. That is, the level of SRBs of the entire group (or subsets thereof) was analyzed, not the pattern of behavior change for any given individual. It is challenging to incorporate RP-based definitions of lapse and relapse into epidemiological research because of the therapeutic, client-centered nature of the RP model, in which the focus of behavior change is on the individual level. Ultimately, lapse and relapse must be defined in terms of the safer-sex goals that individuals set for themselves. Studies that have defined lapse and relapse with the highest RP fidelity have assessed participants' personally set safer-sex rules, and measured the degree to which participants engaged in behaviors that violated those rules (Curtin, Stephens, & Roffman, 1997). Further overview of the applications of lapse and relapse—as well as the full RP model—to the reduction and maintenance of SRBs is provided in the following sections.

Deciding on Safer-Sex Goals

Another fundamental aspect of applying RP approaches to the reduction of SRBs is setting specific goals for safer sex. It is a pragmatic assumption in HIV prevention that once a person becomes sexually active, he or she is not likely to stop being sexually active. Complete abstinence from sex is sometimes considered a viable outcome for adolescents and young people who have not yet initiated sexual intercourse and are in a more amenable stage of life for delaying sexual activity. Among adults, however, complete abstinence is typically not considered a realistic safer-sex goal and is not the focus of reduction interventions for SRBs. A host of strategies exist for HIV-reduction behaviors that target specific sexual acts (e.g., use of barrier contraception; engaging in sexual activities that do not involve exchange of blood, semen, or vaginal secretions; reducing engagement in sexual acts at the highest risk of transmission, such as unprotected anal sex), selection of sexual partners (e.g., monogamy, reducing number of sexual partners, partner testing, enhancing partner communication and sexual negotiation), and addressing intrapersonal and situational antecedents of risky sex (e.g., treating anxiety and depression, reducing alcohol and drug use). Safer-sex goals must be tailored to each individual and must consider the unique circumstances of his or her life. For example, types of partners vary across clients and over time, and a given client may have multiple and varied types of partners (steady/casual/paying). Different partner types may require different strategies. Monogamy and partner testing are more achievable goals with steady or long-term partners, while insistence on the use of barrier protection is a more realistic goal with casual or paying partners. Clients are encouraged to set realistic goals based on their level of willingness, readiness, and ability.

Safer sex includes sexual behaviors that reduce, but do not necessarily eliminate, HIV-transmission risk. Because of differences among anal, vaginal, and oral sex in terms of potential transmission of HIV (i.e., vaginal intercourse typically involves fewer lacerations and less bleeding than does anal intercourse), risk-reduction goals can include engaging in sexual activities that, while still having the potential to transmit HIV, are less likely to do so. For example, based on epidemiological research, Susser, Desvarieux, and Wittkowski (1998) developed the Vaginal Episode Equivalent (VEE) Index, which accounts for differences in the risk of transmission among receptive oral, vaginal, and anal sex acts. According to this index, a client can reduce his or her overall HIV risk by engaging in lower-risk acts (i.e., oral sex) in situations in which they otherwise would have engaged in higher-risk acts (i.e., anal sex). This harm reduction approach acknowledges that behavior change is a process, and that not everyone is able to halt all risky behaviors immediately. Nonetheless, this approach to HIV risk reduction remains controversial because harm reduction is a long-term process that does not necessarily eliminate any and all risk of HIV transmission. Given the extraordinarily grave consequences of HIV transmission, there has been much debate regarding what level of risk, if any, is acceptable (see Ekstrand et al., 1993). In addition, there is much debate surrounding the actual risk level of "safer"-sexual practices such as oral sex (see Caceres & van Griensven, 1994; Newton, 1996; Page-Shafer et al., 2002). Similarly, withdrawal before ejaculation has been considered by some therapists to be a safer-sex behavior (De Vincezi, 1994). However, because failure to withdraw before ejaculation is common and pre-ejaculatory fluids contain HIV, the safety level of withdrawal also has been questioned. Ultimately, safer sex is defined by the standards of the client's community, therapeutic environment, and—most importantly—self. For the purposes of this chapter, safer-sex goals are defined idiographically as any behaviors that will prevent or reduce the risk of HIV transmission and that the client is willing to adopt.

RELAPSE PREVENTION APPLICATIONS
TO REDUCTION OF SEXUALLY RISKY BEHAVIORS

The objectives of RP-based interventions are to prevent occurrence of lapses and relapses through effective coping with high-risk situations, and to promote an overall lifestyle that is resistant to relapse-prone influences. The key components of RP interventions delineated by Marlatt and colleagues (Marlatt, 1996; Marlatt & George, 1984; Marlatt & Gordon, 1980, 1985) include helping the client identify cues and triggers that set the stage for a lapse, building the client's cognitive-behavioral repertoire for dealing with these high-risk situations, and encouraging the client to react to lapses as learning opportunities rather than personal failures. These components of the general RP model apply readily to the reduction of SRBs. In attempting to reduce their SRBs, individuals face high-risk situations in which they are likely to engage in SRBs. When confronted with a high-risk situation, one must generate a cognitive-behavioral coping response, such as negotiating condom use. Failure to enact an effective coping response may result in a lapse into SRBs. If one lapses and engages in a risky sexual behavior, it could lead to self-blame, decreased self-efficacy, and negative affective states, and result in a relapse to prereduction levels of SRBs. Cognitive restructuring of lapses into SRBs as isolated mistakes rather than failures of will and moral fortitude can help to prevent escalation from lapse to relapse. In the following sections, we provide a brief overview of ways in which the RP model can inform strategies for reducing SRBs. These strategies target two pivotal cognitive-behavioral processes that can thwart the lapse–relapse progression: (1) enhancing individuals' awareness of and coping with situations in which they are at high risk of lapse into SRBs, and (2) increasing individuals' ability to manage lapses in such a way that they do not escalate into relapse.

Enhancing Awareness of and Coping with High-Risk Situations

Assessing High-Risk Situations

High-risk situations are those that contain environmental and emotional characteristics that are associated with engaging in SRBs. The analysis of past and preparation for future high-risk situations, in order to prevent lapse, is really the heart of the RP approach. In practice, this generally means a focus on features of particular situations that have served, or are likely to serve, to foster behavioral "slips." Nomothetic research on common potential triggers of SRBs has identified *intrapersonal factors* such as negative emotional states (e.g., stress, anxiety; Folkman, Chesney, Pollack, & Phillips, 1992; Kalichman, Kelly, Morgan, & Rompa, 1997; Kalichman & Weinhardt, 2001) and drug or alcohol use (Kalichman, Kelly, & Rompa, 1997; Kelly, St. Lawrence, & Brasfield, 1991); *interpersonal* factors such as type of relationship (casual/steady) with sexual partner (Misovich, Fisher, & Fisher, 1997); power and control dynamics in the relationship (Canin, Dolcini, & Adler, 1999); and social settings and norms (e.g., frequenting locations known for casual sexual encounters). Although research on common triggers is useful, idiographic assessment of high-risk situations specific to the individual client is essential. With the counselor's guidance a client assesses for potential triggers past situations in which he or she has engaged in SRBs. A client can also self-monitor ongoing sexual behavior for potential triggers. Together the client and therapist assess the client's direct responses in past and ongoing high-risk situations, as well as identify the client's lifestyle factors that may increase exposure to high-risk situations (discussed later). Learning to identify the distal precipitants of SRBs and to recognize proximal cues of high-risk situations provides the client with two tools for identifying and avoiding situations that present an immediate threat. Clients also learn how to prepare for dealing with high-risk situations that they cannot avoid. The therapist and client identify weaknesses in the client's current repertoire of coping responses, and develop strategies for strengthening them.

Coping with High-Risk Situations

The client's coping response to high-risk situations determines whether or not he or she will engage in SRBs. Leaving the situation is often an effective strategy, but not often a realistic one. Whereas many behaviors addressed with RP techniques are amenable to avoidance strategies (e.g., drug users can be encouraged to avoid situations in which drugs are present), the inherently social nature of SRBs limits the client's ability to completely avoid risky situations. As mentioned previously, complete sexual abstinence is not usually a realistic safer-sex goal, and thus clients need to learn a variety of coping strategies when faced with potential sexual interactions.

Here we want to emphasize that, independent of the features of various consensual situations, the incidence of a lapse is essentially the result of a decision on the part of the individual. Figure 12.1 illustrates this point. Although sexual decision making is something of a "black box," we can nonetheless identify processes occurring within the individual—in response to the features of the situation—that are targets for intervention: cognitive, behavioral, affective, and physiological responses. This is wholly consistent with the cognitive-behavioral notion that, while individuals may be power-

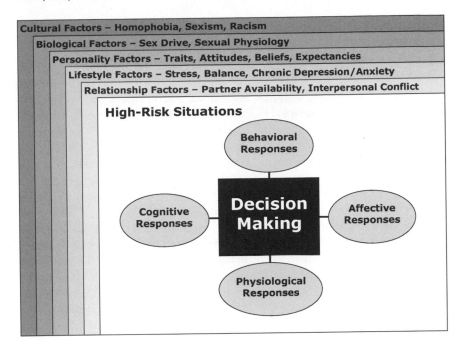

Cultural Factors – Homophobia, Sexism, Racism

Biological Factors – Sex Drive, Sexual Physiology

Personality Factors – Traits, Attitudes, Beliefs, Expectancies

Lifestyle Factors – Stress, Balance, Chronic Depression/Anxiety

Relationship Factors – Partner Availability, Interpersonal Conflict

High-Risk Situations

Behavioral Responses

Cognitive Responses

Decision Making

Affective Responses

Physiological Responses

FIGURE 12.1. Immediate and distal determinants of relapse into sexually risky behaviors.

less to control particular situations, they can certainly learn to control their responses to those situations. Cognitive responses refer to the individual's cognitions that are immediate to the situation, including appraisals of risk, recalling relevant beliefs and expectancies, that is, his or her whole thinking process within that specific situation. Behavioral responses refer to what the person does within that situation, such as saying something or communicating in another way, and engaging in lapse-promoting or lapse-thwarting behaviors. Affective responses refer to the individual's acute emotional state, such as the experience of sexual desire or love, fear or anxiety. Physiological responses refer to what is going on in the body at the time, such as physiological sexual arousal or increased heart rate. It is critical to note that these responses interact dynamically and all potentially factor into the individual's decision making in that situation. For example, being in an acute state of sexual arousal may affect a person's thinking or vice versa. Communicating one's thoughts may allay fear, or fear may stifle communication. In any particular situation, a unique interplay of these proximal, immediate responses, within the context of more distal influences, will determine whether the person lapses or acts according to his or her goals.

Developing Cognitive-Behavioral Skills

Development of coping strategies focuses on building the client's behavioral and cognitive skills for navigating high-risk situations. Cognitive-behavioral skills training can include modeling of effective skills through videotapes or instructor demonstrations, discussion of the model, and client rehearsal of the behavioral skills. A behavioral skill essential to the reduction of SRBs is effective verbal negotiation of safer sex and condom use with sexual partners. Structured role plays have been developed for use in HIV risk reduction programs as assessments of safer-sex communication and negotiation behavioral skills, and as tools for teaching these skills. These role-playing scenarios require clients to negotiate a potentially high-risk social situation using verbal communication skills. Clients' responses to role-played safer-sex negotiation are assessed in terms of their use of specific assertion skills, including acknowledging the role-play partner, communicating in a clear manner, using an "I" statement in the refusal of unsafe sex, providing a reason for refusal, noting the need to be safe, and providing a specific lower-risk alternative sexual activity (Kelly, St. Lawrence, Brasfield, & Hood, 1989; Maisto, Carey, Carey, & Gordon, 2002; Roffman et al., 1998). Cognitive-behavioral skill in the mechanics of condom use is also necessary for successfully enacting protected sex. Clients can rehearse condom use by placing condoms on anatomical models, and receive feedback about correct and incorrect placement. Increased mechanical proficiency at condom use can decrease rates of condom failure (Albert, Warner, Hatcher, Trussell, & Bennett, 1995), as well as reduce participants' inhibitions about discussing and handling condoms (Winter & Goldy, 1993).

On an intrapersonal level, clients can engage in *positive self-talk* when faced with a high-risk situation. Positive self-talk is intended to bolster self-efficacy (discussed later) and decrease anxiety in the face of a potential lapse. In terms of reduction of SRBs, self-talk can include reminders of the positive outcomes of abstaining from SRBs, such as "I will feel much better tomorrow if I don't do anything risky tonight," and endorsement of self-efficacy to reduce SRBs, such as "I am capable of changing my risky sex practices."

Enhancing Self-Efficacy

Building effective coping responses decreases the likelihood of engaging in SRBs through enhancement of *self-efficacy*, which is the belief that one can successfully navigate potentially high-risk situations. Reduction programs for SRBs can use several techniques for increasing self-efficacy, including emphasizing that behavior change is a process of skill acquisition rather than a test of willpower, and breaking down behavior change into smaller,

attainable tasks rather than focusing on overwhelming goals such as abstinence or complete, lifetime elimination of all SRBs. Clients can be encouraged to set short-term, attainable action steps. *Action steps* are circumscribed, incremental steps a client can take to adopt a safer-sex goal
behavior. For example, if one's safer-sex goal is to increase the use of barrier protection during sex, an appropriate action step might be to remember to carry condoms to a planned social event on a given weekend. The
client's successful completion of this action step serves as positive feedback
that he or she will be able to attain safer-sex goals and thereby reduce HIV
risk. If the action step is not fulfilled, the client can identify factors in the
situation that may have acted as barriers to taking the action step, so that
these barriers can be overcome in future attempts.

A client's level and changes in self-efficacy can be assessed using a
number of self-report methods tailored to specific interventions (e.g.,
Langer, Zimmerman, & Cabral, 1994; Roffman et al., 1998), as well as the
multi-item Condom Use Self Efficacy Scale (CUSES; Brafford & Beck,
1991; Brien, Thombs, Mahoney, & Wallnau, 1994). The CUSES items reflect distinct domains of safer-sex self-efficacy, including assertiveness (e.g.,
"I feel confident in my ability to suggest using condoms with a new partner"), partner disapproval (e.g., "If I were to suggest using a condom to a
partner, I would feel afraid that he or she would reject me"), and mechanics (e.g., "I feel confident in my ability to use a condom correctly.")

Changing Outcome Expectancies

Positive-outcome expectancies concern the anticipated, desirable outcomes
of engaging in a behavior, such as expecting to become more sociable after
drinking alcohol. In terms of SRBs, positive-outcome expectancies can include physical pleasure and feelings of intimacy (Roffman et al., 1998).
These expectancies contribute to the likelihood that one will overfocus on
anticipated gratification in a situation of potential SRBs, and overlook negative consequences. This appraisal bias has been labeled the "problem of
immediate gratification" (PIG). Positive-outcome expectancies regarding
risky sex can be addressed through education about the negative health
outcomes of SRBs (e.g., transmission of HIV and other sexually transmitted infections) and through exploring the negative outcomes the client has
actually experienced in the aftermath of engaging in risky sex (e.g., feelings
of regret, guilt, and shame; worry about or actual contraction of sexually
transmitted infections (STIs); concern about endangering partner's health).
In a complementary fashion, outcome expectancies for safer and protected
sexual behavior are important to address (see Albarracin et al., 2000, for
an in-depth analysis of outcome expectancies specific to condom use). Positive safer-sex outcome expectancies can be bolstered by discussions and
activities focusing on the physical pleasure and intimacy that can be at-

tained through protected sex, and through behavior that does not include genital contact, such as holding, touching, massage, and kissing (i.e., eroticization of safer sex).

Lapse Management

The lynchpin of the RP model is the nature of one's emotional and cognitive reaction to an initial lapse from abstinence or moderation. Lapse management aims to halt the lapse behavior as quickly and safely as possible and to combat reactions to the lapse that are likely to lead to relapse. The process leading from lapse to relapse is called the abstinence violation effect (AVE) or, the goal violation effect (GVE; when the goal of treatment is not necessarily abstinence, Larimer & Marlatt, 1990), as is commonly the case in reduction efforts for SRBs. When a lapse occurs, the client can attribute it to either his or her own failure of willpower or inability to cope with a specific, high-risk situation. If one attributes the lapse to a failure of willpower, one is likely to experience negative affect such as guilt, failure, and decreased self-efficacy, which in turn can increase likelihood of engaging in SRBs. Clients can assess their reactions to a lapse in a structured way by identifying the SRBs that violated their goal; listing the central cause of the goal violation; indicating other situational, cognitive, and affective determinants; and describing their personal reactions to the goal violation (Marlatt & Gordon, 1985).

Cognitively Restructuring Causes of the Lapse

RP-based interventions attempt to counteract GVE by helping participants to cognitively restructure the lapse. Cognitive restructuring aims to lessen the GVE by changing the client's attributions of the lapse. The GVE is fostered by attribution of the lapse to causes that are *internal* (e.g., a character flaw), are a *global* influence on aspects of one's life beyond SRBs (e.g., lack of willpower in general), and *stable* across time (e.g., a lifelong moral weakness). Thus, in order to combat the GVE, clients are encouraged to attribute the lapse to causes that are *external* (e.g., an aspect of the situation directly preceding the lapse), *specific* to SRBs (e.g., a flaw in sexual decision making), and *changeable* (e.g., a learned coping skill that can be strengthened). The lapse event is cognitively reframed such that it is not a personal failure with far-reaching, permanent implications, but rather is an opportunity to assess the specific situation in which the lapse occurred and formulate coping responses to deal successfully with similar situations in the future. In this way, guilt and self-blame are avoided, self-efficacy is preserved, and likelihood of relapse into SRBs is made less likely.

The analysis of a lapse can be used as an opportunity to refine the client's cognitive-behavioral repertoire of skills by analyzing the high-risk situation that precipitated the lapse and strengthening corresponding coping skills. For example, assessing the client's negative outcomes from the lapse can be used as a tool for decreasing positive-outcome expectancies about risky sex practices and the PIG. Similarly, analyzing flaws in the client's strategies for verbally negotiating safer sex during the lapse—if relevant—can result in the strengthening of those skills to use in future high-risk situations.

Apparently Irrelevant Decisions

Although it is crucial not to promote self-blame for a lapse, it also is important to challenge rationalization, denial, and minimization of the lapse behavior. This involves an analysis of the covert antecedents and apparently irrelevant decisions (AIDs) that may have contributed to the client entering into a high-risk situation. For example, procrastinating about buying condoms may not seem immediately relevant when a potential sexual encounter does not seem to be on the horizon, but this decision increases the likelihood that the client will be "unable" to use a condom if a sexual encounter unexpectedly occurs. Similarly, engaging in alcohol or drug use prior to sexual encounters is another AID that, upon further reflection, the client may realize provided an excuse for engaging in SRBs.

Distal Determinants of Lapse

In addition to the proximal situational determinants of lapse and relapse, RP emphasizes the influence of more distal precursors to high-risk situations. Retrospective analyses of lapses in high-risk situations tend to be a bit myopic, with good reason; it is critical to understand the "who," "what," "where," "when," and "how" of relapse. A thorough understanding of the "why" may require one to step back further, pan out, and take in the big picture. Here is where distal determinants come into sharper relief. These distal determinants are psychosocial contexts and influences that serve to increase a person's exposure or vulnerability to high-risk situations, such that they may potentiate a lapse or relapse (Larimer, Palmer, & Marlatt, 1999). With regard to sexual risk taking, potential distal determinants include cultural, biological, personality, lifestyle, and relationship factors and can be conceptualized in terms of multiple layers of context or influence, as illustrated in Figure 12.1. The more distal the factor, the more challenging it is to alter directly; however, even the most global factors may wield powerful influences. The salience of different factors may vary depending on aspects of particular situations, but it is useful to examine these multiple, interacting, potential influences on an idiographic level to prepare the client to deal with them whenever they are invoked.

Relationship Factors

The nearest distal determinants to lapse or relapse are relationship factors. Unlike substance abuse, risky sexual behavior cannot occur without a partner. Even one-night stands and anonymous sexual encounters are types of relationships. Thus, relationship factors are of considerable importance. Studies have consistently found that individuals with more sexual partners are more likely to return to risky sex after a period of practicing safer sex (for review, see Donovan et al., 1994). On the other hand, a comprehensive review of sexual risk taking in a variety of populations demonstrated that safer sex is generally practiced less consistently with steady partners than with casual partners (Misovich et al., 1997). Canin et al. (1999) pointed out interpersonal relationship barriers to HIV/STI behavior change, including obstacles related to relationship history (e.g., asserting a desire for condom use in an ongoing relationship where less safe behaviors have been established), obstacles related to power dynamics (e.g., fear of disruption of a valued relationship or fear of a violent response), and obstacles related to communication (e.g., the desire not to appear distrustful toward a partner). RP interventions for sexual risk taking must take relationship factors into consideration and consider relationship dynamics as a context for high-risk situations. Targets for intervention include fostering better communication and conflict resolution skills, negotiating sexual safety in the context of an abusive relationship, and developing healthy relationships with lower-risk partners.

Lifestyle Factors

Marlatt and Gordon (1985) proposed that lifestyle balance was important for the maintenance of behavior change. In the RP model, imbalance is characterized by a preponderance of external demands ("shoulds") at the expense of internally fulfilling or enjoyable activities ("wants"). To a person who is relatively deprived of sources of pleasure as compared to demands, the prospect of sexual pleasure may seem especially appealing, even if it is risky. In the context of imbalance and its associated stress—or chronic stress in general—the individual may be less likely to cope effectively with high-risk situations. Indeed, two studies have reported a relationship between the use of sex to cope with stress and sexual risk taking (Folkman et al., 1992; McKusick, Hoff, Stall, & Coates, 1991). Thus, stress is an important target for intervention, and teaching adaptive stress management techniques may better prepare clients to cope with high-risk situations without engaging in risky sex. Mood may also contribute to the incidence of sexual risk behavior (mood is considered under lifestyle factors because it is presumably fostered by lifestyle factors and less stable than the personality factors discussed later). Although a recent meta-analysis failed to find consistent associations between negative affect and sexual risk taking (Crepaz & Marks, 2001), Bancroft and his colleagues (Bancroft, Janssen, Strong, Carnes, Vukadinovic, & Long, 2003) pointed out that a tendency for negative affect may increase sexual risk taking in some individuals and reduce it in others. In other words, personality factors may moderate the effects of mood on sexual risk taking and vice versa. These authors reported that depressed or anxious mood (as opposed to acute affective states) was associated with increased sexual interest and/or responsiveness in a substantial minority of gay and straight men (Bancroft et al., 2003). These findings suggest that untreated depression or anxiety may facilitate relapse into risky sex and that interventions such as behavioral activation or relaxation to address negative mood may be beneficial for certain groups of clients in the context of RP.

Personality Factors

Personality factors are broadly defined here as stable psychological characteristics of individuals, such as traits, beliefs, attitudes, and expectancies. A large body of research has focused on personality traits as determinants of lapse and relapse. A meta-analysis of 53 studies found that the personality characteristic most reliably found to predict risky sexual behavior, accounting for 64% of the effect sizes, was sensation seeking. Impulsivity, agreeableness, neuroticism, and conscientiousness also produced reliable effects (Hoyle, Fejfar, & Miller, 2000). Although personality traits are generally resistant to change, clinicians can help their clients to understand how such traits may make them more vulnerable to high-risk situations. Certain beliefs have been found to predict risky sex as well. Fatalism (belief that one's own future is dim), belief in a "just world" (where good people are rewarded and bad people are punished), and belief in one's own vulnerability to HIV globally or in particular situations have also been found to be associated with risky sexual practices (Curtin et al., 1997; Hafer, Bogaert, & McMullen, 2001; Kalichman et al., 1997). As discussed earlier, self-efficacy is essentially a belief in one's own ability to effect change, and outcome expectancies are beliefs about what will happen in particular situations. Beliefs are much more amenable to change than personality traits. Classic cognitive-restructuring techniques may be used to challenge and ultimately change beliefs that serve as barriers to safer sexual behavior. Finally, attitudes also fall under the broad umbrella of personality factors that play a role sexual risk taking. Attitudes toward condoms and HIV, as well as more general attitudes toward sex and relationships, are likely to play a role in individuals' sexual risk-taking behavior (Mehryar, 1995; White, Terry, & Hogg, 1994; Williams et al., 2000). Interventions that seek to change attitudes to support safer sex may help to decrease the likelihood of lapse and relapse.

Biological Factors

Biology undoubtedly plays a role in sexual risk taking. Male and female reproductive behaviors are extremely complex biologically, influenced by the brain, neurotransmitters, hormones, and environment. According to Nelson (1995), "understanding the physiological bases of the human sex drive would seem very important if we hope to . . . prevent the spread of sexually transmitted diseases like AIDS. There is something different and possibly unique about sexual motivation as compared with other motivated behaviors that impairs decision-making processes" (p. 204). Unfortunately, funding agencies have been reluctant to provide money for basic research on human sexual behavior, and potential links between sexual physiology and sexual risk taking are not well understood. Bancroft (1999) has proposed a dual-control model of sexual response that may be useful in understanding risky sexual behavior. Sexual arousal per se is an acute state that would potentially function as an immediate, rather than distal, determinant of risky sex; however, individual variability in the biology of sexual response should be considered a potential distal determinant of risky sex. Bancroft's dual-control model posits that the extent of response to a sexual stimulus is determined by a balance between sexual inhibitory and excitatory systems (SIS and SES) within the central nervous system. The model postulates individual variability in the propensity for sexual inhibition, with high propensity producing susceptibility to sexual dysfunction and low propensity promoting high-risk sexual behavior (Bancroft, 1999). Bancroft and his colleagues (2003) have examined the dual-control model of sexual arousal and its effects on sexual risk taking in gay men. The authors found complex relationships among mood, SIS, SES, and sexual risk taking. Because biological factors are for the most part out of an individual's control, the goal of treatment in this regard would be to help the client to understand biological influences and be aware that they may foster lapse or relapse.

Cultural Factors

On the most global level are cultural factors, such as homophobia, sexism, racism, or socioeconomic status. Culture certainly influences one's sense of sexual self, and understanding the cultural meaning of sexual behavior is necessary to understand fully the practice of safer or unsafe sex (Robinson, Bockting, Rosser, Miner, & Coleman, 2002). For example, there has been much recent debate over whether gays and lesbians should be allowed to marry. An important question is what hidden messages are coming through in this debate, especially as they pertain to the expectation of monogamy for homosexual relationships. At the very least, the debate seems to demonstrate that heterosexism and homophobia remain strong. As long as this is the case, the internalization of homophobia among sexual minorities seems likely. Studies have found that internalized homophobia was positively associated with sexual risk-taking (Meyer & Dean, 1998; Stokes & Peterson, 1998) and perceptions of interpersonal barriers to engaging in safer sex (Herek & Glunt, 1995), and negatively associated with self-efficacy for safer sex (Herek & Glunt, 1995). Internalized homophobia was also found to interfere with participants' ability to benefit from preventative interventions (Huebner, Davis, Nemeroff, & Aiken, 2002). As pointed out by Shernoff and Bloom (1991), "a disapproving or conflicted attitude towards one's own sexuality is a poor starting point for taking precautions not to be infected or to infect others" (p. 39). Racism may operate in the same way. There has been little research on the effect of internalized racism on sexual risk taking, but one qualitative study found that Asian and Pacific Islander (API) men who have sex with men tended to feel alienated from both API and gay communities due to the dual stigmas of homophobia and racism. This alienation, in turn, appeared to foster intense needs for closeness as well as API men's willingness to engage in risky sex, often under the influence of drugs or alcohol, to satisfy immediate emotional needs (Nemoto et al., 2003). Sexism is another cultural factor that may influence the implementation and maintenance of safer sexual behavior. Culture-bound power between men and women may limit women's ability to negotiate condom use in relationships (Amaro & Raj, 2000; Holland, Ramazanoglu, Scott, Sharpe, & Thomson, 1992; Kline, Kline, & Oken, 1992). As with biological factors, because cultural factors are out of the individual's control, the clinician's role here would be helping the client to manage his or her reactions to them and understand how they may potentiate a lapse.

COMPREHENSIVE RELAPSE PREVENTION INTERVENTIONS FOR SEXUALLY RISKY BEHAVIORS

In the foregoing sections, we have discussed ways in which RP may be applied to reduce SRBs. We have described specific targets and important areas of focus in designing RP-based interventions. Pioneering research on adapting RP to address the problem of reducing SRBs has integrated many of these approaches and shown the promise of further work on developing RP in this arena. In this section, we describe this pioneering work.

Cognitive-behavioral interventions are the accepted standard for HIV risk reduction interventions; thus, most interventions include components that overlap with those found in the RP model (e.g., cognitive-behavioral skills-building groups). Nonetheless, few reduction programs for SRBs have incorporated the full RP model. In this section, we describe examples of existing comprehensive RP interventions for reduction of SRBs. Roffman and colleagues (Roffman et al., 1997; Roffman et al., 1998) developed, implemented, and evaluated the effectiveness of a 17-session, group RP-based counseling program designed to reduce SRBs for men who have sex with men, as compared to a wait-list control group. As recommended by the RP model, early intervention sessions focused on HIV education, goal setting, motivational enhancement, and group cohesion. Middle sessions moved on to identifying situations at high risk of SRBs, and developing coping strategies for these situations. Behavioral skills training focused on assertive communication skills via role-play exercises and substituting behavioral alternatives for SRBs. Cognitive skills training included positive self-talk and goal setting. Middle sessions also included discussing recent successes and difficulties in avoiding high-risk situations. Final sessions covered maintenance strategies such as cognitively restructuring negative reactions to goal violations, maintaining lifestyle balance, and utilizing social supports.

Prior to and after completion of the 17-session treatment, self-reported sexual activity over the preceding 3-month period was assessed, including total number of occasions of sex (whether protected or not), proportion of protected sex, and total number of male partners. These sexual behavior indices also were assessed during 3-month, 6-month, and 12-month follow-ups after participants completed the 17 weeks of intervention. Proposed mediating variables of the RP model also were assessed prior to and after treatment, including self-efficacy, positive-outcome expectancies, and safer-sex negotiation behavioral skills. Self-efficacy was measured in terms of confidence in not engaging in unprotected sex across a number of high-risk situations (e.g., when drinking alcohol, when feeling depressed), and confidence in engaging in specific strategies to avoid SRBs, such as discussing safer sex with potential partners, refusing to engage in unprotected sex, and reducing overall sexual activity. Positive outcome expectancies were assessed for both protected and unprotected sex, separately (e.g., the degree one expects to feel loved, feel physical pleasure, please partner, and so on, as outcomes of unprotected oral sex, unprotected anal sex, protected oral sex, and protected anal sex, respectively). Safer-sex negotiation behavioral skills were assessed via audiotaped role plays during which participants enacted verbal responses to high-risk situations.

In terms of outcomes for SRBs, treatment participants increased the overall proportion of their sexual activities that were protected and reduced their level of unprotected oral sex. No significant changes were found in level of unprotected anal sex, total amount of sex, or number of male sex partners. Moreover, initial behavior changes found immediately following treatment were maintained at the 3-month follow-up, but eroded to borderline significance at 6 months, and returned to baseline at 12-month follow-up. Results were more promising in terms of effects on the proposed RP mechanisms of behavior change. As compared to controls, treatment participants demonstrated increases in aspects of safer-sex negotiation behavioral skills, increased self-efficacy regarding avoiding unprotected sex across a variety of high-risk situations, and increased self-efficacy regarding using condoms, refusing unsafe sex, and engaging in only safer sex. Treatment participants also reported decreased positive-outcome expectancies for unprotected oral sex, which maps onto treatment participants' self-reported decrease in unprotected oral sex behavior. A trial of a similar, 14-week version of the program also resulted in reduction of risk behaviors and increases in protective behaviors (Roffman, Beadnell, Ryan, & Downey, 1995).

Baker, Beadnell, and colleagues (Baker et al., 2003; Beadnell et al., 1997) developed a 16-week RP intervention for reduction of SRBs in low-income women, based on the program described earlier, and compared clients' outcomes to a health education intervention. Compared to the health education group, women in the RP-based intervention reported acquisition of fewer new STIs during the year following the intervention and greater increases in safer-sex skills. Nonetheless, both groups reported similar decreases in self-reported SRBs (Baker et al., 2003). Although the findings of these example studies do not yet provide unequivocal evidence for the efficacy of RP-based programs in producing reduction of SRBs—particularly in the long term and in comparison to other types of interventions—they do provide support for the feasibility and potential utility of RP-based intervention techniques in reduction interventions for SRBs.

CONCLUSION

Morbidity and mortality associated with the HIV/AIDS exact a heavy toll worldwide. Interventions aimed at reducing SRBs remain the primary approach for containing the epidemic. Among the available psychosocial and cognitive-behavioral interventions, RP offers important advantages. Evolved from the addictions treatment field, RP was specifically formulated to address and solve maintenance problems that arise in behavior change. Also, because it was developed to accommodate nonabstinent treatment goals, RP adapts readily to the sexual domain, where abstinence solutions are largely unrealistic. In theory, RP applications emphasize teaching individuals to understand and cope effectively with situational factors that increase the likelihood of engaging in risky sex. RP also emphasizes enhanced awareness of contextual and background factors that—while they constitute more distal contributors to a person's propensity for risky sex—can affect one's receptivity and vulnerability to risk opportunities. We provided a brief overview of key background considerations and of the rationales and objectives for applying RP constructs and techniques to reduction programs for SRBs. In practice, despite its potential promise and applicability, comprehensive RP interventions have not played a major role in existing reduction programs for SRBs. As was evident in our summary of extant findings, clinical and research evaluations of comprehensive RP-based programs for SRBs have been limited. These data, while decidedly scant, are consistent with the general claim that RP has utility for reduction work with SRBs. However, further clarification and specification about RP's strengths and limitations with regard to explaining and preventing risky sex must await future research. Among the important questions for consideration in future research are the following:

1. Can optimal parameters be identified for establishing stable definitions of SRBs for lapse and relapse, definitions that are comparable across projects and investigators?
2. Can it be reliably established that RP-based reduction programs for SRBs are more or less efficacious and/or effective than alternative programs?
3. Can match variables be identified that predict what types of individuals are most likely to benefit from an RP-based approach?

Until data exist to answer such questions, the utility of applying RP applications to SRB—while interesting and intuitively valuable—will remain a promissory note.

REFERENCES

Adib, S. M., Joseph, J. G., Ostrow, D. G., Tal, M., & Schwartz, S. A. (1991). Relapse to sexual behavior among homosexual men: A 2-year follow-up from the Chicago MACS/CCS. *AIDS, 5,* 757–760.

Albarracin, D., Ho, R. M., McNatt, P. S., Williams, W. R., Rhodes, F., Malotte, C. V., et al. (2000). Structure of outcome beliefs in condom use. *Health Psychology, 19,* 458–468.

Albert, E. A., Warner, D. L., Hatcher, R. A., Trussell, J., & Bennett, C. (1995). Condom use among female commercial sex workers in Nevada's legal brothels. *American Journal of Public Health, 85,* 1514–1520.

Amaro, H., & Raj, A. (2000). On the margin: Power and women's HIV risk reduction strategies. *Sex Roles, 42,* 723–749.

Baker, S. A., Beadnell, B., Stoner, S., Morrison, D. M., Gordon, J., Collier, C., et al. (2003). Skills training versus health education to prevent STDs/HIV in heterosexual women: A randomized controlled trial utilizing biological outcomes. *AIDS Education and Prevention, 15,* 1–14.

Bancroft, J. (1999). Central inhibition of sexual response in the male: A theoretical perspective. *Neuroscience and Biobehavioral Reviews, 23,* 763–784.

Bancroft, J., Janssen, E., Strong, D., Carnes, L., Vukadinovic, Z., & Long, J. S.

(2003). Sexual risk-taking in gay men: The relevance of sexual arousability, mood, and sensation seeking. *Archives of Sexual Behavior, 32*, 555–572.

Beadnell, B., Baker, S., Gordon, J., Collier, C., Morrison, D., & Ryan, R. (1997). Preventing sexually transmitted diseases and HIV in women: Using multiple sources of data to inform intervention design. *Cognitive and Behavioral Practice, 4*, 325–347.

Brafford, L. J., & Beck, K. H. (1991). Development and validation of a condom use self-efficacy scale for college students. *Journal of American College Health, 39*, 219–225.

Brien, T. M., Thombs, D. L., Mahoney, C. A., & Wallnau, L. (1994). Dimensions of self-efficacy among three distinct groups of condom users. *Journal of American College Health, 42*, 197–174.

Brownell, K. D., Marlatt, G. A., Lichtenstein, E., & Wilson, G. T. (1986). Understanding and preventing relapse. *American Psychologist, 41*(7), 765–782.

Caceres, C. F., & van Griensven, G. (1994). Male homosexual transmission of HIV-1. *AIDS, 8*, 1051–1061.

Canin, L., Dolcini, M. M., & Adler, N. E. (1999). Barriers to and facilitators of HIV-STD behavior change: Intrapersonal and relationship-based factors. *Review of General Psychology, 3*, 338–371.

Catania, J. A., Osmond, D., Stall, R. D., Pollack, L., Paul, J. P., Blower, S., et al. (2001). The continuing epidemic among men who have sex with men. *American Journal of Public Health, 91*, 907–914.

Centers for Disease Control and Prevention. (2004). *Global summary of the HIV/ AIDS epidemic, December 2003*. Retrieved on May 5, 2004, from www.who.int/ hiv/pub/epidemiology/en/epi2003_1_full.jpg.

Crepaz, N., & Marks, G. (2001). Are negative affective states associated with HIV sexual risk behaviors? A meta-analytic review. *Health Psychology, 20*, 291–299.

Curtin, L., Stephens, R. S., & Roffman, R. A. (1997). Determinants of relapse and the rule violation effect in predicting safer sex goal violations. *Journal of Applied Social Psychology, 27*, 649–663.

De Vincenzi, I. (1994). A longitudinal study of human immunodeficiency virus transmission by heterosexual partners. *New England Journal of Medicine, 331*, 341–346.

de Wit, J. B. F., van Griensven, G. J. P., Kok, G., & Sandfort, T. G. M. (1993). Why do homosexual men relapse to unsafe sex? Predictors of resumption of unprotected anogenital intercourse with casual partners. *AIDS, 7*, 1113–1118.

Donovan, C., Mearns, C., McEwan, R., & Sugden, N. (1994). A review of the HIV-related sexual behaviour of gay men and men who have sex with men. *AIDS Care, 6*, 605–617.

Ekstrand, M., Stall, R., Kegeles, S., Hays, R., DeMayo, M., & Coates, T. (1993). Safer sex among gay men: What is the ultimate goal? *AIDS, 7*, 281–282.

Folkman, S., Chesney, M. A., Pollack, L., & Phillips, C. (1992). Stress, coping, and high-risk sexual behavior. *Health Psychology, 11*, 218–222.

George, W. H., & Marlatt, G. A. (1989). Introduction. In R. D. Laws (Ed.), *Relapse prevention with sex offenders* (pp. 1–31). New York: Guilford Press.

Hafer, C. L., Bogaert, A. F., & McMullen, S. (2001). Belief in a just world and condom use in a sample of gay and bisexual men. *Journal of Applied Social Psychology, 31*, 1892–1910.

Hart, G., Boulton, M., Fitzpatrick, R., McLean, J., & Dawson, J. (1992). "Relapse" to unsafe sexual behaviour amongst gay men: A critique of recent behavioural HIV/AIDS research. *Sociology of Health and Illness, 14*, 216–232.

Haverkos, H. W., & Battjes, R. J. (1992). Female-to-male transmission of HIV. *Journal of the American Medical Association, 268*, 1855–1856.

Herek, G. M., & Glunt, E. K. (1995). Identity and community among gay and bisexual men in the AIDS era: Preliminary findings from the Sacramento Men's Health Study. In G. M. Herek & B. Greene (Eds.), *Psychological perspectives on lesbian and gay issues: AIDS, identity, and community: The HIV epidemic and lesbian and gay men* (pp. 55–84). Thousand Oaks, CA: Sage.

Holland, J., Ramazanoglu, C., Scott, S., Sharpe, S., & Thomson, R. (1992). Risk, power and the possibility of pleasure: Young women and safer sex. *AIDS Care, 4*, 273–283.

Hoyle, R. H., Fejfar, M. C., & Miller, J. D. (2000). Personality and sexual risk-taking: A quantitative review. *Journal of Personality, 68*, 1203–1231.

Huebner, D. M., Davis, M. C., Nemeroff, C. J., & Aiken, L. S. (2002). The impact of internalized homophobia on HIV preventive interventions. *American Journal of Community Psychology, 30*, 327–348.

Kalichman, S. C. (1998). *Preventing AIDS: A sourcebook for behavioral interventions*. Mahwah, NJ: Erlbaum.

Kalichman, S. C., Kelly, J. A., Morgan, M., & Rompa, D. (1997). Fatalism, current life satisfaction, and risk for HIV infection among gay and bisexual men. *Journal of Consulting and Clinical Psychology, 65*, 542–546.

Kalichman, S. C., Kelly, J. A., & Rompa, D. (1997). Continued high-risk sex among HIV seropositive gay and bisexual men seeking HIV prevention services. *Health Psychology, 16*, 369–373

Kalichman, S. C., & Weinhardt, L. (2001). Negative affect and sexual risk behavior: Comment on Crepaz and Marks. *Health Psychology, 20*, 300–301.

Kelly, J. A., & Kalichman, S. C. (2002). Behavioral research in HIV/AIDS primary and secondary prevention: Recent advances and future directions. *Journal of Consulting and Clinical Psychology, 70*, 626–639.

Kelly, J. A., Kalichman, S. C., Kauth, M. R., Kilgore, H. G., Hood, H. V., Campos, P. E., et al. (1991). Situational factors associated with AIDS risk behavior lapses and coping strategies used by gay men who successfully avoid lapses. *American Journal of Public Health, 81*, 1335–1338.

Kelly, J. A., St. Lawrence, J. S., & Brasfield, T. L. (1991). Predictors of vulnerability to AIDS risk behavior relapse. *Journal of Consulting and Clinical Psychology, 59*, 163–166.

Kelly, J. A., St. Lawrence, J. S., Brasfield, T. L., & Hood, H. V. (1989). Group intervention to reduce AIDS risk behaviors in gay men: Applications of behavioral principles. In V. M. Mays & G. W. Albee (Eds.), *Primary prevention of AIDS: Psychological approaches* (pp. 225–241). Newbury Park, CA: Sage.

Kippax, S., Crawford, J., Davis, M., Rodden, P., & Dowsett, G. (1993). Sustaining safe sex: A longitudinal study of a sample of homosexual men. *AIDS, 7*, 257–263.

Kline, A., Kline, E., & Oken, E. (1992). Minority women and sexual choice in the age of AIDS. *Social Science and Medicine, 34*, 447–457.

Langer, L. M., Zimmerman, R. S., & Cabral, R. J. (1994). Perceived versus actual condom skills among clients at sexually transmitted disease clinics. *Public Health Reports, 109,* 683–687.

Larimer, M. E., & Marlatt, G. A. (1990). Applications of relapse prevention with moderation goals. *Journal of Psychoactive Drugs, 22,* 189–195.

Larimer, M. E., Palmer, R. S., & Marlatt, G. A. (1999). Relapse prevention: An overview of Marlatt's cognitive-behavioral model. *Alcohol Health and Research World, 23,* 151–160.

Maisto, S. A., Carey, M. P., Carey, K. B., & Gordon, C. M. (2002). The effects of alcohol and expectancies on risk perception and behavioral skills relevant to safer sex among heterosexual young women. *Journal of Studies on Alcohol, 63,* 476–486.

Marlatt, G. A. (1996). Taxonomy of high-risk situations for alcohol relapse: Evolution and development of a cognitive-behavioral model of relapse. *Addiction, 91*(Suppl.), 37–50.

Marlatt, G. A., & George, W. H. (1984). Relapse prevention: Introduction and overview of the model. *British Journal of Addiction, 79,* 261–273.

Marlatt, G. A., & Gordon, J. R. (1980). Determinants of relapse: Implications for the maintenance of behavior change. In P. O. Davidson & S. M. Davidson (Eds.), *Behavior medicine: Changing health lifestyles* (pp. 410–452). New York: Brunner/Mazel.

Marlatt, G. A., & Gordon, J. R. (1985). *Relapse prevention: Maintenance strategies in the treatment of addictive behaviors* (1st ed.). New York: Guilford Press.

McKusick, L., Hoff, C. C., Stall, R., & Coates, T. J. (1991). Tailoring AIDS prevention: Differences in behavioral strategies among heterosexual and gay bar patrons in San Francisco. *AIDS Education and Prevention, 3,* 1–9.

Mehryar, A. (1995). Condoms: Awareness, attitudes and use. In J. Cleland & B. Ferry (Eds.), *Sexual behaviour and AIDS in the developing world* (pp. 124–156). London: Taylor & Francis.

Meyer, I. H., & Dean, L. (1998). Internalized homophobia, intimacy, and sexual behavior among gay and bisexual men. In G. M. Herek (Ed.), *Stigma and sexual orientation: Understanding prejudice against lesbians, gay men, and bisexuals* (pp. 160–186). Thousand Oaks, CA: Sage.

Misovich, S. J., Fisher, J. D., & Fisher, W. A. (1997). Close relationships and elevated HIV risk behavior: Evidence and possible underlying psychological processes. *Review of General Psychology, 1,* 72–107.

Nelson, R. J. (1995). *An introduction to behavioral endocrinology.* Sunderland, MA: Sinauer.

Nemoto, T., Operario, D., Soma, T., Bao, D., Vajrabukka, A., & Crisostomo, V. (2003). HIV risk and prevention among Asian/Pacific Islander men who have sex with men: Listen to our stories. *AIDS Education and Prevention, 15*(Suppl. A), 7–20.

Newton, P. (1996). Oral sex: Just how dangerous is it? *Southern Voice, 1,* 9.

Page-Shafer, K., Shiboski, C. H., Osmond, D. H., Dilley, J., McFarland, W., Shiboski, J. D., et al. (2002). Risk of infection attributable to oral sex among men who have sex with men and in the population of men who have sex with men. *AIDS, 16,* 2350–2352.

Perloff, R. M. (2001). *Persuading people to have safer sex: Applications of social science to the AIDS crisis.* Mahwah, NJ: Erlbaum.

Robinson, B. E., Bockting, W. O., Rosser, B. R. S., Miner, M., & Coleman, E. (2002). The sexual health model: Application of a sexological approach to HIV prevention. *Health Education Research*, *17*, 43–57.

Roffman, R. A., Beadnell, B., Ryan, R., & Downy, L. (1995). Telephone group counseling in reducing AIDS risk in gay and bisexual males. In G. A. Lloyd & M. A. Kuszelewicz (Eds.), *HIV disease: Lesbians, gays and the social services* (pp. 145–157). Stroud Glos, UK: Hawthorn Press.

Roffman, R. A., Downey, L., Beadnell, B., Gordon, J. R., Craver, J. N., & Stephens, R. S. (1997). Cognitive-behavioral group counseling to prevent HIV transmission in gay and bisexual men: Factors contributing to successful risk reduction. *Research on Social Work Practice*, *7*, 165–186.

Roffman, R. A., Stephens, R. S., Curtin, L., Gordon, J. R., Craver, J. N., Stern, M., et al. (1998). Relapse prevention as an interventive model for HIV risk reduction in gay and bisexual men. *AIDS Education and Prevention*, *10*, 1–18.

Shernoff, M., & Bloom, D. J. (1991). Designing effective AIDS prevention workshops for gay and bisexual men. *AIDS Education and Prevention*, *3*, 31–46.

Stall, R. D., & Ekstrand, M. (1994). The quantitative/qualitative debate over "relapse" behavior: Comment. *AIDS Care*, *6*, 619–625.

Stall, R., Ekstrand, M., Pollack, L., McKusick, L., & Coates, T. J. (1990). Relapse from safer sex: The next challenge for AIDS prevention efforts. *Journal of Acquired Immune Deficiency Syndrome*, *3*, 1181–1187.

Stall, R. D., Hays, R. B., Waldo, C. R., Ekstrand, M., & McFarland, W. (2000). The gay 90's: A review of research in the 1990s on sexual behavior and HIV risk among men who have sex with men. *AIDS*, *14*(Suppl. 3), 101–114.

Stokes, J. P., & Peterson, J. L. (1998). Homophobia, self-esteem, and risk for HIV among African American men who have sex with men. *AIDS Education and Prevention*, *10*, 278–292.

Stoneburner, R. L., & Low-Beer, D. (2004). Population-level HIV declines and behavioral risk avoidance in Uganda. *Science*, *304*, 714–718.

Susser, E., Desvarieux, M., & Wittkowski, K. M. (1998). Reporting sexual risk behavior for HIV: A practical risk index and a method for improving risk indices. *American Journal of Public Health*, *88*, 671–674.

White, K. M., Terry, D. J., & Hogg, M. A. (1994). Safer sex behavior: The role of attitudes, norms, and control factors. *Journal of Applied Social Psychology*, *24*, 2164–2192.

Williams, M. L., Elwood, W. N., & Bowen, A. M. (2000). Escape from risk: A qualitative exploration of relapse to unprotected anal sex among men who have sex with men. *Journal of Psychology and Human Sexuality*, *11*, 25–49.

Winter, L., & Goldy, A. S. (1993). Effects of prebehavioral cognitive work on adolescents' acceptance of condoms. *Health Psychology*, *12*, 308–312.

Author Index

Subject Index